COMPLETE NURSE'S GUIDE

TO DIABETES CARE

Belinda P. Childs, ARNP, MN, CDE, BC-ADM, Editor

Marjorie Cypress, MSN, RN, C-ANP, CDE, Associate Editor

Geralyn Spollett, MSN, C-ANP, CDE, Associate Editor

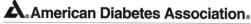
American Diabetes Association.
Cure • Care • Commitment®

Director, Book Publishing, John Fedor; *Managing Editor, Books,* Abe Ogden; *Acquisitions Editor, Professional Books,* Christine Charlip; *Editor,* Gregory L. Guthrie; *Copyeditor,* Wendy M. Martin; *Composition,* Circle Graphics; *Cover Design,* Koncept, Inc.; *Printer,* Port City Press, Inc.

Printed in the United States of America
1 3 5 7 9 10 8 6 4 2

The suggestions and information contained in this publication are generally consistent with the *Clinical Practice Recommendations* and other policies of the American Diabetes Association, but they do not represent the policy or position of the Association or any of its boards or committees. Reasonable steps have been taken to ensure the accuracy of the information presented. However, the American Diabetes Association cannot ensure the safety or efficacy of any product or service described in this publication. Individuals are advised to consult a physician or other appropriate health care professional before undertaking any diet or exercise program or taking any medication referred to in this publication. Professionals must use and apply their own professional judgment, experience, and training and should not rely solely on the information contained in this publication before prescribing any diet, exercise, or medication. The American Diabetes Association—its officers, directors, employees, volunteers, and members—assumes no responsibility or liability for personal or other injury, loss, or damage that may result from the suggestions or information in this publication.

☉ The paper in this publication meets the requirements of the ANSI Standard Z39.48-1992 (permanence of paper).

ADA titles may be purchased for business or promotional use or for special sales. To purchase this book in large quantities, or for custom editions of this book with your logo, contact Lee Romano Sequeira, Special Sales & Promotions, at the address below, or at LRomano@diabetes.org or call 703-299-2046.

American Diabetes Association
1701 North Beauregard Street
Alexandria, Virginia 22311

Library of Congress Cataloging-in-Publication Data

Complete nurse's guide to diabetes care / Belinda P. Childs, editor; Marjorie Cypress and Geralyn Spollett, associate editors.
    p. ; cm.
  Includes bibliographical references and index.
  ISBN 1-58040-200-3 (alk. paper)
  1. Diabetes—Nursing.
  [DNLM: 1. Diabetes Mellitus—nursing. 2. Nursing Care—methods. WY 155 C737 2005] I. Childs, Belinda. II. Cypress, Marjorie. III. Spollett, Geralyn. IV. American Diabetes Association.

RC660.C515 2005
616.4'620231—dc22

2005003561

Contents

COMPLICATIONS

DIABETES CARE AND MANAGEMENT

SPECIAL POPULATIONS

DISEASES AND TREATMENTS THAT AFFECT DIABETES

DIABETES CARE IN COMMUNITY SETTINGS

Preface

A FEW WORDS ABOUT WHAT THIS GUIDE HOLDS FOR YOU

As you begin your evening shift at the local hospital, you meet Denver. He is well known to you, not only for his frequent admissions to the hospital but also because he was your band teacher in high school. He always has a joke to share. Today, he is admitted because of shortness of breath. This proud World War II veteran, a man who cherishes his wife of 56 years, has congestive heart failure.

Denver was diagnosed with diabetes nearly 20 years ago and, at age 85, has been on insulin for over 10 years. He has developed all of the complications of diabetes. He sees a diabetes specialist. Denver and his wife have attended a diabetes education program. Five years ago, he had cardiac bypass surgery. His kidneys are failing. He has had chronic foot ulcers. One month ago, a pacemaker was placed, and just 3 weeks ago, he started hemodialysis.

Denver has recuperated after several hospitalizations in a skilled nursing care facility but has always returned home. Today he lives with his wife. A home health nurse comes to their house twice daily to assist his wife in daily care. He has a primary care physician and receives additional care from several specialty physicians, but the VA hospital that provides his medications, home equipment, and medical supervision is 60 miles away. Through all this, Denver continues to love life, his wife, his family and especially his grandchildren, music, and God.

Denver has experienced all of the devastating complications of a disease that has taken three of his six siblings. He and his family have needed diabetes care and support at home, in the nursing home, in the hospital, and at the clinic. In every one of these settings, nurses have participated and provided expert care. Yet, exceptional as this care may have been, they were not always knowledgeable about diabetes.

This book is dedicated to Denver Childs, my husband's father, my second dad.

Denver is the face of diabetes. Diabetes is a devastating disease that has become a worldwide epidemic. The prevalence of type 1 diabetes has remained steady, whereas the incidence of type 2 diabetes is growing at epidemic proportions. One million individuals are diagnosed with diabetes annually. Currently, 18 million Americans have diabetes, 6.3% of the population. Thirteen million are known to have the disease, and 5.2 million are undiagnosed. Another 41 million have either impaired glucose tolerance or impaired fasting glucose (1), a state that has recently been named pre-diabetes. Individuals with pre-diabetes may be able to prevent the development of full-blown diabetes, as was shown in the Diabetes Prevention Program, by increasing activity and decreasing weight. This epidemic is being driven by our sedentary lifestyles and increasing rates of obesity. Today, even our children are developing type 2 diabetes at an alarming rate, and one in three children will develop diabetes in his or her lifetime.

Diabetes is the leading cause of cardiovascular disease, kidney disease, amputation, and blindness and occurs more often in Latinos, Native Americans, and African Americans. It costs $132 billion annually (2).

This devastating disease affects millions of people. Nurses take care of people with diabetes every day, no matter where we work. Diabetes affects the rate of recovery from all of the other diseases that the individual with diabetes may encounter. It is therefore imperative that all nurses be knowledgeable about diabetes. Nurses have always played an important role in the care of a person with diabetes, and they will continue to be an essential part of the health care team.

There are diabetes educators, diabetes nurse specialists, and diabetes education programs across the country, but they are few compared to the number of individuals with diabetes. To improve outcomes for individuals with diabetes, we believe it is important for all nurses to have a good understanding of diabetes care and education. All nurses must be knowledgeable about diabetes, regardless of their setting. It is my hope that this book will be a valuable resource for nurses in all settings as they care for patients with diabetes. The nurse must have information that is up to date and easily accessible when they are providing patient care. My co-editors, Marjorie Cypress, MSN, RN, C-ANP, CDE, and Geralyn Spollett, MSN, C-ANP, CDE, and I asked many of the leading experts in diabetes to contribute to this book. The majority are nurses. It is a book for nurses written by nurses. It is our hope that through this effort, patients may be diagnosed earlier, care may be improved in all settings, and diabetes may even be prevented by the actions of nurses.

In 1973, the American Association of Diabetes Educators (AADE) was founded (3). This organization provides training and information for the diabetes educator. Their membership includes nurses, dietitians, pharmacists, social workers, psychologists, physicians, exercise specialists, and others interested in diabetes education. This group recognized the need for a specialty certification examination. The National Certification Board for Diabetes Educators (NCBDE) bestows the title of Certified Diabetes Educator (CDE) on those who pass the examination, which has been offered by the NCBDE since 1986 (4). More information is available in the RESOURCES section of this book. At present, there are over 10,000 CDEs, and the AADE has more than 10,000 members. As of 1 January 2005, the number of CDEs documenting a discipline of RN, NP, or CNS was 7,877, or 56% nurse CDEs (there are 13,987 CDEs as of 1 January 2005) (S. Traficano, NCBDE, personal communication, 1 January 2005).

In 2002, the first diabetes specialty certification through the American Academy for Nurse Credentialing was administered. This certification recognizes nurses, dietitians, and pharmacists with master's degrees who have met the eligibility criteria for advanced practice providers and passed an exam. The certification is designated as Board Certified–Advanced Diabetes Management (BC-ADM).

Since 1986, the American Diabetes Association (ADA) has recognized diabetes education programs that meet the criteria for recognition (5). In many cases, ADA Recognition is required for insurance and Medicare reimbursement. Over 1,800 programs in more than 2,700 sites throughout the U.S. are recognized by the ADA.

Diabetes Spectrum is a journal published by the ADA that translates research into practice for the diabetes care specialist. The readership consists of nurses, dietitians, psychologists, social workers, pharmacists, physician's assistants, nurse practitioners, and physicians.

Many resources are available for patients and professionals alike. This book has an extensive RESOURCES section to assist the health care professional and individual with diabetes in gaining the most up-to-date information.

Knowledge is a key to success whether you are a health care professional, a person with diabetes, or a family member of someone with diabetes. The advances in the understanding of diabetes and treatment strategies change almost daily. This is an exciting time to be caring for individuals with diabetes. Science is adding to our knowledge about obesity-related hormones. New hormones such as amylin are being identified. Fat is now being considered an endocrine organ that produces hormones that affect one's ability to regulate food intake. We have new insulin delivery systems and are nearing the day when we will have a continuous glucose sensor. New insulins and other medications for diabetes therapy are becoming available at a breakthrough pace.

Nursing can be challenging for many reasons, from long working hours and staffing issues to complexity of care. But it can also be one of the highlights of one's life. There is no greater satisfaction than making a difference in a person's life and outcome. Advocating for a person with diabetes is a joy. In helping patients accept the challenges before them, guiding someone toward financial support for medication, referring a family to a support group, or providing hope to the child newly diagnosed with diabetes, you make a difference. Consider yourself a coach. You, the nurse, are providing strategies that assist the individual with

---

Current Knowledge on Diabetes

- Type 2 diabetes can be prevented with changes in lifestyle
- The complications of diabetes can be delayed or prevented with
  - Optimal glucose control (glycated hemoglobin A_{1c} <7.0%) and early, aggressive treatments
  - Management of lipids
    - □ HDL cholesterol >40 mg/dl
    - □ LDL cholesterol <100 mg/dl (<70 mg/dl for those with diabetes and overt cardiovascular disease)
    - □ Triglycerides <150 mg/dl
  - Management of blood pressure
    - □ <130/80 mmHg
- Smoking cessation is imperative
- One aspirin per day reduces myocardial infarctions and strokes

These recommendations are taken from the ADA Clinical Practice Recommendations, which are updated annually (6).

diabetes live each day to its fullest. It takes all of us to support individuals with diabetes and their families.

This book has been designed and developed to be used as a resource guide. It is organized into sections. These sections are Fundamentals of Diabetes Care, Complications, Key Aspects in Diabetes Management, Specific Patient Groups, Diseases and Treatments That Affect Diabetes, Diabetes Care in Community Settings, and Resources. Each chapter features helpful Practical Points, implications for nursing practice that are interspersed throughout, and a summary, which is provided at the end.

Thank you for your interest in diabetes. I encourage you to be an enthusiastic coach for the person with diabetes and hope that the *Complete Nurse's Guide to Diabetes Care* will support you in your work and lifelong learning.

Belinda P. Childs, ARNP, MN, CDE, BC-ADM
Editor

REFERENCES

1. Centers for Disease Control and Prevention: National diabetes fact sheet: United States, 2003 [Internet]. Available from http://www.cdc.gov/diabetes/pubs/estimates.htm. Accessed 16 October 2004
2. American Diabetes Association: Economic costs of diabetes in the U.S. in 2002. *Diabetes Care* 26:917-932, 2003
3. American Association of Diabetes Educators: About AADE [Internet], 2003. Available from http://www.aadenet.org/AboutAADE/index.html. Accessed 1 January 2005
4. National Certification Board for Diabetes Educators: About NCBDE certification [Internet]. Available from http://www.ncbde.org/about.html. Accessed 1 January 2005
5. American Diabetes Association: Recognition programs [Internet]. Available from http://www.diabetes.org/for-health-professionals-and-scientists/recognition.jsp. Accessed 1 January 2005
6. American Diabetes Association: Clinical practice recommendations. *Diabetes Care* 28 (Suppl. 1):S1–S79, 2005

About the Editors

Belinda P. Childs, ARNP, MN, CDE, BC-ADM, is a diabetes nurse specialist at Mid-America Diabetes Associates in Wichita, KS. She received her bachelor's and master's degrees in nursing from Wichita State University. She has worked with Drs. Richard and Diana Guthrie for over 25 years. She is the clinic and research coordinator for the practice and provides diabetes care and education for children, adults, and their families. She has authored several book chapters and journal articles and has done numerous presentations. She is currently the editor of *Diabetes Spectrum*, a publication of the American Diabetes Association (2001–2005). Lindy is an adjunct faculty member and instructor in the Department of Nursing at Wichita State University. She is a past President, Health Care & Education, of the American Diabetes Association. When she is not studying diabetes, she is spending time with her husband of nearly 30 years. She has two young adult children, Allison and Brandon, and is the co-founder and chair of the Parish Nursing Ministry at her church.

Marjorie Cypress, MSN, RN, C-ANP, CDE, is an adult nurse practitioner in Albuquerque, NM. She received her bachelor's degree from C.W. Post College, her MSN from State University of New York at Stony Brook, and is currently enrolled in the Nursing PhD program at the University of New Mexico. She has worked in diabetes management and in education of patients and health care professionals for over 20 years in New York and New Mexico. She has authored articles in professional and patient diabetes journals and has done numerous presentations. She has served on national committees for the American Diabetes Association (ADA) and the American Association of Diabetes Educators (AADE) and has served as chair of the National Certification Board for Diabetes Educators. Marjorie is on the editorial boards for *Diabetes Spectrum* and the Program Publications department for the ADA, serves on the Professional Practice Committees for the ADA and AADE, and is the recipient of the ADA's 2004 Outstanding Educator in Diabetes award.

Geralyn Spollett, MSN, C-ANP, CDE, is an adult nurse practitioner and associate director at the Yale Diabetes Center, affiliated with the Yale School of Medicine Faculty Practice. She received her BSN from Fairfield University and MSN from

Boston College. During her 10 years at the Yale School of Nursing, she taught in the diabetes care concentration, conducted research in type 2 diabetes in African-American women, and lectured nationally and internationally on diabetes management from a nurse practitioner perspective. Geri has served as associate editor for *Diabetes Spectrum* and written for many of the leading nursing- and diabetes-related journals. She is an active member of the American Diabetes Association, currently serving on its board of directors and the American Association of Diabetes Educators. She has also served as chair of the National Certification Board for Diabetes Educators.

Acknowledgments

We thank all of the authors who contributed to this book. We would also like to thank our colleagues at Mid-America Diabetes Associates and Yale University who have supported us in this endeavor. We are especially indebted to the Guthries for their everlasting impact on thousands of diabetes care providers and patients across the U.S. and internationally. They had a vision and believed that their calling was to promote the importance of diabetes self-management and patient and professional education throughout their lives.

The American Diabetes Association must be noted for recognizing the need for a comprehensive book dedicated to the role of the nurse in providing care for people with diabetes. A heartfelt thank you goes to the dedicated American Diabetes Association staff, who provided countless hours, enthusiastic energy, and incredible expertise in making this book a reality. In particular, Christine Charlip and Greg Guthrie deserve recognition.

We gratefully acknowledge those who took on the critical and significant task of reviewing this book: Nathaniel Clark, MD; Dolly Daniel, RN BC, BSN, CDE; Clara Schneider, MS, RD, RN, LD, CDE; and Suzanne Strowig, MSN, RN.

We also thank our families for their support and understanding as we hovered over our desks and did not always pay fair attention to them. Without their love, support, and guidance, we would not have been able to undertake this endeavor.

And finally, we are grateful to those who live with diabetes for all that they have taught us over our lifetimes.

Belinda P. Childs, ARNP, MN, CDE, BC-ADM
Marjorie Cypress, MSN, RN, C-ANP, CDE
Geralyn Spollett, MSN, C-ANP, CDE

FUNDAMENTALS OF DIABETES CARE

1. Diagnosis and Classification

MARJORIE CYPRESS, MSN, RN, C-ANP, CDE, AND
JEREMY GLEESON, MD, FACP, CDE

D iabetes is a group of related conditions, each resulting in elevated blood glucose levels. Insulin, a hormone secreted by β-cells in the pancreatic islets, is mainly responsible for controlling blood glucose levels. Diabetes may result from defects in insulin secretion or action or a combination of both factors. Regardless of the underlying cause, the diagnosis of diabetes is straightforward and based on elevation of blood glucose alone.

Chronic hyperglycemia is associated with several diabetes complications—most notably damage to the eyes, kidneys, and nerves, as well as other organs. These complications appear to be direct consequences of blood glucose elevation. Importantly, patients with diabetes are also at much higher risk for cardiovascular diseases, such as heart attack and stroke. Symptoms of diabetes, all caused by elevated blood glucose, include polyuria, polydipsia, weight loss, blurred vision, and dry mouth. Many people, usually with milder elevations in blood glucose, have no symptoms at all, and the diagnosis may be first suspected on routine measurements of blood glucose or on an incidental finding of glucose in the urine. Sometimes, diagnosis occurs when there is already evidence of chronic diabetes complications such as vascular disease or neuropathy. The onset of diabetes is generally insidious. Because many patients, especially those with type 2 diabetes, are free of symptoms, they may remain undiagnosed for prolonged periods.

CLASSIFICATION OF DIABETES

There are several distinct forms of diabetes. The most common forms of diabetes are designated type 1, type 2, and gestational. Type 1 diabetes is caused by an absolute deficiency of insulin secretion, whereas type 2 diabetes is caused by a combination of insulin resistance and a relative, progressive decrease in insulin secretion. Approximately 90% of patients with diabetes have type 2 diabetes. Diabetes first diagnosed in pregnancy is designated gestational diabetes mellitus (GDM); most patients with GDM have features in common with type 2 diabetes. Type 1 and type 2 diabetes encompass the vast majority of patients with diabetes. Rarer forms of diabetes include genetic defects in β-cell function, pancreatic diseases, various endocrine diseases, and drug-induced diabetes. The terms *insulin-dependent diabetes mellitus* and *non-insulin-dependent diabetes mellitus*, for type 1 and type 2 diabetes, respectively, are no longer used, to avoid patient misclassification. Many patients with type 2 diabetes "depend" on insulin for glucose control.

EPIDEMIOLOGY

The incidence of diabetes is increasing at an alarming rate. The World Health Organization has estimated that the number of individuals diagnosed with diabetes worldwide has grown from 30 million in 1985 to 177 million in 2000 (1). In 2003, the Centers for Disease Control and Prevention estimated that 18.2 million people in the U.S. (6.3% of the total population) have diabetes, 13 million diagnosed and 5.2 million undiagnosed. Approximately 90% of those with undiagnosed diabetes have type 2 (2). The prevalence of diagnosed diabetes increased 33% between 1990 and 1998 among all races, ethnicities, ages, and weight classes (3). Over the past 20 years, the number of people in the U.S. reported to have diabetes has more than doubled. This is believed to be related to the increasing rates of obesity and higher prevalence of sedentary lifestyle among Americans and the rapidly growing high-risk populations of Native Americans, Hispanics/Latinos, non-Hispanic blacks, African Americans, and Pacific Islanders (2). In those <20 years of age, 1 of 400 have diabetes. Although historically diagnoses of diabetes in children have been almost exclusively of type 1, the incidence of the development of type 2 diabetes in children has increased significantly. There are no accurate statistics yet on this relatively new phenomenon, but there have been reports that as many as 8–45% of children with newly diagnosed diabetes have type 2 diabetes (4,5).

In the U.S., type 2 diabetes is more common in minority populations. From an international perspective, however, an increased risk for type 2 diabetes is seen in many diverse ethnic groups. Typically, type 2 diabetes increases when susceptible populations adopt a westernized lifestyle with increased caloric intake and reduced physical activity.

GDM occurs more frequently in African American, Hispanic/Latino, and Native American populations. Approximately 4% of all pregnancies in the U.S. result in GDM, but the prevalence rate ranges from 1 to 14% depending on the population studied (5). Although GDM is glucose intolerance during pregnancy, 5–10% of women with GDM are discovered to have type 2 diabetes, and women with a history of GDM have a 20–50% chance of developing diabetes over the next 5–10 years (2).

High-Risk Ethnicities and Type 2 Diabetes

Non-Hispanic blacks/African Americans. A total of 11.4% of all non-Hispanic blacks ≥20 years of age have diabetes. The risk of type 2 diabetes is 1.6 times that for non-Hispanic whites (2).

Hispanic/Latino Americans. An estimated 8.2% of Hispanics ≥20 years of age have type 2 diabetes. Hispanic/Latino Americans are 1.5 times more likely to have diabetes than non-Hispanic whites. Mexican Americans have a risk for diabetes more than twice that of non-Hispanics, and Puerto Ricans are 1.8 times more likely to have diabetes than non-Hispanic whites (2).

Native Americans/Alaska Natives. Native Americans/Alaska Natives have the highest risk of developing type 2 diabetes (2.3 times that of non-Hispanic whites), and it is estimated that 14.9% of this population ≥20 years of age has type 2 diabetes. Among all Native Americans, Alaska Natives have the least risk (8.2%), whereas Native Americans in the southeastern U.S. (27.8%) and in southern Arizona (27.8%) have the highest risk of developing diabetes (2).

DIAGNOSING DIABETES

The recommended screening and diagnostic test for diabetes (Table 1.1) is to measure fasting plasma glucose (6,7). Individuals suspected of having diabetes and those with high risk factors (Table 1.2), even though asymptomatic, should be tested for diabetes. Adults over the age of 45 years should be screened every 3 years. Screening should occur more often (every 1–2 years) in patients with any of the following:

- overweight (body mass index [BMI] ≥25 kg/m²)
- history of GDM or delivery of a baby weighing >9 lb
- history of vascular disease
- first-degree relative with diabetes
- high-risk ethnic group
- previously found to have impaired glucose tolerance or impaired fasting glucose

Table 1.1 Criteria for Diagnosing Diabetes

In nonpregnant adults	Testing for type 2 diabetes in children
Symptoms of diabetes and casual plasma glucose ≥200 mg/dl (≥11.1 mmol/l). Casual is defined as any time of day without regard to time since last meal. The classic symptoms of diabetes include polyuria, polydipsia, and unexplained weight loss.	Overweight (BMI >85th percentile for age and sex, weight for height >85th percentile, or weight >12–30% of ideal for height)
OR	PLUS
Fasting plasma glucose ≥126 mg/dl (≥7 mmol/l). Fasting is defined as no caloric intake for at least 8 h.	Any two of the following risk factors: Family history of type 2 diabetes in first- or second-degree relative Race/ethnicity (Native American, African American, Latino, Asian American, Pacific Islander)
OR	Signs of insulin resistance or conditions associated with insulin resistance (acanthosis nigricans, hypertension, dyslipidemia, or polycystic ovary syndrome)
2-h plasma glucose ≥200 mg/dl (≥11.1 mmol/l) during an OGTT. The test should be performed using a glucose load containing the equivalent of 75 g anhydrous glucose dissolved in water.	Age of initiation: age 10 years or at onset of puberty Frequency: every 2 years Test: fasting plasma glucose preferred

From the American Diabetes Association (6). OGTT, oral glucose tolerance test.
These criteria should be confirmed by repeat testing on a different day. Clinical judgment should be used for diabetes in high-risk patients who do not meet these criteria.

Table 1.2 Risk Factors for Type 2 Diabetes

Age ≥45 years
Overweight (BMI ≥25 kg/m²; may not be correct for all ethnic groups)
Family history of diabetes (e.g., parents or siblings with diabetes)
Habitual physical inactivity
Race/ethnicity (e.g., African Americans, Hispanic Americans, Native Americans, Alaskan Americans, and Pacific Islanders)
Previously identified as having impaired glucose tolerance or impaired fasting glucose
History of GDM or delivery of a baby weighing >9 lb
Hypertension (≥140/90 mmHg in adults)
HDL cholesterol ≤35 mg/dl and/or triglyceride level ≥250 mg/dl
Polycystic ovary syndrome
History of vascular disease

From the American Diabetes Association (6).

- history of vascular disease
- signs of insulin resistance, such as acanthosis nigricans, hypertension, dyslipidemia, or polycystic ovary syndrome

Diabetes may also be diagnosed based on an oral glucose tolerance test (OGTT) (Table 1.1), but this test is not routinely recommended in clinical practice because evaluating fasting plasma glucose is simpler and more convenient. A 75-g OGTT is used in nonpregnant individuals, and a 100-g OGTT is used to screen for GDM (see below) in the U.S. Use of the glycated hemoglobin A_{1c} (A1C) measurement, which is a standard test for monitoring glucose control in patients with diabetes, is not currently recommended for establishing the diagnosis of diabetes. In clinical practice, however, a markedly elevated A1C is virtually diagnostic of diabetes.

Pre-Diabetes

Individuals who do not meet the criteria for diabetes but who clearly have abnormal glucose levels as evidenced by a fasting plasma glucose >100 mg/dl (>5.6 mmol/l) but <126 mg/dl (<7 mmol/l) (impaired fasting glucose) or an OGTT 2-h postglucose level ≥140 mg/dl (≥7.8 mmol/l) and <200 mg/dl (<11.1 mmol/l) (impaired glucose tolerance) are considered to have pre-diabetes. As suggested by the term *pre-diabetes*, these individuals have a very high risk of subsequent diabetes. See Table 1.3 for diagnostic criteria, including pre-diabetes.

Diagnosing GDM

If possible, a patient's risk for GDM should be determined before conception, but certainly at the onset of the diagnosis of pregnancy. Women who are obese or have a prior history of GDM, a family history of diabetes, or glycosuria should have glucose screening done as soon as possible. Other women who are of average risk, older than age 25 years, overweight, or a member of a high-risk ethnic group or have a history of poor obstetrical outcomes (e.g., spontaneous abortion, congenital malformation, fetal macrosomia) should be screened for GDM at 24–28 weeks' gestation. Screening for GDM is performed with a glucose challenge or OGTT (Table 1.4). The diagnosis of GDM can be made with either a 100-g OGTT as

Table 1.3 Diagnostic Criteria

Normoglycemia	Pre-Diabetes	Diabetes
FPG ≤100 mg/dl (≤5.6 mmol/l) 2-h PG <140 (<7.8 mmol/l)	FPG >100 mg/dl (>5.6 mmol/l) 2-h PG ≥140 mg/dl (≥7.8 mmol/l) and <200 mg/dl (11.1 mmol/l)	FPG ≥126 mg/dl (≥7 mmol/l) 2-h PG ≥200 mg/dl (≥11.1 mmol/l) plus symptoms of diabetes and casual plasma glucose concentration (random) ≥200 mg/dl (≥11.1 mmol/l)

FPG, fasting plasma glucose; PG, plasma glucose.

the initial test or a two-step screening approach that begins with a 50-g glucose challenge, followed by the 100-g OGTT if the postchallenge glucose is >130 mg/dl (>7.2 mmol/l). Using a cutoff of ≥130 mg/dl, this two-step screening approach identifies 90% of women with GDM (6).

It is important to be aware that overt type 2 diabetes may manifest early in pregnancy because of weight gain and the increasing insulin resistance of pregnancy. Abnormal blood glucose levels before the 24- to 28-week period of pregnancy suggest a diagnosis of type 2 diabetes or pre-diabetes as opposed to typical GDM. Regardless, because the diagnosis of GDM is a risk factor for the development of diabetes, women with abnormal blood glucose levels should be screened for diabetes 6 weeks postpartum and continue to be followed and screened for the development of pre-diabetes or diabetes (9).

Table 1.4 GDM Diagnosis

Diagnosis of GDM with a 100-g oral glucose load

Time	mg/dl (mmol/l)
Fasting	≥95 (5.3)
1 h	≥180 (10)
2 h	≥155 (8.6)
3 h	≥140 (7.8)

Diagnosis of GDM with a 75-g oral glucose load

Time	mg/dl (mmol/l)
Fasting	≥95 (5.3)
1 h	≥180 (10)
2 h	≥155 (8.6)

From the American Diabetes Association (8). Two or more of the venous plasma concentrations must be met or exceeded for a positive diagnosis. The test should be done in the morning after an overnight fast of 8–14 h and after at least 3 days of unrestricted diet (≥150 g carbohydrate/day) and unlimited physical activity. The person should remain seated and should not smoke throughout the test.

PATHOGENESIS OF DIABETES

Type 1 Diabetes

The pathogenesis of type 1 diabetes is divided into autoimmune-mediated diabetes and idiopathic diabetes. In autoimmune-mediated diabetes, insulin-producing β-cells are destroyed by an autoimmune-mediated process. Typically, β-cells are totally destroyed, but in some patients, destruction is incomplete, resulting in residual insulin production. The rate of destruction is variable. In children, it is often rapid, whereas in adults, it may take several years. Antibody markers are usually seen. These include islet cell antibodies, insulin autoantibodies, and antibodies to glutamic acid decarboxylase (GAD), among others. Antibodies that are present early in the course of diabetes may subsequently become undetectable. There are well-recognized associations with several genes in the HLA (human leukocyte antigen) loci, including both predisposing and protective genes. Patients with type 1 diabetes have increased incidences of other autoimmune diseases, including Hashimoto's thyroiditis, Graves' disease, pernicious anemia, vitiligo, celiac disease, and Addison's disease.

There is a less common form of type 1 diabetes known as idiopathic diabetes, in which there is no evidence of autoimmune disease and immune markers are absent. This appears to be inherited, but the cause is unknown. Idiopathic diabetes is more common in those of African or Asian ethnic origin and is characterized by episodic ketoacidosis and varying degrees of insulin deficiency. The need for insulin replacement is intermittent—it comes and goes.

Type 2 Diabetes

The pathogenesis of type 2 diabetes is complex. Type 2 diabetes develops progressively, with the pathogenic abnormalities already present in the phase of prediabetes. Virtually all patients have insulin resistance combined with varying degrees of insulin deficiency. Typically, this is a relative, not absolute, insulin deficiency. Early in the course of type 2 diabetes, insulin secretion may be increased in relation to individuals without diabetes; however, it is always deficient in terms of the amount required to overcome the patient's insulin resistance. Later in the course of type 2 diabetes, insulin deficiency is often more pronounced.

The progressive decline in β-cell function over several years, regardless of type of therapy, was demonstrated in the U.K. Prospective Diabetes Study (UKPDS) (10), wherein the ability to maintain A1C levels continued to decrease markedly throughout the 9 years of follow-up, even when the researchers controlled for adherence issues such as diet, exercise, and medication. This progression of insulin deficiency is reflected in the treatment required by patients with type 2 diabetes. Many patients with type 2 diabetes, therefore, will go on to require insulin therapy either in combination with oral agents or as monotherapy.

Type 2 diabetes shows a strong familial tendency. There are likely to be multiple genes involved, but none has been clearly identified. Obesity and sedentary lifestyle are major risk factors for type 2 diabetes. Obesity, particularly abdominal obesity, increases insulin resistance and the risk for type 2 diabetes. Genetic factors, i.e., those unrelated to obesity, also contribute to insulin resistance. Clearly, though, many obese individuals do not develop type 2 diabetes. They presumably have adequate β-cell function to produce sufficient insulin to overcome the insulin resistance. Even with insulin resistance, diabetes will usually not develop unless there is a concomitant defect in β-cell function resulting in a deficiency of insulin secretion. Weight loss in overweight patients with diabetes improves insulin resistance but usually does not fully restore insulin sensitivity.

GDM

Diabetes that is first recognized in pregnancy is classified as GDM, although most patients with GDM share pathogenic features in common with type 2 diabetes. The insulin resistance of pregnancy leads to hyperglycemia in susceptible women that often resolves after delivery but may recur in subsequent pregnancies. Consistent with this pathogenesis, women who had GDM are at increased risk of developing diabetes later in life and should be screened for the subsequent development of diabetes throughout their lives. Any form of diabetes, including type 1 diabetes, can be first recognized in pregnancy and would be technically included in the definition of GDM (8).

Maturity-Onset Diabetes of the Young

Although the genes that underlie type 2 diabetes have not been identified, various genetic defects have been recognized that cause more rare forms of diabetes. Several genetic defects in β-cell function are known to result in diabetes at an early age. They cause impaired insulin secretion without insulin resistance. At least three specific gene mutations have been identified; they are all inherited in an autosomal-dominant fashion. These rare forms of diabetes have been called maturity-onset diabetes of the young (MODY). This term, however, should not be applied to the more common type 2 diabetes that, unfortunately, is occurring more frequently in children and adolescents.

Other Causes of Diabetes

Diabetes may be seen in diseases of the exocrine pancreas, such as cystic fibrosis. Various endocrine diseases such as Cushing's syndrome, acromegaly, and pheochromocytoma can cause diabetes. Drug-induced diabetes is an important clinical problem. Corticosteroid drugs are the most frequent cause of hyperglycemia in clinical practice, but numerous other drugs can impair insulin action and precipitate diabetes. Most likely, these drugs are not the sole cause of diabetes but unmask hyperglycemia in individuals already at risk (6). See CHAPTER 28 for additional information.

CLINICAL FEATURES OF TYPE 1 AND TYPE 2 DIABETES

Most often, type 1 diabetes occurs in children and young adults but may also occur in individuals of any age. The rate of β-cell destruction varies; it is typically more rapid in younger individuals, who frequently present with severe symptomatic hyperglycemia or sometimes diabetic ketoacidosis. This suggests severe insulin deficiency. Insulin therapy is required for survival in these patients. Patients with a slower progression of β-cell destruction may retain some insulin secretion for many years and may present with only modest asymptomatic hyperglycemia. As the disease progresses, they require insulin for survival and are at risk for ketoacidosis. Patients with type 1 diabetes are not typically obese at diagnosis; however, obesity at the time of diagnosis does not exclude a diagnosis of type 1 diabetes.

The clinical presentation of type 2 diabetes is even more variable than that of type 1 diabetes. Because the insulin deficiency is only relative, many of these patients can be treated without insulin, at least initially. Most patients with type 2 diabetes are obese or overweight with increased abdominal adiposity. It is most commonly seen in adults, but is also increasingly being seen in adolescents and children, usually in association with obesity. Symptoms may be mild or nonexistent in many patients with type 2 diabetes. Although diabetic ketoacidosis is characteristically associated with type 1 diabetes, it may be seen in rare cases in which patients with type 2 diabetes are under severe physical stress, such as major infection. This is quite different from the situation in type 1 diabetes, where patients are ketosis prone and may develop ketoacidosis rapidly by simply omitting insulin.

Although it may be easy to distinguish the classic presentations of type 1 diabetes seen in a lean child with weight loss and ketoacidosis or those of type 2 diabetes seen in an obese older adult with no symptoms and mildly elevated glucose levels, other individuals may be difficult to classify in the initial stages of the disease process. Overlap between the two common forms of diabetes does exist. It may not be clear whether a middle-aged adult with onset of fasting hyperglycemia has type 2 diabetes or a slowly evolving form of type 1 diabetes. In addition, an individual with a clear history of type 1 diabetes may subsequently become obese and develop additional features associated with insulin resistance that are common in patients with type 2 diabetes. Some patients who develop diabetes in adulthood, and who may initially appear to have type 2 diabetes, may have a form of autoimmune diabetes. These individuals are usually leaner than the typical patient with type 2 diabetes. Insulin deficiency may develop more rapidly than in a typical type 2 diabetes patient but more slowly than in a child with type 1 diabetes. Some of these patients may have autoimmune markers such as anti-GAD antibodies, indicating autoimmune β-cell destruction as the cause of their diabetes. The term *latent autoimmune diabetes of adulthood* (LADA) has been applied to this group. They are frequently misdiagnosed as having type 2 diabetes and may respond to insulin secretagogues for a limited period of time. However, as they become more insulin deficient, the hyperglycemia and symptoms become more pronounced. They may exhibit ketonuria, and insulin is the only appropriate treatment.

The development of type 2 diabetes in children and adolescents is a rapidly increasing clinical problem. These individuals are usually obese and most often belong to ethnic groups with a high incidence of type 2 diabetes. No longer is age of onset a reliable indicator of the type of diabetes present.

PRACTICAL POINT

Carefully assessing all patients with new-onset hyperglycemia to determine whether they are insulin deficient or insulin resistant is critical for deciding the safest and most effective treatment plan.

SUMMARY

The diagnosis of diabetes is made strictly by the blood glucose test. Therapy is initiated based on the level of blood glucose and the type of diabetes diagnosed. Nurses in all settings have the opportunity to identify patients who are at risk for diabetes, have pre-diabetes, and have diabetes. Studies indicate that early diagnosis

Clues to Determining Type of Diabetes

Type 1 Diabetes	Type 2 Diabetes
Usually lean	Usually overweight or obese
May not have a family history	Almost always has a family history
May not be a member of a high-risk group	Often a member of a high-risk ethnic group
Ketosis prone	Not ketosis prone
Onset slow to rapid (3–4 weeks)	Onset usually slow and progressive
Usually young but can be any age	Usually over age 30 years, but can occur in youth
	May have history of GDM or delivery of baby >9 lb
	May have associated complications, such as hypertension, atherogenic dyslipidemia, cardiovascular disease, or risk factors
	Markers for insulin resistance

and aggressive therapy will delay and possibly prevent the complications of diabetes. Nurses therefore have the opportunity to counsel, refer, and promote healthy behaviors among individuals with diabetes and pre-diabetes and those at high risk for diabetes.

REFERENCES

1. World Health Organization: Diabetes: the cost of diabetes [Internet], 2002. Available from http://www.who.int/mediacentre/factsheets/fs236/en/. Accessed 5 January 2005
2. Centers for Disease Control and Prevention: *National Diabetes Fact Sheet: General Information and National Estimates on Diabetes in the United States.* Atlanta, GA, Centers for Disease Control and Prevention, 2003
3. Mokdad AH, Ford ES, Bowman BA, Nelson DE, Engelgau MM, Vinicor F, Marks JS: Diabetes trends in the U.S.: 1990–1998. *Diabetes Care* 23: 1278–1283, 2000
4. American Diabetes Association: Type 2 diabetes in children and adolescents (Consensus Statement). *Diabetes Care* 23:381–389, 2000
5. Fagot Campagna A: Emerging type 2 diabetes mellitus in children: epidemiological evidence. *J Pediatr Endocrinol Metab* 13 (Suppl. 6):1395–1402, 2000
6. American Diabetes Association: Diagnosis and classification of diabetes mellitus (Position Statement). *Diabetes Care* 28 (Suppl. 1):S37–S42, 2005

7. American Diabetes Association: Screening for type 2 diabetes (Position Statement). *Diabetes Care* 27 (Suppl. 1):S11–S14, 2004

8. American Diabetes Association: Gestational diabetes mellitus (Position Statement). *Diabetes Care* 27 (Suppl. 1):S88–S90, 2004

9. American Diabetes Association: Standards of medical care in diabetes (Position Statement). *Diabetes Care* 28 (Suppl. 1):S4–S36, 2005

10. UK Prospective Diabetes Study Group: Overview of 6 years' therapy of type II diabetes: a progressive disease. *Diabetes* 44:1249–1258, 1995

Ms. Cypress is an Adult Nurse Practitioner and Certified Diabetes Educator in Albuquerque, NM. Dr. Gleeson is Chair of the Division of Endocrinology and Medical Director of the Diabetes Program at Lovelace Sandia Health Systems, Albuquerque, NM.

2. Prevention and Risk Reduction

MARJORIE CYPRESS, MSN, RN, C-ANP, CDE, AND
JEREMY GLEESON, MD, FACP, CDE

Primary prevention of diabetes should be a focus of all health care professionals. Unfortunately, this does not always occur. Interventions to recognize high-risk individuals and strategies to decrease the risk of diabetes and diabetes-related complications should be considered an essential part of medical and nursing care.

COMMUNITY SCREENING

Community blood glucose screening is not recommended. However, with the large number of people with undiagnosed diabetes, screening for diabetes and pre-diabetes may be an effective strategy for diabetes prevention and diabetes control. Community blood glucose screening, as is often done at health fairs and shopping malls, is difficult to evaluate, is subject to wide variability and inaccuracies, and has been challenged as to its cost-effectiveness as well as its sensitivity and specificity (1,2). Yet, community screening in the form of risk factor assessment to identify individuals who have multiple risk factors for developing type 2 diabetes may be beneficial. The Diabetes Detection Initiative is a program started in 2004 to identify high-risk individuals through risk factor assessment, random capillary blood glucose testing, and, if appropriate, diagnostic testing (3). Community risk factor screening can also provide the opportunity to heighten awareness of diabetes, identify high-risk individuals, refer them for appropriate testing, and promote early intervention of prevention strategies.

PREVENTING DIABETES

Attempts to prevent type 1 diabetes have been largely unsuccessful. The large, multicenter Diabetes Prevention Trial (4) in type 1 diabetes sought to prevent the development of type 1 diabetes in people at high risk by using low-dose injected, as well as oral, insulin. These interventions proved ineffective.

Several studies that focused on preventing type 2 diabetes have had more success (5–7). In the U.S., the Diabetes Prevention Program (7) demonstrated that type 2 diabetes could be either prevented or delayed in a population of people identified to have increased risk of diabetes or pre-diabetes.

This study, a controlled trial conducted in 27 sites in the U.S. and Canada, randomly assigned 3,234 participants ages 25–85 years to either an intensive lifestyle intervention consisting of a weight-loss diet and 150 min of exercise a week, a medication intervention group (metformin), or a control group. The results showed that individuals in the lifestyle intervention group who lost an average of 7% of their body weight and exercised an average of 150 min/week had a 58% decrease in the risk for developing type 2 diabetes. There was a 31% decrease in the risk for developing type 2 diabetes among individuals in the metformin group. The lifestyle group was most successful in decreasing the risk of developing diabetes in the population >60 years of age. Of note is that 45% of the study population was made up of high-risk minority groups. This landmark study has affected how we treat patients diagnosed with pre-diabetes and those at high risk for developing type 2 diabetes.

Heart Disease and Diabetes

People with diabetes are at risk for chronic microvascular and macrovascular complications; ~80% die of cardiovascular disease. It has been demonstrated that people with diabetes and no prior history of myocardial infarction have a risk of dying from heart disease comparable to those who have had a myocardial infarction but do not have diabetes (8). As a result, the National Cholesterol Education Program (NCEP) lists diabetes as a coronary disease risk factor equivalent in the Adult Treatment Practice guidelines (9).

Metabolic Syndrome

Many people with and without type 2 diabetes have a constellation of cardiac risk factors, including abdominal obesity, hypertension, dyslipidemia, and coagulation abnormalities. Several of these conditions are grouped together and termed the *metabolic syndrome*. This clustering of risk factors is specifically seen in individuals with high triglyceride and low HDL cholesterol levels, hyperinsulinemia, hypertension, and insulin resistance. They may or may not have pre-diabetes, but the syndrome is highly predictive of cardiovascular disease. It has been estimated that the metabolic syndrome is present in ~20% of the U.S. population (10). Two definitions for the metabolic syndrome currently exist: one from the NCEP Adult Treatment Panel (ATP) III (9) and one from the World Health Organization (WHO) (11) (Table 2.1). In a study by Ford and Giles (12) comparing the prevalence of the metabolic syndrome using both definitions, a similar prevalence was found (ATP III 23.9% and WHO 25.1%). However, among various ethnic subpopulations, the two definitions differed in terms of identifying individuals with and without the metabolic syndrome, e.g., African American men were identified to have a 24.9% estimated prevalence using WHO criteria and a 16.5% prevalence using ATP III criteria. Although it appears that a more universally accepted definition is needed, these estimates underscore the critical problem of increasing morbidity and mortality in the U.S. related to this syndrome. Prevention, therefore, requires aggressive management of all of these risk factors.

DIABETES PREVENTION STRATEGIES

Prevention strategies can be divided into primary and secondary prevention. In individuals who have already been diagnosed with diabetes, strategies should be aimed at preventing cardiovascular disease and other complications of diabetes. In

Table 2.1 Metabolic Syndrome Definitions

ATP III criteria

Three or more of the following:

1. Abdominal obesity: waist circumference >102 cm or >40 in for men and >88 cm or >35 in for women
2. Hypertriglyceridemia: ≥150 mg/dl (1.695 mmol/l)
3. Low HDL cholesterol: <40 mg/dl (1.036 mmol/l) in men and <50 mg/dl (1.295 mmol/l) in women
4. High blood pressure: ≥130/85 mmHg
5. High fasting glucose: ≥110 mg/dl (≥6 mmol/l)

WHO criteria

Presence of diabetes, impaired glucose tolerance, impaired fasting glucose, or insulin resistance plus two or more of the following abnormalities:

1. High blood pressure: ≥160/90 mmHg
2. Hyperlipidemia: triglyceride concentration >150 mg/dl (1.695 mmol/l) and/or HDL cholesterol <35 mg/dl (0.9 mmol/l) in men and <39 mg/dl (1.0 mmol/l) in women
3. Central obesity: waist-to-hip ratio of >0.90 in men or >0.85 in women and/or BMI >30 kg/m^2
4. Microalbuminuria: urinary albumin excretion rate ≥20 μg/min or an albumin-to-creatinine ratio ≥20 mg/g

---

individuals with pre-diabetes, the metabolic syndrome, or a high risk for developing type 2 diabetes, the focus is on preventing the onset of the disease and associated cardiovascular disease (Table 2.2).

ABCs of Diabetes Management

For individuals with type 2 diabetes, the American Diabetes Association (ADA) has advocated the ABCs of diabetes management (13) (see also "For Great Diabetes Care, Remember Your ABCs!", a patient handout in RESOURCES). This plan focuses on targets for blood glucose control via the glycated hemoglobin A$_{1c}$ (A1C) test, blood pressure control, and lipid management.

A is for A1C. The A1C test is the assay done to evaluate glucose control over the preceding 2–4 months. The current goal for A1C recommended by the ADA is <7% (4–6% is normal on most assays); some advocate lower levels. A1C should be tested routinely, approximately every 3 months.

B is for blood pressure. Hypertension management frequently requires multiple medications. Angiotensin-converting enzyme (ACE) inhibitors or angiotensin receptor blockers (ARBs) are recommended first-choice antihypertensive drugs in patients with diabetes. Other classes of agents, such as thiazide diuretics, β-blockers, and calcium-channel blockers, may be added to reach the target of <130/80 mmHg.

Table 2.2 Recommendations for Preventing or Delaying Diabetes

- Individuals at high risk should be educated about the benefits of modest weight loss and regular physical activity.
  - Medical nutrition therapy: Reduce fat, especially saturated fat; increase dietary fiber; control calories.
  - Physical activity: Perform ≥30 min of moderate-intensity exercise or activity a day, 5–7 days a week.
- Screen high-risk individuals with risk factors for pre-diabetes or with diagnosed pre-diabetes (BMI >25 kg/m², family history of diabetes, member of a high-risk ethnic group, history of giving birth to a baby >9 lb, history of impaired glucose tolerance or glycosuria, history of GDM).
  - If normal, re-screen at 3-year intervals or more frequently if indicated.
  - If abnormal, confirm test on another day.
- Counsel all individuals with pre-diabetes on weight loss, if needed, and physical activity. Refer to a dietitian for education and follow-up.
- Assess for other cardiovascular risk factors.
  - Stop smoking.
  - Control blood pressure.
  - Manage lipid levels.
- Recommend or refer for appropriate treatment, e.g., smoking cessation program, primary care provider for control of hypertension and dyslipidemia, dietitian, CDE, exercise physiologist, community resources, mental health specialist, etc.
- Consider drug therapy (metformin) for diabetes prevention in some individuals and evaluate whether there is a need for aspirin therapy.

C is for cholesterol. The atherogenic dyslipidemia associated with diabetes is typically a low HDL cholesterol level, a high triglyceride level, and an LDL cholesterol level that is not markedly elevated. In fact, studies have shown that patients with type 2 diabetes have lower LDL levels than the population at large. Cholesterol-lowering drugs (statins) have been shown to be effective in reducing cardiovascular disease in patients with diabetes. A recent study suggested that all patients with diabetes at high cardiac risk, regardless of LDL level, may benefit from these drugs (14). Lipid levels should be tested at least annually.

Current ADA Recommendations for Lipid Management

- *People aged >40 years, without overt cardiovascular disease (CVD):* statin therapy with goals of LDL cholesterol <100 mg/dl and total cholesterol ≥135 mg/dl
- *People aged <40 years, without CVD but at risk, and who do not achieve lipid goals with lifestyle modification:* pharmacological therapy with an LDL cholesterol goal of <100 mg/dl
- *People with diabetes and overt CVD:* high-dose statin therapy with an LDL cholesterol goal of <70 mg/dl

From ADA (15).

Aspirin Therapy

There is evidence that aspirin therapy can reduce the risk of cardiovascular events in individuals with diabetes without a diagnosis of cardiovascular disease and in individuals who have already been diagnosed with cardiovascular disease. Recommendations from ADA for primary and secondary prevention of coronary heart disease for individuals aged >30 years are 81–325 mg/day enteric aspirin, unless contraindicated (16).

Because it is well known that lifestyle changes can decrease the risk for developing type 2 diabetes, improve lipids, improve blood pressure, lower weight, and generally decrease risk for cardiovascular events, identifying high-risk individuals and intervening with prevention strategies is of utmost importance (Table 2.2). Screening, counseling, monitoring, and perhaps drug therapy may be indicated.

Lifestyle Interventions

Lifestyle interventions, specifically medical nutrition therapy and physical activity, are effective in helping people lower their risks for developing diabetes, hypertension, dyslipidemia, and heart disease. They are key management strategies for all patients.

Medical nutrition therapy should focus on decreasing the total intake of fat, particularly saturated fat, and increasing the intake of whole grains and dietary fiber. It is important to incorporate individual circumstances, health status, preferences, and cultural and ethnic considerations (17). There is no standard nutrition plan, neither is there an "ADA diet" applicable to all individuals with diabetes (17). However, healthy eating and striving to reach a healthy body weight (BMI 18.5–24.9 kg/m^2) should be the focus of medical nutrition therapy. It is important to set achievable and maintainable weight loss goals (18).

Physical activity should be universally encouraged. The Centers for Disease Control and Prevention, the American College of Sports Medicine, and Healthy People 2010 all recommend moderate-intensity physical activity for 30 min/day for 5 days a week or vigorous-intensity physical activity for 20 min/day for at least 3 days a week (19). Starting to exercise or increasing physical activity to 20 or 30 min/day may be too difficult a goal initially. Advise sedentary people to begin increasing their physical activity gradually. Walking 10 min several times a day may be easier for some people than trying to walk for 30–40 min at a time. Exercise can be a variety of activities. Assessing individual preferences, physical ability, and safety is appropriate when choosing the type of exercise. Stress the importance of adequate hydration while doing any type of physical activity.

Smoking Cessation

Cigarette smoking and diabetes markedly increase the risk for vascular disease. The risks of smoking may be well known, but it is important that health care providers continue to urge individuals who smoke to stop and to educate people who smoke about the increased risks of cardiovascular disease. All smokers should be asked about their readiness to stop smoking and be referred to smoking cessation programs (20,21). In addition, health care providers should advise all individuals with diabetes or risk factors for diabetes and vascular diseases not to start smoking.

Alcohol

Carefully assess alcohol consumption and counsel people on the dangers of excessive alcohol intake. Aside from being high in calories, stimulating appetite, and perhaps being contraindicated with certain medications, excessive alcohol consumption is associated with other social and health problems. Modest alcohol intake (1–2 drinks/day [one drink is the equivalent of 5 oz of wine, 12 oz of light beer, or 1.5 oz of 80-proof distilled spirits]) may be incorporated into the nutrition plan for individuals who choose to drink. There is some evidence that modest alcohol intake may reduce cardiovascular risk (22).

Immunizations

Individuals with diabetes, especially those with vascular complications, are at high risk for morbidity and mortality associated with influenza and pneumococcal disease. Patient education regarding the need for vaccinations is necessary. Individuals with diabetes who are age ≥6 months should receive an influenza vaccine every fall. A pneumococcal vaccination is recommended for individuals <65 years of age, and a one-time revaccination is recommended for individuals ≥65 years of age if the vaccine was administered >5 years previously. Revaccination may also be advised in individuals with diabetes who suffer from renal disease or other immunocompromised states (23).

Periodic Medical Visits

It is often challenging to convince individuals who feel healthy to see their health care providers for routine visits. However, individuals with multiple risk factors need regular evaluation and management. A person with a chronic illness may need to be seen three to four times a year. Health care providers must emphasize the need for regular screening and evaluation not only in these individuals, but in their family members as well. Identification of individuals at high risk for diabetes and cardiovascular disease may be effectively done when patients come in accompanied by a family member who has obvious risk factors. Education regarding the risks of developing type 2 diabetes should be done at that time, and those family members should be referred for further evaluation.

Individual health care beliefs may present a barrier to preventive care if individuals at high risk do not perceive themselves as susceptible to illness. It is the duty of the health care team to be cognizant of the health care beliefs of the individuals they see. The health care team should work together to identify, screen, and diagnose high-risk individuals so that early intervention strategies can be initiated.

PRACTICAL POINT

ABCs of Diabetes
- A1C <7.0%
- Blood pressure <130/80 mmHg
- LDL cholesterol <70 mg/dl
- Triglycerides <150 mg/dl
- HDL cholesterol >40 mg/dl (men) and >50 mg/dl (women)

SUMMARY

Primary and secondary prevention is essential in the prevention of diabetes and the potential complications of diabetes. Interventions to recognize high-risk individuals and strategies to decrease the risk of diabetes and diabetes-related complications should be considered an essential part of nursing care. Every January, the ADA publishes the updated Standards of Medical Care in Diabetes based on the latest research findings. The Standards can be accessed on the Internet at www.diabetes.org.

REFERENCES

1. Rolka DB, Narayan KM, Thompson TJ, Goldman D, Lindenmayer J, Alich K, Bacall D, Benjamin EM, Lamb B, Stuart DO, Engelgau MM: Performance of recommended screening tests for undiagnosed diabetes and dysglycemia. *Diabetes Care* 24:1899–1903, 2001
2. Tabaei BP, Burke R, Constance A, Hare J, May-Aldrich G, Parker SA, Scott A, Stys A, Chickering J, Herman WH: Community-based screening for diabetes in Michigan. *Diabetes Care* 26:668–670, 2003
3. Diabetes Detection Initiative (DDI) web site. Available from http://www.ndep.nih.gov/ddi. Accessed 10 January 2005
4. Diabetes Prevention Trial—Type 1 Diabetes Study Group: Effects of insulin in relatives of patients with type 1 diabetes mellitus. *N Engl J Med* 346:1685–1691, 2002
5. Pan XR, Li GW, Hu YH, Wang JX, Yang WY, An ZX, Hu ZX, Lin J, Xiao JZ, Cao HB, Liu PA, Jiang XG, Jiang YY, Wang JP, Zheng H, Zhang H, Bennett PH, Howard BV: Effects of diet and exercise in preventing NIDDM in people with impaired glucose tolerance: the Da Qing IGT and Diabetes Study. *Diabetes Care* 20:537–544, 1997
6. Tuomilehto J, Lindstrom J, Eriksson JG, Valle TT, Hamalainen H, Ilanne-Parikka P, Keinanen-Kiukaanniemi S, Laakso M, Louheranta A, Rastas M, Salminen V, Uusitupa M, Finnish Diabetes Prevention Study Group: Prevention of type 2 diabetes mellitus by changes in lifestyle among subjects with impaired glucose tolerance. *N Engl J Med* 344:1343–1350, 2001
7. Diabetes Prevention Program Research Group: Reduction in the incidence of type 2 diabetes with lifestyle intervention or metformin. *N Engl J Med* 346:393–403, 2002
8. Haffner SM, Lehto S, Ronnemaa T, Pyorala K, Laakso M: Mortality from coronary heart disease in subjects with type 2 diabetes and in nondiabetic subjects with and without prior myocardial infarction. *N Engl J Med* 339:229–234, 1998
9. Expert Panel on the Detection, Education, and Treatment of High Blood Cholesterol in Adults: Executive summary of the third report of the National Cholesterol Education Program (NCEP) Expert Panel on Detection, Education, and Treatment of High Blood Cholesterol in Adults (Adult Treatment Panel III). *JAMA* 285:2486–2497, 2001
10. Park Y, Zhu S, Palaniappan L, Heshka S, Carnethon MR, Heymsfeld SB: The metabolic syndrome: prevalence and associated risk factor findings in the US population from the Third National Health and Nutrition Examination Survey, 1988–1994. *Arch Intern Med* 163:427–436, 2003
11. Alberti KG, Zimmet PZ: Definition, diagnosis and classification of diabetes mellitus and its complications. Part 1. Diagnosis and classification of dia-

betes mellitus, provisional report of a WHO consultation. *Diabet Med* 15: 539–553, 1998

12. Ford ES, Giles WH: A comparison of the prevalence of the metabolic syndrome using two proposed definitions. *Diabetes Care* 26:575–581, 2003

13. Abbate S: Expanded ABCs of diabetes. *Clinical Diabetes* 21:128–133, 2003

14. Heart Protection Study Collaborative Group: MRC/BHF Heart Protection Study of cholesterol lowering with simvastatin in 20,536 high risk individuals: a randomized placebo controlled trial. *Lancet* 260:7–22, 2002

15. American Diabetes Association: Standards of medical care in diabetes (Position Statement). *Diabetes Care* 28 (Suppl. 1):S4–S36, 2005

16. American Diabetes Association: Aspirin therapy in diabetes (Position Statement). *Diabetes Care* 27 (Suppl. 1):S72–S73, 2003

17. American Diabetes Association: Nutrition principles and recommendations in diabetes (Position Statement). *Diabetes Care* 27 (Suppl. 1):S36–S46, 2004

18. Klein S, Sheard NF, Pi-Sunyer X, Daly A, Wylie-Rossett J, Kulkarni K, Clark NG: Weight management through lifestyle modification for the prevention and management of type 2 diabetes: rationale and strategies. *Diabetes Care* 27:2067–2073, 2004

19. Centers for Disease Control and Prevention: *Physical Activity Guidelines.* Atlanta, GA, Centers for Disease Control and Prevention, 2003

20. American Diabetes Association: Smoking and diabetes (Position Statement). *Diabetes Care* 27 (Suppl. 1):S74–S75, 2004

21. Haire-Joshu D, Glasgow RE, Tibbs TL: Smoking and diabetes. *Diabetes Care* 22:1887–1898, 1999

22. Rimm E, Williams P, Fosher K, Criqui M, Stampfer J: Moderate alcohol intake and lower risk of coronary heart disease: meta-analysis of effect on lipids and haemostatic factors. *Br Med J* 319:1523–1528, 1999

23. American Diabetes Association: Influenza and pneumococcal immunization in diabetes (Position Statement). *Diabetes Care* 27 (Suppl. 1):S111–S113, 2004

Ms. Cypress is an Adult Nurse Practitioner and Certified Diabetes Educator in Albuquerque, NM. Dr. Gleeson is Chair of the Division of Endocrinology and Medical Director of the Diabetes Program at Lovelace Sandia Health Systems, Albuquerque, NM.

3. Healthy Lifestyle Changes: Food and Physical Activity

ANNE DALY, MS, RD, BC-ADM, CDE

TWIN EPIDEMICS: DIABETES AND OBESITY

Recent evidence demonstrates the unfolding of a diabetes epidemic in the U.S. According to two reports from the Centers for Disease Control and Prevention, from 1990 to 1998, the number of people with diabetes increased by 33% (1), and from 1998 to 1999, this incidence grew by another 6% (2). Of particular concern is that type 2 diabetes is being diagnosed at alarming rates in children and adolescents (3). Simultaneously, from 1991 to 1999, there was a 57% increase in the incidence of obesity in the U.S. (4,5). This increasing incidence of obesity is thought to be the primary culprit in the diabetes epidemic, bolstered by the growth of population groups with high incidences of type 2 diabetes and the aging of the American population.

How do we address these epidemics? Improving health—particularly blood glucose and lipid levels, blood pressure, and body weight—through food choices and physical activity is the basis of all recommendations for the treatment and prevention of diabetes. Most important, supporting people with diabetes in achieving lifestyle-related goals and maintaining healthy lifestyles requires the coordinated effort of a team that includes physicians, nurses, registered dietitians (RDs), and diabetes educators.

ROLE OF LIFESTYLE CHANGES IN DIABETES PREVENTION

Evidence is building that lifestyle changes, especially healthy eating and physical activity, are beneficial for people with impaired glucose tolerance, or pre-diabetes, and insulin resistance. In fact, the Diabetes Prevention Program (DPP) ended a year early because even modest lifestyle changes—eating less fat, losing 7% of body weight, and exercising 150 min weekly—dramatically and conclusively reduced the development of type 2 diabetes for people who were most at risk (6). The DPP, with 3,234 participants at 27 medical centers, was the largest and first in the U.S. to include 45% of participants from the ethnic groups at highest risk to develop diabetes—African Americans, Native Americans, Hispanics/Latinos, Asians, and Pacific Islanders. The study had three intervention arms: an intensive lifestyle group, a metformin group, and a control group using standard lifestyle intervention plus placebo. Results showed a 58% reduction in progression to diabetes among people in the intensive lifestyle group compared with the control group, and the metformin group experienced a 31% reduction in progression to diabetes. The highest reduction in progression to diabetes in the intensive lifestyle group (71%) was achieved among people age ≥60 years.

Education and concerted support from a health care team were key elements of the DPP. Participants in the intensive lifestyle group attended 16 group sessions within the first 24 weeks in which a structured core curriculum was used. After the core curriculum was delivered, participants met with their case manager monthly. Participants in the standard treatment group received written information and one 20- to 30-min individual session with their case manager. Participants in the standard treatment group were encouraged to follow the food pyramid and the equivalent of the National Cholesterol Education Program (Step 1) diet (7).

The DPP results are consistent with earlier reports of the Finnish Diabetes Prevention Study, a smaller study that involved a single ethnic group (8). In that study, the intervention group received detailed and individualized counseling aimed at reducing weight, reducing total intake of fat and saturated fat, and increasing fiber, along with personal guidance on increasing physical activity. This counseling was provided in seven sessions with a nutritionist during the first year and one session every 3 months during the study. The control group received general oral and written information about diet (a two-page leaflet) and physical activity at annual visits. The incidence of diabetes in the intervention group was reduced by 58%, a rate identical to the U.S. study. The study investigators concluded that although pessimism is commonly expressed with regard to the challenge of inducing lifestyle change in overweight and sedentary people, this pessimism is unwarranted.

The conclusions of these major studies are remarkably consistent, and the clinical implications are clear: type 2 diabetes is not inevitable, individuals at high risk to develop diabetes can be identified, and with early lifestyle intervention, diabetes can be delayed, if not prevented (6,8). Because the burden resulting from diabetes complications is enormous, an effort to prevent and/or delay diabetes is worthwhile. Policymakers and health care systems must develop low-cost ways to promote physical activity and weight loss. Health care providers need to be more aggressive with nutrition and exercise therapies. In most clinical settings, weight management is not considered a primary intervention for the prevention or treatment of type 2 diabetes. However, a recent meta-analysis concluded that weight management may be the most important therapeutic task for managing obese individuals with type 2 diabetes (9). Early referral for lifestyle advice—either to prevent the development of diabetes or as soon as possible after the diagnosis of diabetes—is essential. Nutrition therapy is most effective in the initial phases of type 2 diabetes when insulin resistance is likely to be the greatest (10).

ROLE OF DIABETES NUTRITIONAL CARE IN LIFESTYLE CHANGE

Over the past decade, along with changes in the medications used for treating diabetes have come changes in medical nutrition therapy (MNT) and behavior-change strategies. Gone are the days when the primary nutrition messages for people with diabetes were to limit sugar intake and follow a "diabetic diet" with a specified calorie level. Before 1994, American Diabetes Association (ADA) nutrition recommendations attempted to define ideal macronutrient percentages for a diabetes nutrition prescription. Although individualization was a basic principle, it had to be done within the confines of the nutrition prescription.

Now, instead of a rigid nutrition prescription, MNT is based on an assessment of lifestyle changes that would assist the person with diabetes in achieving and maintaining clinical goals, but is focused on changes the person with diabetes is able and willing to make (11). Studies have shown that a positive approach—focusing on "to do" behaviors rather than "not to do" behaviors—is more effective in producing improved clinical outcomes (12) and weight loss (13). Table 3.1 illustrates the paradigm shift that has occurred in nutrition therapy.

Table 3.1 Outdated Versus Updated Diabetes Nutrition Recommendations

Outdated	Updated
MNT is a calculated ADA diet with calculated calories and percentages of carbohydrate, protein, and fat.	There is no one ADA diet for all people with diabetes. An ADA diet can only be defined as an individualized food plan based on assessment, therapy goals, and meal planning approaches that meet patients' needs. The use of diet sheets or a one-time "diet instruction" is rarely effective to change eating habits. For people to make lifestyle changes that result in positive clinical outcomes requires education and counseling in both nutrition and physical activity with support over time.
Ideal body weight (per Metropolitan Life Insurance) is the goal.	Even modest weight loss (5–7% starting body weight) can improve glucose, lipids, and insulin resistance. Participation in a structured and intensive maintenance program improves long-term weight maintenance.
Sugars and sweets are forbidden because they are rapidly digested and absorbed and cause blood glucose levels to go higher than do starches.	Evidence from many clinical studies has demonstrated that sugars do not increase glycemia more than isocaloric amounts of starch.
Protein is recommended because it slows the absorption of carbohydrates and prevents hypoglycemia.	Ingested protein does not slow the absorption of carbohydrate and neither does adding protein prevent/assist in the treatment of hypoglycemia.
"When diet and exercise fail, add medications." The implication: no need to pay attention to lifestyle.	Diet doesn't fail, the pancreas does. Type 2 diabetes is a progressive disease. MNT should continue to be an essential part of the treatment plan. Patients can "eat their way through" any medications they are given.

The Process of MNT

MNT is the service provided by an RD that, when implemented properly, consists of a four-step process.

1. An individual assessment
2. Goal setting
3. Intervention
4. Evaluation

MNT is effective in diabetes management (14,15). Evidence from randomized controlled trials, observational studies, and meta-analyses has shown that MNT improves metabolic outcomes such as blood glucose and glycated hemoglobin A_{1c} (A1C) in people with diabetes (Table 3.2).

Dietitians have found it helpful to prioritize nutrition advice based on an individualized assessment. Patients often choose small, gradual changes in lifestyle, and it is essential that lifestyle goals be changes that the patient is willing and likely to be able to make. Choosing just one or two primary behavior-change areas is suggested initially so as not to overwhelm the patient. Focusing on specific "how to" steps is helpful for successful behavior change (see also "Resources for People Who Want to Lose Weight," a patient handout in RESOURCES). Providing the patients with a written copy of the goals is recommended.

Once an assessment has been completed and clinical and behavioral goals agreed upon with the patient, a nutrition intervention strategy is selected. This might include selecting a meal-planning strategy as well as a specific education resource for the patient to use. No single strategy or method can be recommended because various methods have been tested and demonstrated to facilitate attainment of nutrition goals. During initial phases of education (survival), simplified resources, such as the Food Guide Pyramid, that can illustrate basic nutrition guidelines are recommended. There are basic diabetes nutrition messages that are associated with improved outcomes:

Eat similar amounts of carbohydrate. To control blood glucose levels, the first priority is to eat consistent amounts of carbohydrate at meals and to eat at similar

---

Table 3.2 Lessons Learned from Nutritional Outcomes Research

- Nutrition therapy does not fail—it is essential for optimal diabetes management. The β-cells of the pancreas fail.
- In the U.K. Prospective Diabetes Study (UKPDS), intensive nutrition therapy provided by dietitians decreased A1C levels by ~2%.
- Other studies have shown that nutrition therapy provided by registered dietitians lowers A1C by 1–2% and fasting plasma glucose levels by 50–100 mg/dl (2.8–5.6 mmol/l).
- The UKPDS revealed that type 2 diabetes is a progressive disorder, and therapy—medication(s) combined with nutrition therapy—needs to be intensified over time.
- The focus of lifestyle interventions should be on improving blood glucose control, lipids, and blood pressure.
    - Teach patients which foods contain carbohydrate, emphasize portion sizes, and specify the number of servings for meals and snacks.
    - Encourage 30 min of physical activity on most days of the week.
    - Monitor blood glucose, lipids, and blood pressure to determine effectiveness of therapy.

It is important when developing behavioral goals with patients that the goals be attainable and very specific regarding the type, frequency, and duration of the behavior. For example:

- "I will decrease the number of fast food meals I eat to one a week for the next 2 months."
- "I will walk 20 min, 5 days a week, for the next month."
- "I will increase the amount of green vegetables I eat to at least two servings a day for the next month."
- "I will replace lard with canola oil in my cooking for the next 3 months."

Be sure to follow up with patients to evaluate their progress toward meeting their goals or to help them identify barriers and develop new goals.

times of day. Carbohydrate is the primary predictor of postprandial blood glucose levels because carbohydrate in foods raises blood glucose levels fastest and the most after eating. This does not mean foods containing carbohydrate should be eliminated, simply controlled and consistent. Foods that contain carbohydrate are among the healthiest foods—starches, whole grains, fruits, vegetables, and milk. An adult typically needs between three and five carbohydrate servings (starches, fruits, milk, or yogurt) per meal. One serving is equal to 15 g carbohydrate. Non-starchy vegetables contain smaller amounts of carbohydrate and are encouraged because they provide good nutrition and volume. Distribution of carbohydrate foods is difficult for many patients, especially those who skip breakfast. When a person with diabetes eats only one or two meals per day or drinks large volumes of regular soda or fruit juice, simply changing to three spaced meals and using calorie-free beverages can improve blood glucose significantly.

Practice portion control. In our "super-sized" world, reasonable portion sizes are essential for optimal glucose and weight control. Encourage people to continue to eat the foods they enjoy, but to eat smaller portions. An RD can help people with diabetes learn what portions are appropriate for them. Meanwhile, asking patients to fill their plates only once without going back for seconds can lower caloric intake and blood glucose levels.

Skim the fats. Fat is loaded with calories, and all fats (except omega-3s) may be associated with insulin resistance. A reduction in fat helps with weight loss and maintenance and improves lipid levels. Fat is found in salad dressing, margarine, oil, chips, fried foods, and more. Saturated fat is found in meats, whole milk, other full-fat dairy foods, butter, and coconut, palm, and hydrogenated oils. *Trans* fats are found in processed foods and baked goods, shortening, and some fast food items, such as French fries. In 2006, food labels will be required to include *trans* fats, making it easier to identify these foods. Urge patients to cut down on calories and eat "heart healthy" by skimming the fat and calories without reducing the amount of food at a meal. Increasing fruits and vegetables to at least seven servings total per day is an excellent way to add volume to meals but decrease calorie and dietary fat at the same time. This is an example of where using a positive approach, focusing on "to do" behaviors, rather than "not to do" behaviors, can be effective. In essence, more fruits and vegetables becomes a "back door" way of decreasing fat.

Engage in adequate physical activity. Ideally, patients should accumulate a total of 30 min of physical activity most days of the week, similar to the newest public health recommendations (16) as well as the Surgeon General's report on physical activity and health (17). Being active helps improve blood glucose levels, lowers risk of mortality, and improves insulin sensitivity. It may also improve other common metabolic abnormalities of insulin resistance including hypertension, hyperlipidemia, and atherosclerosis. Encourage patients to identify activities they can enjoy safely and can realistically include in their schedule. In the case of children and adolescents, encourage a reduction in time spent doing sedentary activities.

Get to or stay at a healthy weight. Encourage patients to maintain a healthy weight. Overweight patients who lose as little as 10 lb can have significant improvements in blood glucose, blood pressure, and lipids and can also decrease insulin resistance. This message is one of the most helpful that patients can hear. Discuss what reasonable body weight and weight loss goals would be for each individual's situation. Recording food intake along with blood glucose levels often helps reduce caloric intake and promotes weight loss.

Subsequently, more complex approaches, such as calorie or carbohydrate counting, *Exchange Lists for Meal Planning*, adjusting insulin using insulin-to-carbohydrate ratios, or even medically supervised very-low-calorie diets, may be appropriate. Offering a variety of nutrition interventions provides greater flexibility and choices to the person with diabetes and is especially useful for individuals who have been discouraged or frustrated by previous nutrition instruction methods. Although the approach that best meets the individual needs of the client is ideally chosen, the choice of a food plan is also influenced by the RD's experience with different strategies. This means the RD needs a "toolbox" of approaches for supporting patients in structured lifestyle change to promote weight loss (Table 3.3), with close monitoring of outcomes to determine whether goals are being met. These approaches are used in multicenter clinical trials and have been found to be effective.

Many printed resources are available to support nutrition interventions. The ADA and American Dietetic Association co-published nine diabetes resources, designed to reflect the 2002 ADA nutrition recommendations (11) and the American Dietetic Association's evidence-based guides for practice for type 1 diabetes, type 2 diabetes (18), and gestational diabetes; updated nutrient composition data; consumer trends; and feedback from educators (19). These resources include the following titles:

- *The First Step in Diabetes Meal Planning* (English and Spanish)
- *Healthy Food Choices*
- *Eating Healthy with Diabetes: Easy Reading Guide*
- *Exchange Lists for Meal Planning* (English and Spanish)
- *Exchange Lists for Weight Management*
- *Basic Carbohydrate Counting*
- *Advanced Carbohydrate Counting*

These publications can be ordered from the ADA at 800-232-6733 or http://store.diabetes.org.

Table 3.3 Toolbox Approaches to Structured Lifestyle Changes to Promote Weight Loss and Problem Solving

- Increase frequency of contact with health care provider
- Review self-monitoring skills (e.g., records of food, activity, weight, blood glucose levels, medications)
- Change self-monitoring approach
- Provide recipes
- Assign calorie goal or lower fat/calorie goal
- Refer to RD for structured meal plans
- Involve significant other(s)
- Conduct small group visits
- Schedule meeting with behavioral therapist
- Use meal replacements for one to two meals per day
- Try calorie/fat-controlled frozen entrees
- RD-led grocery store visit
- Loan self-help materials
- Provide motivational strategy/incentive/contract
- Refer to a dietitian, fitness club, etc., for additional coaching

---

What About the Glycemic Index?

The glycemic index (GI) is a method for classifying carbohydrates based on their blood glucose response. The GI is formally defined as the incremental area under the blood glucose curve (AUC) after the consumption of 50 g carbohydrate from a test food divided by the AUC after eating a similar amount of a control food (generally white bread or glucose).

The use of diets with a low GI in the management of diabetes is controversial, with contrasting recommendations around the world. Findings of randomized controlled trials have been mixed; some studies have shown statistically significant improvements, whereas others have not (20). As a result, the issue of the GI has been fraught with controversy and has polarized the opinion of leading experts.

After reviewing the evidence, the ADA concluded that the total amount of available carbohydrate is more important than the source (starch or sugar) or type (low or high GI), and although low-GI foods may reduce postprandial hyperglycemia, there was not sufficient evidence to recommend use of low-GI diets as a primary strategy in food/meal planning (11). Rather, the use of GI is raised as an additional technique beyond considering the total amount of carbohydrate alone (21). Primary nutrition interventions documented to have the greatest impact on metabolic outcomes should be selected.

- In the case of type 1 diabetes, outcomes from adjusting insulin based on the carbohydrate content of the meal would appear to be a better primary strategy than a low-GI diet (22).
- For type 2 diabetes, primary nutrition interventions should focus on behavioral strategies such as reduced calorie intake, modest weight loss, and basic carbohydrate counting.

These strategies have been demonstrated to produce better outcomes than a low-GI diet approach. For instance, using a moderate-carbohydrate approach reduced A1C by ~20% compared with 7.4% from the low-GI diet (22). Information on glycemic responses of foods can perhaps best be used for fine-tuning glycemic control.

What About High-Protein, Low-Carbohydrate Diets ("Atkins") for People with Diabetes?

The bottom line is that the jury is still out on the Atkins diet and other high-protein, low-carbohydrate meal plans, particularly for individuals with diabetes. A recent ADA statement strongly advises against recommending low-carbohydrate diets and cautions against restricting carbohydrate to <130 g/day (21).

A systematic review of the efficacy and safety of low-carbohydrate eating plans concluded that there is insufficient evidence to make recommendations for or against the use of low-carbohydrate meal plans (23). Authors have also concluded that more careful studies of people with and without diabetes and with and without lipid abnormalities are needed to more fully describe the effects of lower-carbohydrate eating plans on lipids, GIs, and ketogenesis. Research supported by the National Institutes of Health is underway that should provide more objective data on the long-term effects of such eating plans.

It is true that high-protein, low-carbohydrate eating plans produce substantial initial weight loss—partly because of fluid loss and partly because people end up eating fewer calories because of the limited choices and the effect of ketones to decrease appetite. However, these eating plans do not appear effective for long-term weight maintenance (24). Major concerns about the safety of these plans in people with diabetes include potential progression of cardiovascular disease, cancer, osteoporosis, gout, and renal disease. Nutrition concerns include loss of water-soluble vitamins with diuresis; inadequate fiber, calcium, and B vitamins; and depletion of glycogen stores. Until more evidence becomes available about the safety and efficacy of high-protein, low-carbohydrate eating plans, they should not be recommended to individuals with diabetes. If clients with diabetes choose to follow low-carbohydrate diets and truly adhere to the recommended guidelines, adjustments of glucose-targeted medication may be necessary. Regular blood glucose monitoring should be recommended, along with guidelines for when to call the health care provider.

ROLE OF PHYSICAL ACTIVITY IN RISK FACTOR REDUCTION

The possible benefits of physical activity for patients with type 2 diabetes are substantial. Several long-term studies have demonstrated a consistent beneficial effect of regular physical activity on carbohydrate metabolism and insulin sensitivity. Improvements in A1C are most marked in patients with mild type 2 diabetes and in individuals who are likely to be the most insulin resistant (25).

Multiple epidemiological studies have shown an inverse relationship between physical activity and the risk of coronary heart disease (CHD). Sedentary individuals have almost twice the risk of CHD as those performing high-intensity activity. However, the optimal level of activity for preventing CHD is unclear. In some studies, the reduction in risk from increased levels of activity appeared to be linear up to a certain level, above which there was no further benefit; in others, the effect was restricted to the highest categories of total energy expenditure (26).

Physical activity decreases cardiovascular risk through a number of mechanisms:

- decreased blood pressure
- increased HDL cholesterol level
- decreased triglyceride level
- reduced weight
- increased fibrinolysis in response to thrombotic stimuli
- increased insulin sensitivity and potentially improved blood glucose levels
- reduced susceptibility to serious ventricular arrhythmias
- associated behavioral changes, e.g., smoking cessation, healthier eating, stress reduction
- psychological benefits, e.g., decreased depression and anxiety.

Aerobic activity benefits the cardiovascular system by decreasing heart rate and increasing stroke volume at rest and during physical activity and increasing cardiac output. Physical activity of moderate intensity is usually recommended for people with known coronary artery disease (CAD) in the absence of ischemia or significant arrhythmias. Physical activity of moderate intensity is also generally recommended for the person with hypertension. This level of activity can be targeted to 60–80% of maximum heart rate, which corresponds to 50–75% of the maximum oxygen consumption. High-intensity activity should be minimized because it can cause a significant rise in blood pressure.

Physical activity reduces blood pressure by 5–10 mmHg in some people, and its effects are usually noted within 10 weeks of training. Before starting a physical activity program, people with hypertension require adequate blood pressure control because physical activity causes acute increases in systolic pressure and this increase can be exaggerated in diabetes. The blood pressure response to physical activity should be monitored initially, and adjustments in therapy should be made accordingly.

Before increasing usual patterns of physical activity or beginning an exercise program, the person with diabetes should undergo a detailed medical evaluation with appropriate diagnostic studies. He or she may require an exercise stress test (see below). Physical activity should be performed on most days of the week or at least four times per week, with each session lasting between 30 and 60 min. Physical activity at regular intervals has been noted to decrease the risk of myocardial infarction. Sedentary individuals experience a higher relative risk of myocardial infarction after an episode of heavy exertion compared with individuals who engage in physical activity five or more times per week.

In addition to cardiovascular disease, sedentary lifestyles are closely associated with obesity. Physical activity is a potent physiological stimulus of lipolysis, which results in the release of free fatty acids from triglycerides stored in fat for use as an energy source by muscle. Therefore, physical activity increases energy expenditure, which results in a negative calorie balance, adding potential for weight loss to occur. Although physical activity alone may produce a 2–3% reduction in BMI, it is more effective when used as an adjunct to MNT (27). Multiple studies have shown that once weight loss has been accomplished, physical activity is the primary predictor of weight maintenance. Without increasing physical activity, often weight loss is temporary.

Getting Started with Physical Activity

Walking is the most commonly prescribed activity and the most likely to be successful because of both safety and accessibility. Almost anyone can participate in brisk walking, and when pedometers are used, the individual has feedback concerning the number of steps or miles walked. Monitoring physical activity data is useful for shaping this behavior in small, simple steps. Individuals might begin by walking for 5–10 min 3 days/week and gradually increase duration, frequency, and intensity of walking to the target level. The DPP intervention included 150 min/week of medium-intensity activity. Proponents of counting steps advocate 4,000 steps per day initially and suggest increasing to 10,000 steps daily over a 6-month period. The National Weight Control Registry, a group of successful weight maintainers, reports participants engage in an average of 2,800 calories of physical activity weekly (28).

Getting started with a physical activity program is not easy, and keeping one going can be even more difficult. The use of written goal-oriented plans is associated with success. Other factors that promote increased physical activity are

- doing some activity daily
- doing some activity before noon
- having a home option, e.g., treadmill, neighborhood walking route
- using multiple, short bouts of exercise (≤20 min)
- doing multiple types of activities
- follow-up with a case manager/coach.

Exercise Stress Tests

The use of stress tests is recommended for some people with type 1 or type 2 diabetes because they have at least twice the morbidity and mortality related to myocardial infarction as the general population. In addition, many studies indicate that the incidence of asymptomatic CAD or CAD associated with atypical symptoms is higher in the diabetes population. A 10% prevalence of occult clinically significant CAD in the typical clinic population with type 2 diabetes without classic symptoms of ischemia is probably a conservative estimate (26). One of the most feared risks of initiating an activity program is that of inducing sudden death secondary to an arrhythmia or ischemic event. This is most likely to occur when CAD is already diagnosed.

Therefore, before starting a physical activity program of moderate intensity (e.g., walking at a rate of ≥3 mph) to high intensity, ADA recommendations for type 2 diabetes suggest that previously sedentary individuals >35 years of age or sedentary individuals of any age with duration of diabetes >10 years undergo stress testing. In addition, the presence of nephropathy, autonomic neuropathy, or peripheral vascular disease indicates the need for stress testing. The clearest example of groups of people for whom stress testing would be more useful are those with a prior coronary event and those with nontraditional risk factors (i.e., autonomic neuropathy, peripheral arterial disease, proteinuria, and azotemia) (26).

Little is known about the risks of physical activity training in individuals with type 1 diabetes because most research is conducted in people with type 2 diabetes. Until additional information is available, anyone with the onset of type 1 diabetes in childhood or adolescence who is over the age of 35 years or who has diabetes for >15 years should be considered a high-risk patient.

ROLE RESPONSIBILITIES

Both the ADA (11) and the Institute of Medicine (29) state that because of the complexity of nutrition issues, it is recommended that an RD, knowledgeable and skilled in implementing nutrition therapy into diabetes management and

Table 3.4 Nurse and RD Responsibilities Related to MNT

Nurse's responsibilities

1. Refer patient to an RD for MNT.
2. Provide referral data: diabetes treatment regimen, laboratory values for A1C, glucose values, cholesterol fractions, blood pressure, and presence of microalbuminuria; medical goals for patient care; medical history; medications that affect MNT; and clearance for physical activity.
3. Collaborate with the patient to establish medical treatment goals.
4. Provide and reinforce basic nutrition messages.
5. Reinforce the importance of working with an RD on nutrition self-management.

RD's responsibilities

1. Obtain referral data and treatment goals before the initial nutrition intervention.
2. Obtain and assess information about patient's eating habits, activity, self-monitoring of blood glucose levels, cultural and ethnic background, psychosocial and economic issues, and support system(s).
3. Assess patient's knowledge, age, skill level, readiness to change, and goals.
4. In partnership with the patient, select and implement appropriate nutrition prescription and use appropriate teaching tools to provide education on food, meal planning, and self-management.
5. Evaluate the effectiveness of MNT based on treatment targets and adjust MNT as needed.
6. Make recommendations to the nurse based on the outcomes of nutrition interventions and communicate progress/outcomes of nutrition interventions; communicate progress/outcomes to all team members.
7. Plan for follow-up and ongoing education.

education, be the team member providing MNT. However, it is essential that all team members be knowledgeable about nutrition therapy and be supportive of the person with diabetes who needs to make lifestyle changes. Table 3.4 lists nurse and other health care professional and dietitian responsibilities related to MNT.

SUMMARY

The evidence for more aggressive treatment of diabetes using nutrition and physical activity is growing. To best meet the challenge and manage the diabetes epidemic in the U.S., all health care professionals must accept expanding role responsibilities. To effectively help people with diabetes achieve behavior change, it is important to recognize the person with diabetes as the most important person on the health care team. Nurses should encourage small, gradual changes in just one or two behaviors and emphasize the "to do" behaviors rather than "not to do" behaviors. These strategies are associated with improved behavioral and clinical outcomes. Teaching strategies that help the person become his or her own manager of behavior change are likely to result in the most lasting change. The nurse should be knowledgeable of community resources to refer the patient for additional nutritional services such as diabetes self-management programs and dietitians in the community (see RESOURCES for some of these services and programs).

REFERENCES

1. Mokdad AH, Ford ES, Bowman BA, Nelson DE, Engelgau MM, Vinicor F: Diabetes trends in the U.S.: 1990–1998. *Diabetes Care* 23:1278–1283, 2000
2. Mokdad AH, Ford ES, Bowman BA, Nelson DC, Engelgau MM, Vinicor F, Marks JS: The continuing increase of diabetes in the U.S. (Letter). *Diabetes Care* 24:412, 2001
3. Alberti G, Zimmet P, Shaw J, Bloomgarden Z, Kaufman F, Silink M: Type 2 diabetes in the young: the evolving epidemic: the International Diabetes Federation Consensus Workshop (Consensus Statement). *Diabetes Care* 27:1798–1811, 2004
4. Mokdad AH, Serdula MK, Dietz WH, Bowman BA, Marks JH: The spread of the obesity epidemic in the United States (Letter). *JAMA* 282:1519–1522, 1999
5. U.S. Department of Health and Human Services: *The Surgeon General's Call to Action to Prevent and Decrease Overweight and Obesity.* Washington, DC, Govt. Printing Office, 2001 (DHHS publ. no. 017-001-00551-7)
6. Diabetes Prevention Program Research Group: Reduction in the incidence of type 2 diabetes with lifestyle intervention or metformin. *N Engl J Med* 346:393–401, 2002
7. Expert Panel on Detection, Evaluation, and Treatment of High Blood Cholesterol in Adults: Cholesterol Education Program (Adult Treatment Panel III): Executive Summary of the Third Report of the National Cholesterol Education Program. *JAMA* 285:2486–2497, 2001
8. Finnish Diabetes Prevention Study Group: Prevention of type 2 diabetes mellitus by changes in lifestyle among subjects with impaired glucose tolerance. *N Engl J Med* 344:1343–1350, 2001
9. Anderson JW, Kendall C, Jenkins DJ: Importance of weight management in type 2 diabetes: review with meta-analyses of clinical studies. *J Am Coll Nutr* 22:331–339, 2003
10. Franz M, Green-Pastors J, Warshaw H, Daly A: Does diet fail? *Clinical Diabetes* 18:162–168, 2000
11. American Diabetes Association: Nutrition principles and recommendations in diabetes (Position Statement). *Diabetes Care* 27 (Suppl. 1):S36–S46, 2004
12. Nicholson AS, Sklar M, Barnard ND, Gore S, Sullivan R, Browning S: Toward improved management of NIDDM: a randomized, controlled, pilot intervention using a low fat, vegetarian diet. *Prev Med* 29:87–91, 1999
13. Epstein LH, Gordy CC, Raynor HA, Beddome M, Kilanowski CK, Paluch R: Increasing fruit and vegetable intake and decreasing fat and sugar intake in families at risk for childhood obesity. *Obes Res* 9:171–178, 2001
14. Pastors JG, Warshaw H, Daly A, Franz M, Kulkarni K: The evidence for the effectiveness of medical nutrition therapy in diabetes management. *Diabetes Care* 25:608–613, 2002
15. Pastors JG, Franz M, Warshaw H, Daly A, Arnold M: How effective is medical nutrition therapy in diabetes care? *J Am Diet Assoc* 103:827–831, 2003
16. Pate RR, Pratt M, Blair SN, Haskell Wl, Macera CA, Bouchard C, Buckner D, Caspersen CJ, Ettinger W, Heath GW, King A, Kriska AM, Leon AS, Marcus BH, Morris J, Paffenbarger R, Patrick K, Pollock M, Ripper JM, Sallis J, Wilmore JH: Physical activity and public health: recommendations from the Centers for Disease Control and Prevention and the American College of Sports Medicine. *JAMA* 273:402–407, 1995

17. Centers for Disease Control and Prevention, National Center for Chronic Disease Prevention and Health Promotion: *Physical Activity and Health: A Report of the Surgeon General.* Washington, DC, U.S. Department of Health and Human Services, President's Council on Physical Fitness and Sports, 1996

18. American Dietetic Association: *ADA Medical Nutrition Therapy Evidence Based Guidelines for Practice for Type 1 and Type 2 Diabetes.* Chicago, IL, American Dietetic Association, 2001

19. Daly A, Franz M, Holzmeister LA, Kulkarni K, O'Connell B, Wheeler M: New diabetes nutrition resources. *J Am Diet Assoc* 103:832–834, 2003

20. Brand-Miller J, Hayne S, Petocz P, Calagiuri S: Low–glycemic index diets in the management of diabetes. *Diabetes Care* 26:2261–2267, 2003

21. Sheard NF, Clark NG, Brand-Miller JC, Franz MJ, Pi-Sunyer FX, Mayer-Davis E, Kulkarni K, Geil: Dietary carbohydrate (amount and type) in prevention and management of diabetes. *Diabetes Care* 27:2266–2271, 2004

22. Franz M: The glycemic index: not the most effective nutrition therapy intervention (Editorial). *Diabetes Care* 26:2466–2468, 2003

23. Bravata DM, Sanders L, Kuang J, Krumholz HM, Olkin I, Gardner CD, Brafada D: Efficacy and safety of low-carbohydrate diets: a systematic review. *JAMA* 289:1837–1850, 2003

24. Friedman MR, King J, Kennedy E: Popular diets: a scientific review. *Obes Res* 9 (Suppl. 1):1S–40S, 2001

25. American Diabetes Association: Physical activity/exercise and diabetes mellitus (Position Statement). *Diabetes Care* 27 (Suppl. 1):S58–S62, 2004

26. Wannamethee SG, Shaper AG: Physical activity in the prevention of cardiovascular disease: an epidemiological perspective. *Sports Med* 31:101–114, 2001

27. Pi-Sunyer FX, Becker DM, Bouchard C, et al.: NHLBI Obesity Education Initiative Expert Panel on the Identification, Evaluation, and Treatment of Overweight and Obesity in Adults: *Obes Res* 6 (Suppl. 2):51S–209S, 1998

28. McGuire MT, Wing RR, Klem ML, Seagle HM, Hill JO: Long-term maintenance of weight loss: do people who lose weight through various weight loss methods use different behaviors to maintain their weight? *Int J Obes* 22: 572–577, 1998

29. Institute of Medicine: *The Role of Nutrition in Maintaining Health in the Nation's Elderly: Evaluating Coverage of Nutrition Services for the Medicare Population.* Washington, DC, National Academy Press, 2000, p. 118–131

Ms. Daly is the Director of Nutrition and Diabetes Education at the Springfield Diabetes and Endocrine Center, Springfield, IL.

4. Treatment Strategies for Type 1 Diabetes

BELINDA P. CHILDS, ARNP, MN, CDE, BC-ADM, AND
DAVIDA KRUGER, ARNP, MSN, BC-ADM

Type 1 diabetes is a complex, multihormonal disease. Insulin has been the primary treatment for type 1 diabetes. However, to successfully manage type 1 diabetes, individuals must integrate several diabetes treatment components into their lifestyle, including insulin action times, food intake, and physical activity. The role of the other regulatory hormones, such as glucagon and amylin, is also important. The individual with type 1 diabetes and the health care provider must share an understanding of the disease process and available treatment strategies and collaborate in determining the best treatment choices.

EPIDEMIOLOGY

The incidence of type 1 diabetes in the U.S. in people <20 years of age is estimated at 18.2/100,000 per year. For those ≥20 years of age, the incidence is estimated at 9.2/100,000. This statistic represents 29,713 new cases per year or an estimated total of 300,000–500,000 people with type 1 diabetes. The risk for type 1 diabetes is higher for whites than for African Americans or Hispanics/Latinos (1).

Autoimmune type 1 diabetes has multiple genetic predispositions and is also related to poorly defined environmental factors. People with type 1 diabetes are prone to other autoimmune disorders such as Graves' disease, Hashimoto's thyroiditis, vitiligo, pernicious anemia, and celiac disease. Evidence also supports an increased risk for multiple sclerosis in those with type 1 diabetes.

The genes that confer susceptibility for type 1 diabetes are located in the HLA (human leukocyte antigen) region of chromosome 6. Genetically susceptible individuals who also have autoantibodies to islet cell antigens, insulin, and GAD (glutamic acid decarboxylase) are at greatest risk of developing type 1 diabetes (2). Tests are available to identify those at risk, but lacking a way to prevent type 1 diabetes, testing is typically not done. Many individuals were screened as part of the Diabetes Prevention Trial—Type 1, which attempted unsuccessfully to prevent type 1 diabetes in those at risk with insulin therapy. The follow-up study is called Type 1 Diabetes TrialNet. Information can be obtained online at www.niddk.nih.gov/patient/NIH2-TrialNet-Fact-Sheet.htm.

PATHOPHYSIOLOGY

Type 1 diabetes occurs most frequently in children and young adults but can be diagnosed at any age, even in the eighth and ninth decade. As stated in CHAPTER 1, there are two types of type 1 diabetes: immune mediated and idiopathic, the former being much more common. The etiology of type 1 diabetes remains unclear, but the key is insulin deficiency due to the failure of the β-cell to produce adequate insulin to control blood glucose levels. Type 1 diabetes has been referred to in the past as *insulin-dependent diabetes* and *juvenile-onset diabetes*.

Other hormones are involved in glucose regulation, including glucagon, somatostatin, and amylin (Fig. 4.1). Glucagon, produced by the α-cells in the islets of Langerhans, plays a major role in sustaining plasma glucose production. Glucagon maintains the basal blood glucose within a normal range during fasting. In the nondiabetic milieu, if the glucose level falls below normal, glucagon is

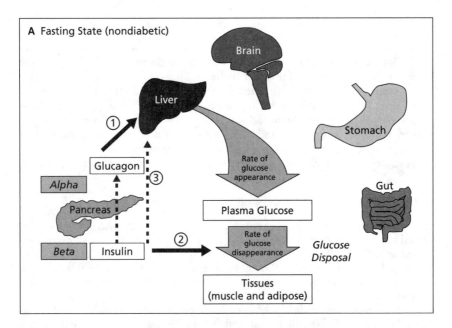

Figure 4.1 Glucose homeostasis: role of insulin and glucagon. *A:* For nondiabetic individuals in the fasting state, plasma glucose is derived from glycogenolysis under the direction of glucagon (1). Basal levels of insulin control glucose disposal (2). Insulin's role in suppressing gluconeogenesis and glycogenolysis is minimal due to low insulin secretion in the fasting state (3). *B:* For individuals with diabetes in the fasting state, plasma glucose is derived from glycogenolysis and gluconeogenesis (1) under the direction of glucagon (2). Exogenous insulin (3) influences the rate of peripheral glucose disappearance (4) and, because of its deficiency in the portal circulation, does not properly regulate the degree to which hepatic gluconeogenesis and glycogenolysis occur (5). *From* Aronoff et al. (Ref. 3).

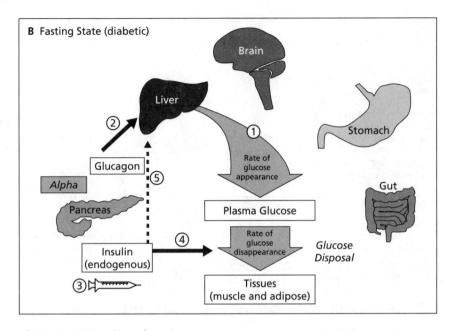

Figure 4.1 *Continued.*

released, which in turn triggers hepatic glucose to be released from the liver (glucogenolysis). The blood glucose level returns to normal. This glucose release is not needed after a meal. Normally, glucagon is suppressed by the effect of insulin on the liver, and glucagon is almost totally suppressed after a meal. In diabetes, there is an inadequate suppression of postprandial glucagon (hyperglucagonemia), resulting in increased hepatic glucose production (gluconeogenesis). Exogenous insulin is unable to restore normal postprandial insulin concentrations in the portal vein or suppress the postprandial glucagon secretion. This results in an abnormal glucagon-to-insulin ratio and results in the release of hepatic glucose and, ultimately, hyperglycemia (3). Somatostatin, which is produced by the δ-cells in the islets of Langerhans, also plays a role in the regulation of insulin and glucagon release.

Amylin is the most recently identified regulatory hormone (discovered in 1987) and is co-secreted by the β-cells with insulin. It appears to play a role in postprandial glucose regulation by reducing excess glucagon in the postprandial period and regulating gastric emptying from the stomach to the small intestines. Amylin also appears to have an effect on satiety.

Glucose homeostasis is complex. In addition to the above-mentioned hormones, several exocrine hormones also play a role in glucose uptake by the gut. Currently identified hormones are glucagon-like peptide-1 (GLP-1) and glucagon-like peptide (GLP) (3).

DIAGNOSIS

Although the symptoms of diabetes (Table 4.1) can arise suddenly, the disease is considered to have an insidious onset. In the past, most patients newly diagnosed

Table 4.1 Symptoms of Type 1 Diabetes

Polyuria—increased urination
Polyphagia—increased appetite
Polydipsia—increased thirst
Unexplained weight loss
In children, bedwetting
Yeast infections
Flushed skin
Fruity breath
Severe abdominal pain
Nausea and/or vomiting
Lethargy

with type 1 diabetes were hospitalized with ketoacidosis, but today, most are identified by symptoms and early glucose testing before becoming ill. Insulin can be started as an outpatient unless the patient is a young child or meets the criteria for hospitalization (see CHAPTER 31).

THE IMPORTANCE OF OPTIMAL GLUCOSE CONTROL

Insulin is the principle treatment for hyperglycemia associated with type 1 diabetes. There are many insulin options and strategies allowing for more physiological (closer to natural) insulin replacement. Insulin delivery methods include syringes, pens, injectors, and insulin pumps. It is vital that both health care providers and individuals with diabetes understand the options available for achieving optimal glucose control. Although hypoglycemia remains the limiting factor in the achievement of euglycemia, when analog insulins are used, the risk of hypoglycemia is reduced and postprandial glucose control is improved.

The findings of the Diabetes Control and Complications Trial (DCCT) left no doubt that glucose control reduces the likelihood of developing the microvascular complications of diabetes (4). Data from the DCCT show that the risk of the development of microvascular complications as reduces as hemoglobin A_{1c} (A1C) nears the normal level. Any lowering of A1C and blood glucose level decreases the risk of developing microvascular complications.

The Epidemiology of Diabetes Interventions and Complications (EDIC) study has demonstrated a beneficial effect of optimal glucose control 7 to 8 years after the study completion. A cohort of 1,349 patients who participated in the DCCT has been followed since the completion of the DCCT. Those who had near-normal glycemia during the DCCT continue to have less albumin excretion and reduced incidence of hypertension when compared with the less well-controlled group, regardless of their current glucose control (5).

BASAL-BOLUS INSULIN THERAPY

In the nondiabetic individual, nature carefully controls blood glucose levels within a very narrow range. This is accomplished by the continuous secretion of a small amount of insulin, termed *basal insulin*, at a relatively constant level, i.e., it never "peaks." Superimposed on the basal insulin is a bolus of insulin that the body secretes with each feeding. Fig. 4.2 shows normal physiology.

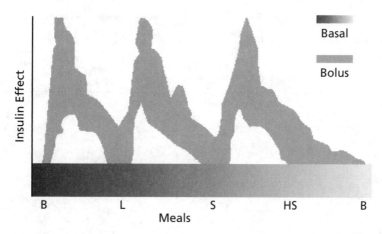

Figure 4.2 Physiologic insulin secretion. B, breakfast; L, lunch; S, supper; HS, bedtime.

It is possible to closely mimic the pattern of basal and bolus insulin using exogenous insulin. One option is to use a continuous subcutaneous insulin infusion (CSII) pump, which can be programmed to release basal insulin at chosen rates, plus bolus insulin controlled by the pump wearer (see CHAPTER 24 for further information on CSII). Multiple daily injections using a long-acting (peakless or nearly peakless) insulin analog plus a rapid-acting insulin analog to cover meals also allow physiological basal-bolus insulin therapy. To maximize the advantages of these approaches, it is important for both patient and provider to understand not only the basal-bolus concept but also the action times of the various insulins (Table 4.2).

Insulin Timing and Action

There are four general categories of insulin based on action times:

- rapid acting: insulins lispro, aspart, and glulisine, which are genetically engineered insulin analogs
- short acting: regular soluble insulin
- intermediate acting: NPH, an isophane insulin, and lente, an insulin-zinc suspension
- long acting: insulin glargine, a genetically engineered analog, and ultralente, an extended-release insulin-zinc suspension

Table 4.2 summarizes the action profiles, i.e., the time to onset, time to peak action, and duration of action, of these preparations. The values shown are for human insulin. Pork insulin is still available, but most patients use genetically engineered human insulin.

For most individuals with type 1 diabetes, a basal-bolus approach to management is the best choice. The basal insulin reduces hepatic glucose production, keeping it in equilibrium with the use of basal glucose by the brain and other tissue. After meals, bolus (prandial) insulin secretion stimulates glucose use and storage while inhibiting hepatic glucose output, thereby limiting the meal-related

Table 4.2 Insulin Action Times

	Onset (h)	Peak (h)	Effective duration (h)
Rapid acting			
Insulin lispro (analog)*	0.25–0.5	0.5–2.5	≤5
Insulin aspart (analog)*	<0.20	1–3	3–5
Insulin glulisine (analog; a.k.a., Apidra)			
Short acting			
Regular (soluble)	0.5–1	2–3	3–6
Intermediate acting			
NPH (isophane)	2–4	4–10	10–16
Lente (insulin zinc suspension)	3–4	4–12	12–18
Long acting			
Ultralente (extended insulin zinc suspension)	6–10	10–16	18–20
Insulin glargine (analog)	2–4	Peakless	20–24
Combinations			
50% NPH, 50% regular	0.5–1	Dual	10–16
70% NPH, 30% regular	0.5–1	Dual	10–16
70% NPA, 30% aspart	<0.25	Dual	10–16
75% NPL, 25% lispro	<0.25	Dual	10–16

*Per manufacturers' data; other data indicate equivalent pharmacodynamic effect (Plank J, Wutte A, Brunner G, Siebenhofer A, Semlitsch B, Sommer R, Hirschberger S, Pieber TR: Direct comparison of insulin aspart and insulin lispro in patients with type 1 diabetes. *Diabetes Care* 25:2053–2057, 2002).

glucose excursion. Individuals with type 1 diabetes lack both basal and bolus insulin production. The basal-bolus approach allows for the most flexible lifestyle.

One basal-bolus strategy is to use glargine as the basal insulin and insulin lispro or aspart as the bolus insulin (Fig. 4.3). Usually, 40–60% of the total daily insulin dose is for basal needs and the remaining would go to the bolus doses, divided based on meal content and composition. Glargine can be given at any time of day but should be given at a consistent time of day, e.g., in the morning or at bedtime. Alternatively, NPH in two or three doses per day can be used to provide basal needs. Ultralente can be used as basal insulin, but its absorption is variable and unpredictable.

Insulin mixtures are also available. Premixed insulins do not allow flexibility in eating and physical activity times and are usually not the best choice in type 1 diabetes. Carefully instruct patients about the onset of action of insulin and time of administration. Premixed 70/30 NPH/regular should be taken 30 min before eating, whereas a 70/30 NPA/aspart (or 75/25 NPL/lispro) dose is administered with the meal.

Education and caution to ensure accurate dosing are needed when patients are asked to mix insulins themselves. The rule is to draw the clear insulin, i.e., regular, lispro, or aspart, before the cloudy insulin, i.e., NPH, lente, or ultralente. The dose should be given within 2–10 min of mixing. The exception is glargine, which cannot be mixed with any insulin or drawn into a syringe that contained any other insulin due to its acidic nature (pH 4.2). Also, glargine should be administered immediately after being drawn into a syringe (6), unlike some insulins, which can

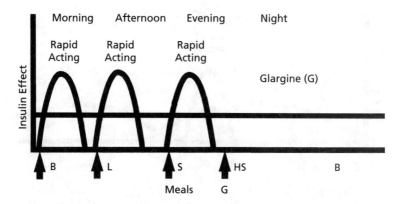

Figure 4.3 Representation of idealized insulin effect provided by three daily injections of rapid-acting insulin with an evening injection of insulin glargine. B, breakfast; L, lunch; S, supper; HS, bedtime.

be stored in syringes and refrigerated for up to 30 days (7). Lente and ultralente should not be mixed and stored in a syringe. If glargine or any other clear insulin has particles or has become cloudy, a new vial should be used and the contaminated vial discarded.

PRACTICAL POINT

For reproducibility and to ensure equivalent dosing, it is important to follow the same day-to-day routine when measuring, mixing, and administering insulin.

Starting Insulin

Starting doses of insulin are best calculated based on body weight. The initial dose is usually 0.5–1.5 units/kg body wt/day. The starting dose is determined within this range by the degree of ketosis with which the patient presents, not the blood glucose level. Most individuals with type 1 diabetes have some level of ketosis and may have initially been treated with intravenous insulin and rehydrated (see CHAPTER 7). Others may be identified early in the disease process and simply need insulin replacement, which will mean a lower starting dose.

Children and adolescents with newly diagnosed type 1 diabetes usually have some degree of ketosis or acidosis and thus are very insulin deficient and require high doses of insulin. Children also have a higher metabolic rate than adults and therefore a higher clearance rate of drugs, e.g., insulin. Growth hormones can cause elevated blood glucose levels. Children require higher doses of most insulins, as well as other medications, than adults. Children and adolescents who develop diabetic ketoacidosis (DKA) are usually treated with low-dose intravenous insulin.

When a patient is stable and ready for subcutaneous insulin, start with a dose of 1–2 units/kg/day, reserving the lower doses for patients who have hyperglycemia and little or no ketosis, and the highest dose for patients who have or have had DKA. Children should be fed to satiety (usually 40–60 kcal/kg/day) to

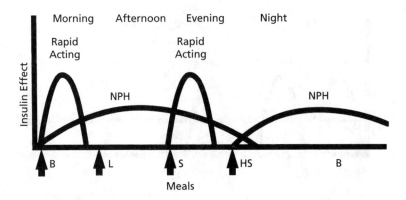

Figure 4.4 Representation of a split mix of NPH and rapid-acting insulin at breakfast, rapid-acting insulin at the evening meal, and NPH at bedtime. B, breakfast; L, lunch; S, supper; HS, bedtime. *From* Bode (Ed.) (2).

replenish their lost stores of body nutrients and given enough insulin to control blood glucose levels and restore anabolism to regain lost weight.

Insulin is divided between a rapid-acting insulin, which is administered with meals, and a longer-acting insulin, such as glargine, administered at bedtime. About 40–60% of the total daily insulin requirement should be given as glargine and the remaining given as aspart or lispro. Mealtime aspart/lispro is dosed according to meal size, except that the largest dose per calorie/carbohydrate is normally given with breakfast because of the large amount of growth hormone secreted in the early hours of the day in growing children. In children, especially toddlers, aspart or lispro can be given after the meal and the dose adjusted by how much the child has actually eaten.

Regimens using a split mix of NPH and lispro or aspart can be used in patients with type 1 diabetes (Fig. 4.4). Approximately 56–60% would be given as a breakfast dose or mixed insulin NPH/lispro; 15–20% would be given as a supper dose of regular, lispro, or aspart at the evening meal; and 15–20% NPH at 10:00 P.M. As noted, it is important to eat meals as the insulin is peaking. Snacks are likely necessary during midmorning and midafternoon and at bedtime. It will be important during the adjustment phase to monitor 3:00 A.M. blood glucose levels to prevent nocturnal hypoglycemia.

SELF-MONITORING OF BLOOD GLUCOSE

Self-monitoring of blood glucose (SMBG) is essential to diabetes control regardless of the treatment strategies. Commonly, patients are told to monitor their blood glucose levels before meals and at bedtime. This is done so that insulin can be adjusted on a sliding scale or algorithm according to the blood glucose level at the time. Regardless of the insulin tactics used, this method is retrospective. The calculated change corrects a previous error, which may then overlap another insulin dose and cause hypoglycemia later. This is particularly true when longer-acting insulins are used.

For example, using a sliding scale with a patient taking mixed regular and NPH insulins could potentially cause significant afternoon hypoglycemia. The morning NPH insulin may be working well, but adding extra regular insulin at noon because the prelunch blood glucose level was high will result in an overlap with the duration of the NPH and may cause afternoon hypoglycemia. The next logical action would be to decrease the evening insulin dose because the presupper blood glucose level was low, which will result in a high bedtime blood glucose level. As is evident, this becomes a vicious cycle. In contrast, the pattern management approach is proactive.

Using SMBG for Pattern Management

Pattern management is the method of choice for making any insulin dose adjustments but is essential when using basal-bolus insulin therapy with rapid- and long-acting insulin. With pattern management, blood glucose level is checked at fasting and 2 h postprandially. If the values are >200 mg/dl (11.1 mmol/l) or ketones are present in the urine, supplements or a correction dose can be given immediately. Unless the blood glucose is very high, it is better to observe a 2- to 3-day pattern and then make the change based on the pattern. Correction doses may be given based on the premeal blood glucose as long as it is noted.

Changes in insulin doses are then made according to the type of insulin involved. The fasting blood glucose level is a reflection of the glargine or bedtime insulin, and if it is too high or too low over a 2- to 3-day period, the glargine dose should be adjusted accordingly. Many sliding scales are based on a set of standing orders for all patients regardless of weight or insulin sensitivity. Of note, the change should be within 10–20% of the existing dose. If a percentage of the existing dose is used as the adjustment guide, the individual's insulin sensitivity and weight have been taken into consideration. One size does not fit all in insulin management or adjustment. The blood glucose level after breakfast is used to adjust the prebreakfast rapid-acting insulin dose, the level after lunch is used to adjust the lunchtime insulin dose, and the level after the evening meal is used to adjust the premeal insulin dose. Again, changes are made every 2–3 days in 10–20% increments until the measured values are in the target range agreed to by the patient and/or family. The American Diabetes Association (ADA) goals of therapy are fasting plasma glucose 90–130 mg/dl (5.0–7.2 mmol/l), postprandial plasma glucose <180 mg/dl (<10.0 mmol/l), and A1C <7% (8).

Optimal pattern management uses several days of SMBG records, whether handwritten or downloaded from the meter. However, written records with detailed journaling of factors such as specific food, emotions, and physical activity help the individual with diabetes learn problem-solving skills. Downloaded meter information will require supplemental information about the individual's food plan, medication, activity, and treatment of hypoglycemia. Adjustments in medication, meals, or activity must be based on accurate information. The other key for downloaded information is regular downloading, e.g., weekly. If the meter is only downloaded at the health care provider's office, the individual with diabetes is missing the opportunity to make regular adjustments to his or her meal plan, exercise, and medication. Glucose monitoring is a tool for the individual with diabetes.

Correcting Hyperglycemia

Correctional doses of insulin can be given, but care should be taken to avoid overtreating with insulin. If one overtreats hyperglycemia with too much or too

Table 4.3 Correction Factors

1,500 Rule	1,800 Rule
Insulin dose: 40 units 70/30 breakfast, 15 units aspart at supper, and 15 units NPH at 10:00 P.M. 12 units of aspart before each meal and 38 units of NPH at bedtime. Total dose = 70 units divided into 1,500 = 21; therefore, 1 unit of aspart will drop the blood glucose about 21 mg/dl. If the blood glucose is >200 mg/dl (>11.1 mmol/l) before the evening meal, give an extra 5 units aspart to decrease the blood glucose to 100 mg/dl (55.6 mmol/l).	Insulin dose: 3–5 units lispro with each meal and 10 units glargine at 8:00 P.M. Total dose = ~20 units divided into 1,800 = ~90; therefore, 1 unit will drop the blood glucose by 90 mg/dl (5 mmol/l). If blood glucose is >200 mg/dl (>11.1 mmol/l) before the evening meal, add 1 unit lispro with the evening dose to decrease the glucose to 110 mg/dl (6.1 mmol/l).

frequent insulin, one increases the risk of hypoglycemia. The resultant hypoglycemia may then be overtreated with food, which could result in hyperglycemia and insulin being supplemented again. This is referred to as the sliding-scale effect. The level of hyperglycemia at which a patient corrects may vary between individuals and should be decided by the patient and provider. Extreme caution should be used if using a correction bolus with split-mixed insulin.

For patients who are on intermediate- or long-acting insulin, there is no single value in adjusting it to correct for a high premeal glucose level. In this case, 10% of the total insulin dose may be supplemented as rapid-acting insulin. Another method is to use the rule of 1,500 or 1,800 (Table 4.3). This method involves dividing the total daily dose of insulin, including rapid- and long-acting insulins, into 1,500 (in adults who are not extremely insulin sensitive) or 1,800 (in children and adult patients who are insulin sensitive) (9,10). In this way, the patient with diabetes can determine approximately how many milligrams 1 unit of insulin will lower his or her blood glucose. Correction doses should be used cautiously. Food and activity can also be adjusted to alter blood glucose.

Correcting Hypoglycemia

With basal-bolus insulin therapy, the 15-g/15-min rule becomes important. This rule suggests that to treat hypoglycemia, the individual with diabetes should take 15 g glucose, wait 15 min, recheck, and, if necessary, retreat with an additional 15 g glucose. In the past, we often taught individuals with diabetes to follow up treatment with a complex carbohydrate/protein snack. However, this may not be necessary. It will depend on the time of day in which the hypoglycemia occurs. If the reaction occurs during the peak of the NPH action, an additional snack may be required to prevent recurrent hypoglycemia (Table 4.4) (see also CHAPTER 7).

Patients converting from a regimen in which frequent and/or prolonged hypoglycemia existed may find that elevated blood glucose levels will occur after treatment if low blood glucose levels are treated the same way as in their previous regimen. This will be particularly true if these patients eat a high-calorie/high-fat food such as chocolate, in which case they might experience blood glucose levels ≥300 mg/dl (≥16.6 mmol/l). Assumptions might be made that the high glucose levels that followed the low glucose levels are due to the Somogyi effect, when it is most likely related to the type of treatment or to overtreatment of low blood

Table 4.4 Quick Tips for Treating Hypoglycemia

Glargine and Rapid-Acting Insulin Analog	Split-Mixed or Multiple-Dose Regimen Using Intermediate- and Rapid- or Short-Acting Insulins
If <70 mg/dl (<3.9 mmol/l), treat with 15 g carbohydrate (three to four glucose tablets, 1/2 cup juice or sugared soda, 1 cup skim milk). Recheck in 15 min; if <70 mg/dl (<3.9 mmol/l), repeat the above treatment. If >3 h since the last dose of rapid-acting insulin, no additional treatment is necessary. If <3 h since the last dose of rapid-acting insulin, follow with a snack of 75–100 calories.	If ≥70 mg/dl (≥3.9 mmol/l) and symptomatic, treat with a carbohydrate and protein snack. If <70 mg/dl (<3.9 mmol/l), treat with 15 carbohydrate (three to four glucose tablets, 1/2 cup juice or sugared soda, 1 cup skim milk). Recheck in 15 min; if <70 mg/dl (3.9 mmol/l), repeat the above treatment. Follow with a carbohydrate and protein snack if >30 min until next planned snack or meal.

glucose. The Somogyi phenomenon has been defined as a counterregulatory effect in response to hypoglycemia in which the liver releases glucose and the result is high blood glucose. There is debate as to whether this phenomenon exists. If it does exist, it occurs infrequently.

Food Plan Considerations

Using the basal-bolus regimen provides greater flexibility in lifestyle and schedule for patients with diabetes (Table 4.5). Rapid-acting insulin can be adjusted based on the carbohydrate consumption at any given time. Snacks may not be required, as is often the case with the split-mix regimens. However, snacks may be eaten, if desired, without compromising glucose control if carbohydrates are counted and supplemented with insulin. This is a benefit for many children and adults who have been frustrated by a strict eating schedule, such as at bedtime, that requires that they eat even when they are not hungry. A general guideline is that additional insulin is

Table 4.5 Quick Tips for Meal Planning

Glargine and Rapid-Acting Insulin Analog	Split-Mixed or Multiple-Dose Regimen Using Intermediate- and Short- or Rapid-Acting Insulins
Total calories divided into three meals and no snacks. Snacks of 75–120 calories (15–20 carbs) usually acceptable without extra insulin. If the snack is >75–120 calories (15–20 carbs), additional rapid-acting insulin may need to be administered. Children will likely need snacks to avoid hypoglycemia. Insulin doses need to be determined based on postprandial blood glucose levels. Individualization is the key.	Three meals and three snacks will likely be needed with a split-mix regimen. This method was designed to match the peaks of the available insulins but limits meal variability, especially with premixed insulin.

not needed if the snack is <120 calories/20 g carbohydrate, but any food containing >120 calories/20 g carbohydrate may require additional insulin (11).

The key to achieving the greater flexibility in meal timing and portions afforded by basal-bolus therapy is learning to count carbohydrate intake and match insulin doses appropriately. This can be taught in the course of medical nutrition therapy delivered by an RD (see CHAPTER 3). Often, the first step in learning carbohydrate counting is eating consistent amounts of carbohydrates and calories. Advanced carbohydrate counting includes determining the individual's insulin-to-carbohydrate ratios and insulin sensitivity factor and how to appropriately use these factors. The ability to be flexible with the timing and quantity of meals has had a major impact on glucose control as well as the ability to control weight.

Exercise Considerations

Typically, exercise lowers blood glucose levels. The individual with diabetes will need to either increase caloric intake or decrease insulin with additional physical activity. With a basal-bolus regimen, the patient may lower either the basal or the bolus insulin. If the exercise is anticipated and occurs within 3 h of the rapid-acting dose, the patient can decrease the premeal dose or ingest more calories/carbohydrates. SMBG to detect postexercise hypoglycemia is needed for up to 36 h after the activity (12). The intermediate- or long-acting dose can be decreased if a prolonged activity, such as an active vacation, or intense physical activity, such as skiing or yard work, is planned. The keys are to individualize the plan and to carefully monitor blood glucose.

INSULIN STORAGE AND ADMINISTRATION

Typically, insulin does not need to be refrigerated but should not be exposed to extremes in temperature. All insulin products have varying durations of stability once opened and used unrefrigerated. The stability varies from 14 to 28 days depending on the product and whether it is in a vial or an insulin pen. Marking the vial or syringe with the date it should be discarded ensures use before expiration.

Patients should be alert to unexpected changes in blood glucose levels. Unexplained increases should prompt a patient to verify that their insulin is not outdated, has not been exposed to direct sunlight or excessive heat (>86°F for most, >96°F for aspart), or has not been frozen (6).

Insulins that are in suspension (cloudy) should be gently rolled a minimum of 20 times before use. This should be done with consistency because some of the variable absorption of the suspended insulin is related to inconsistent mixing of the suspension. Drawing up a dose and then laying the syringe down before injection requires that the filled syringe be remixed by gentle rolling before administration.

Manufacturers of disposable syringes and pen needles recommend that these devices only be used once. One potential issue, which arises with reuse of syringes or needles, is the inability to guarantee sterility. Most insulin preparations have bacteriostatic additives that inhibit the growth of bacteria commonly found on the skin. Nevertheless, syringe/needle reuse may carry an increased risk of infection for some individuals. Patients with poor personal hygiene, an acute concurrent illness, open wounds on the hands, or decreased resistance to infection for any reason should not reuse a syringe or pen needle.

Some patients find it practical to reuse syringes/needles. Certainly, a needle should be discarded if it is noticeably dull or deformed or if it has come into contact with any surface other than skin. If needle reuse is planned, the needle must be recapped after each use. Also, with just one injection, tips of the newer, smaller (30- and 31-gauge) needles can become bent into a hook form that can lacerate tissue or break off, leaving needle fragments in the skin. The medical consequences of these findings are unknown but may increase lipodystrophy or have other adverse effects. In addition to the dulling of the fine needle after puncturing the bottle and the skin, lubrication is lost and the next injection can be painful. Advise patients who are reusing needles to inspect injection sites for redness or swelling and consult their health care provider before initiating the practice and if signs of skin inflammation are detected.

Insulin may be injected into the subcutaneous tissue of the upper arm and the anterior and lateral aspects of the thigh, buttocks, and abdomen (with the exception of a circle within a 2-inch radius around the navel). Intramuscular injection is not recommended for routine injections, although it can be given under some circumstances, e.g., DKA or dehydration, because the rate of absorption is faster. Exercise increases the rate of absorption from injection sites, probably by increasing blood flow to the skin and perhaps also by local actions.

Site selection should take into consideration the variable absorption between sites. The abdomen has the fastest rate of absorption, followed by the arms, thighs, and buttocks. Rotating within one area (e.g., rotating injections systematically within the abdomen), rather than rotating to a different area with each injection, decreases variability in insulin absorption from day to day. However, glargine is reported to be consistent in absorption regardless of injection site.

Insulin Injection Tips

- Select a site that has no lipohypertrophy or scar tissue.
- Use the anatomical region for selected injections, e.g., all morning shots in the abdomen, evening meal injection in the arm, bedtime injection in the thigh.
- Use insulin that is at room temperature.
- Make sure no air bubbles remain in the syringe before injection.
- Day-to-day use of topical alcohol is not required. If used, wait until alcohol has evaporated completely before injection.
- Keep muscles in the injection area relaxed, not tense, when injecting.
- Penetrate the skin quickly.
- Do not change the needle's direction during insertion or withdrawal.
- Count to 5 to ensure that all insulin is delivered through a small-gauge needle; count to 10 if using an insulin pen.
- Do not wipe the needle with alcohol. Recap carefully.

Rotation of the injection site is also important to prevent lipohypertrophy or lipoatrophy. Lipohypertrophy is a buildup of fat at the injection site. Lipoatrophy is a loss of fat that causes dipping of the tissue at injection sites. Hypertrophy and atrophy can occur with overuse of an injection site. Some patients are more prone to lipohypertrophy and lipoatrophy. Both were more common with insulins from animals and are less common with the new insulin preparations. Areas of hypertrophy usually lead to slower inconsistent absorption. Autoimmunity to the insulin may play a role in the development of lipohypertrophies and lipoatrophies. If a patient has hypertrophied injection sites, precautions should be taken to prevent hypoglycemia when insulin is injected into a new site because a dramatic decrease in insulin requirements and hypoglycemia may be seen. In addition, unexplained hypoglycemia may occur if insulin is consistently injected into a hypertrophied area.

INSULIN DELIVERY SYSTEMS

In addition to syringes with needles, insulin pens and other delivery devices are available today. Insulin pens are not only convenient, but individuals are more likely to deliver accurate doses with insulin pens. Patients may be able to see the numbers on the dial or screen better than on a syringe and manipulate a dialing mechanism more easily than a syringe plunger. Also, when beginning insulin, an anxious patient is often less threatened by an insulin pen than a needle, syringe, and vial. The smaller volume of insulin that needs to be carried around, compared with a vial and syringe, means that there is less exposure of the insulin to the elements of daily living. The cartridges in the pens hold 150–300 units each. Insulin pens are available with replaceable cartridges or as disposable pens. Three important patient education points are that

- the needles should be removed after each use
- caution needs to be taken to make sure that there is no air in the cartridge
- the needle should remain in the skin for the count of 10 to ensure that all the insulin has been delivered before removing the needle.

Pen needles should be removed immediately after injection. The needle provides an opening into the sterile chamber, permitting an entry for bacteria and/or leakage of insulin. In the case of cloudy suspension, the concentration may be altered by leakage of fluid when insulin is not fully suspended.

Air injectors are available, but they are costly and frequently not covered by insurance. Many people with type 1 diabetes, from children to elders, use CSII with an insulin pump. Learning to use an insulin pump successfully requires a program of user education and frequent support from the health care team (see CHAPTER 24).

SUMMARY

Near-physiological glucose control is achievable in type 1 diabetes with a motivated individual and a knowledgeable health care team. An insulin regimen can be crafted to match each individual's lifestyle. To achieve optimal glucose control requires that the individual become active in self-managing his or her disease and that the health care team provide coaching and support. When the person with diabetes understands insulin action times and his or her individualized response to insulin as well as the effects of the food plan, physical activity, and emotions and is willing to monitor blood glucose levels regularly, he or she has the ability to optimally manage hyperglycemia and hypoglycemia.

Future Treatments

Only continued research will reveal the prevention and cure for type 1 diabetes. Although pancreas transplantations are sometimes an option, they are usually performed only if the individual with diabetes also needs a kidney, and there are not enough donor organs to treat everyone with type 1 diabetes. The pancreas is difficult to transplant, and 10–20% of transplants fail within the first year. In addition, there are risks associated with the need for antirejection medications (13,14).

Islet transplantations are another potential cure under investigation. A multicenter clinical trial is finding that up to 50% of transplant recipients remain free of the need for exogenous insulin for 1 year after receiving islet cells. Major obstacles are islet cell rejection, a limited supply of islets, and the risk of long-term use of antirejection medications (15).

Investigations of other new therapies center on amylin (pramlintide), a neuroendocrine hormone regulator of insulin action co-secreted with insulin, as well as incretin hormones from the gut that regulate glucose; new insulin analogs; and new insulin delivery systems, such as a portable, possibly implanted, closed-loop insulin delivery system that would both sense glucose levels and release appropriate amounts of insulin.

REFERENCES

1. LaPorte RE, Matsushima M, Chang Y-F: Prevalence and incidence of insulin-dependent diabetes. In *Diabetes in America.* 2nd ed. Harris MI, Cowie CC, Stern MP, Boyko EJ, Reiber GE, Bennett PH, Eds. Washington, DC, U.S. Govt. Printing Office, 1995 (NIH publ. no. 95-1468), p. 36–47
2. Bode BW (Ed.): *Medical Management of Type 1 Diabetes.* 4th ed. Alexandria, VA, American Diabetes Association, 2004
3. Aronoff SL, Berkowitz K, Shreiner B, Want L: Glucose metabolism and regulation: beyond insulin and glucagon. *Diabetes Spectrum* 17:183–190, 2004
4. Diabetes Control and Complications Trial Research Group: The effect of intensive treatment of diabetes on the development and progression of long-term complications in insulin dependent diabetes mellitus. *N Engl J Med* 329:977–986, 1993
5. DCCT/EDIC Writing Group: Sustained effect of intensive treatment of type 1 diabetes mellitus on development and progression of diabetic nephropathy. *JAMA* 290:2159–2167, 2003
6. Grajower MM, Fraser CG, Holcombe ML, Daugherty ML, Harris WC, Felippis OM, Santiago OM, Clark NG: How long should insulin be used once a vial is opened? (Editorial). *Diabetes Care* 26:2665–2669, 2003
7. American Diabetes Association: Insulin administration (Position Statement). *Diabetes Care* 27 (Suppl. 1):106–109, 2004
8. American Diabetes Association: Standards of medical care in diabetes (Position Statement). *Diabetes Care* 28 (Suppl. 1):S4–S36, 2005

9. Warshaw HS, Kulkarni K: *Complete Guide to Carb Counting.* Alexandria, VA, American Diabetes Association, 2001, p. 148–149

10. Hinnen DH, Guthrie DW, Childs BP, Friesen J, Rhiley D, Guthrie RA: Pattern management of blood glucose. In *Core Curriculum for Diabetes Education: Diabetes Management Therapies.* Franz M, Ed. Chicago, IL, American Association of Diabetes Educators, 2003, p. 220–221

11. Guthrie RA, Childs BP, Guthrie DW: Rapid and long acting insulin analogs: strategies for patient use. Monograph. 2nd ed. Wichita, KS, Quontum Press, August 2004

12. American Diabetes Association: Physical activity/exercise and diabetes (Position Statement). *Diabetes Care* 27 (Suppl. 1):S58–S62, 2004

13. National Institute of Diabetes and Digestive and Kidney Diseases: Pancreatic islet transplantation [Internet]. Available from http://diabetes.niddk.nih.gov/dm/pubs/pancreaticislet/index.htm. Accessed 16 November 2004

14. American Diabetes Association: Pancreas transplantation [Internet]. Available from http://www.diabetes.org/type-1-diabetes/pancreas-transplants.jsp. Accessed 16 November 2004

15. American Diabetes Association: Islet transplantation [Internet]. Available from http://www.diabetes.org/type-1-diabetes/islet-transplants.jsp. Accessed 16 November 2004

Ms. Childs is a Diabetes Nurse Specialist at Mid-America Diabetes Associates, Wichita, KS. Ms. Kruger is a Certified Nurse Practitioner at Henry Ford Health Systems, Detroit, MI.

5. Treatment Strategies for Type 2 Diabetes

ANDREA ZALDIVAR, MS, C-ANP, CDE, AND
JANE JEFFRIE SELEY, MPH, MSN, GNP, CDE

The majority of patients encountered over the course of a nursing career will have type 2 diabetes, which affects 90–95% of all people with diabetes. Because hyperglycemia develops slowly over time, many people are asymptomatic and may have had type 2 diabetes for up to 10 years before diagnosis and may already have diabetes complications (1,2). Type 2 diabetes is most common in obese individuals who are ≥45 years of age, but due to the increasing rate of obesity, we now see type 2 diabetes in children as young as age 10 years (3,4). The public health ramifications of a formerly adult disease affecting children and adolescents remains to be seen. Whether a nurse chooses to work with adults or children, he or she should become familiar and comfortable with the early identification and management of type 2 diabetes.

If glucose is to be used or stored efficiently in the body, the pancreas must secrete sufficient insulin that is used properly by the body. In type 2 diabetes, this altered process represents two main defects. As in type 1 diabetes, patients with type 2 diabetes are deficient in insulin production. In type 2 diabetes, however, the deficiency is relative because some insulin is still produced in the pancreas (5). In addition to insulin deficiency, there appears to be a problem of increased insulin resistance in the muscle, adipose cells, and liver (6). Overproduction of glucose by the liver appears to coexist in individuals with type 2 diabetes (6), along with decreased insulin secretion and increased insulin resistance. A good strategy to use when treating patients with type 2 diabetes is to select medications that address both defects.

TREATING INSULIN DEFICIENCY

Oral Medications

Health care providers who treat people with diabetes today are fortunate to have a large arsenal of medications to assist in treating the insulin deficiency found in type 2 diabetes. A class of long-acting insulin secretagogues known as sulfonylureas has been in existence since the 1950s and is often the first choice of pharmacologic treatment in type 2 diabetes (Table 5.1). Sulfonylureas, which stimulate the β-cells in the pancreas to produce more insulin, appear to work quickly in reducing blood glucose levels.

When sulfonylureas were first introduced, health care providers were often disappointed with the unpredictable way in which they stimulated the β-cells to secrete insulin. The first generation of sulfonylureas often encouraged insulin secretion when insulin was not needed, resulting in hypoglycemia. Fortunately, the newer, or second-generation, sulfonylureas cause less hypoglycemia than their predecessors by stimulating insulin secretion in response to meals (6). Weight gain and hypoglycemia continue to be potential side effects of this class of medication (7).

The U.K. Prospective Diabetes Study (UKPDS) documented a progressive decline in β-cell function in individuals with type 2 diabetes commencing years before the actual diagnosis of diabetes and continuing throughout the person's life regardless of mode of treatment (8). For sulfonylureas to be effective, they require functioning β-cells and therefore are most useful in the earlier stages of type 2 diabetes. Over time, sulfonylureas become less effective, and other medication will be needed to achieve glycemic targets.

Meglitinides are short-acting insulin secretagogues that are taken just before a meal (Table 5.1). Meglitinides are more sensitive than sulfonylureas to being activated in the presence of hyperglycemia or a meal. For this reason, meglitinides appear to produce less hypoglycemia. Meglitinides should be taken immediately before a meal and omitted if the meal is skipped. This group of medications works well in individuals with unpredictable eating patterns because the dose can be varied according to the size of the meal or not taken if the meal is missed. At the same time, because meglitinides are taken before every meal, they may not be the best choice

---

Table 5.1 Medications that Increase Insulin Secretion

Sulfonylureas stimulate insulin secretion in the pancreatic β-cells.

Second generation:
Glyburide/DiaBeta, Micronase, Glynase Prestabs (1.25–10 mg), Glipizide/Glucotrol, Glucotrol XL (2.5–20 mg), Glimepiride/Amaryl (1–4 mg)

Notes:
- Taken before meals
- Hypoglycemia is the most common side effect
- Contraindicated during pregnancy or in people allergic to sulfa

Meglitinides stimulate insulin production in the pancreatic β-cells (shorter acting than sulfonylureas).

Repaglinide/Prandin (0.5–16 mg), Nateglinide/Starlix (60–120 mg × 3 days)

Notes:
- Taken just before meals and omitted if a meal is missed
- Hypoglycemia is the most common side effect
- Can be titrated according to meal size
- Contraindicated during pregnancy

for patients who have trouble remembering to take their medications. Meglitinides, like sulfonylureas, are not recommended for use during pregnancy (8).

Insulin Therapy in Type 2 Diabetes

Because type 2 diabetes is chronic and progressive, β-cell function is decreased by at least 50% at diagnosis and by 75% 6 years later (9). β-Cell function may also be impaired temporarily in the case of severe hyperglycemia known as glucose toxicity (6). In either case, insulin therapy should be considered whenever optimal glucose control, i.e., glycated hemoglobin A_{1c} (A1C) <7%, cannot be reached to decrease the risk of long-term microvascular complications (9). The decision to initiate insulin therapy should be made based on glycemic control, not patient and provider readiness. Whenever insulin is mentioned, it is not uncommon for patients to plead for more time to eat better, exercise more, and improve their glycemic control. It should be stressed that the initiation of insulin is not intended to punish patients for not taking care of themselves; rather, it is simply necessary to achieve glycemic control. Many patients express a fear of weight gain and hypoglycemia while on insulin.

Weight gain as a result of initiating insulin therapy is a valid concern for the patient with type 2 diabetes and his or her health care provider. As glycemic control improves, glycosuria decreases and calories once wasted by the body are now stored as fat. Intermittent overinsulinization may result in hypoglycemia that leads to hunger and an increase in caloric consumption (10). Weight gain can be minimized with attention to carbohydrate counting and increased physical activity as insulin therapy is advanced. Concurrent use of metformin along with insulin therapy has also been shown to minimize weight gain (11,12). If still effective, sulfonylureas combined with insulin can lower the insulin dose by 25–50% with less weight gain (10). In two separate studies, both bedtime administration of NPH instead of daytime NPH and use of insulin glargine instead of NPH yielded less weight gain (10).

Many patients verbalize a fear of the actual act of injecting the insulin and the increased risk of hypoglycemia with insulin therapy. In reality, the rates of severe hypoglycemia in type 2 diabetes are low. The Kumamoto study, for example, showed an average A1C of 7.1% for the tightly controlled group and the same rate of mild hypoglycemia as that of the conventional therapy group, which had a mean A1C of 9.4% (13). Nurses can be influential in helping patients understand the benefits of insulin therapy and the ease of use and increased accuracy with new delivery devices such as insulin pens (10,14). Patient education regarding the signs, symptoms, and especially prevention of hypoglycemia can help allay fears. In addition, showing patients an insulin syringe or pen and needle and asking them to try an injection usually is met with surprise at how tiny the needle actually is and how little pain is experienced.

> **PRACTICAL POINT**
>
> Insulin therapy should never be used as a threat. The natural progression of the disease tells us that most people with type 2 diabetes will need insulin eventually, regardless of previous therapies.

The initiation of insulin therapy is often delayed because of both patient and provider resistance. Health care providers often bargain with patients and place insulin initiation on the backburner because insulin training involves considerable time and effort in a busy practice setting. Insulin is often used as a threat to patients rather than a valuable tool. The reality is that the longer a person lives with type 2 diabetes, the fewer functioning β-cells they have, and the need for insulin becomes inevitable over time (6). We must prepare patients for this by talking about insulin in a positive way.

The rationale for starting insulin for a patient with type 2 diabetes is initially different from that in the case of type 1 diabetes. This is because the pancreas in type 2 diabetes patients may still be able to "help" by producing some insulin. The current philosophy is to use a simple and easy-to-follow regimen, keeping the oral agents the same and adding a single injection of insulin once daily, usually at bedtime (13). The current options include a long-acting basal insulin such as glargine, an intermediate-acting insulin such as NPH, or a premixed insulin such as 70/30 and 75/25 (6). Glargine can be given either in the morning or at bedtime, depending on patient preference. Although the single injection of NPH is often given at bedtime, it could also be given before breakfast or before supper depending on the patient's lifestyle or preferences and the insulin chosen. The premixed insulins are best given before meals, such as before breakfast and before supper. Because of insulin resistance, insulin dose requirements in type 2 diabetes are often much higher than in type 1 diabetes (10). The important thing to remember is that there is no one treatment regimen for all patients but rather that individualized regimens should be designed or tailored to a patient's particular needs.

As type 2 diabetes progresses, more intensive insulin regimens will be needed to achieve the same glycemic goals (insulin treatment is more fully covered in CHAPTER 4). Basal-bolus regimens such as those used in type 1 diabetes will help patients reach glycemic targets when oral agents fail (10). The use of exogenous insulin administered in a way that mimics normal physiology will help reduce the chance of long-term complications (13). Once insulin therapy is agreed upon, it is important that the patient receive extensive patient education beyond lifestyle interventions, including training in

- proper administration of insulin
- site selection and rotation
- time-action profile(s) of insulin
- disposal and reuse of syringes and pen needles
- hypoglycemia treatment and prevention
- blood glucose monitoring targets
- sick-day management

In addition, the patient should be followed closely and taught to adjust the insulin, if possible, as needed to achieve optimal glycemic control. The patient expects improvement with insulin therapy, and it is up to the provider to facilitate success by both optimizing therapy and encouraging patient self-management.

TREATING INSULIN RESISTANCE

Early in the progression of the disease, a person with type 2 diabetes experiences resistance to insulin in the liver as well as in the adipose and muscle cells (6). When insulin resistance is present, more insulin is required to lower glucose levels. Initially, an individual may be able to adequately compensate and produce sufficient insulin to meet the body's metabolic needs. He or she may experience a period of increased insulin production or "hyperinsulinemia" before having overt diabetes.

Although the exact mechanism is unknown, hyperinsulinemia is thought to be a possible cause of macrovascular risk factors, including dyslipidemia and hypertension (6). Whether referred to as the metabolic syndrome, dysmetabolic syndrome, syndrome X, or the insulin resistance syndrome, the characteristics of hypertension, dyslipidemia, and central obesity put the individual with type 2 diabetes at higher risk for developing cardiovascular disease (6,15). The UKPDS highlighted the need to tightly control both hypertension and lipids in individuals with type 2 diabetes to decrease the occurrence of cardiovascular events. This study further showed that control of blood pressure and lipids might require the use of multiple medications (8).

Insulin resistance in the liver, muscle, and adipose cells appears first, then worsens with the progression of type 2 diabetes (16). Eventually the pancreas cannot keep up with the increased demands of extra insulin to compensate for the insulin resistance, and glucose control becomes challenged. Insulin resistance can be decreased through weight loss, physical activity, and the use of insulin sensitizers such as biguanides and thiazolidinediones (7,15).

Medications that Treat Insulin Resistance

Medications that treat insulin resistance act primarily on the liver (biguanides) or in the muscle and adipose cells (thiazolidinediones) (Table 5.2). Because of their

---

Table 5.2 Medications that Reduce Insulin Resistance

Biguanides suppress glucose production in the liver and decrease insulin resistance.

Metformin/Glucophage, Glucophage XR, Fortamet/Riomet (500–1,000 mg)

Notes:
- Taken with meals
- Gastrointestinal complaints are the most common side effect
- Should be stopped the day of any procedure using iodinated contrast media or major surgical procedures and restarted 48 h later if renal function has been confirmed to be adequate and stable
- Contraindicated
  - during pregnancy
  - in renal disease (serum creatinine ≥1.5 mg/dl in men and ≥1.4 mg/dl in women, or abnormal creatinine clearance)
  - in liver dysfunction
  - in congestive heart failure
  - with history of alcohol abuse
  - in acute or chronic metabolic acidosis
- If age >80 years, confirm normal renal function with creatinine clearance test before initiating therapy and monitor closely

Thiazolidinediones decrease insulin resistance in adipose and muscle cells.

Pioglitazone/Actos (15–45 mg), Rosiglitazone/Avandia (4–8 mg)

Notes:
- Usually taken once daily with the first meal (rosiglitazone may be given once or twice daily)
- Weight gain and fluid retention are the most common side effects
- Contraindicated during pregnancy
- Use with caution in liver disease; liver function tests should be done before initiating therapy and according to the prescriber's discretion (the authors recommend quarterly for the first year), and then annually
- Contraindicated in patients with New York Heart Association (NYHA) Class III and IV cardiac status; observe patients for signs and symptoms of heart failure, especially increased shortness of breath, edema, and weight gain

See also "Oral Agents" in RESOURCES.

ability to target insulin resistance in these two areas, biguanides and thiazolidine-diones can be taken together to produce a greater effect (7).

Biguanides work to control diabetes by decreasing glucose production in the liver (particularly during the night), thus lowering fasting blood glucose levels. Also, biguanides lower peripheral insulin resistance, although to a lesser extent. Lactic acidosis, though rare, is a potential risk of this category of medication. Any individuals who are predisposed to lactic acidosis, such as binge drinkers and people with impaired renal function (creatinine ≥1.5 mg/dl in men and ≥1.4 mg/dl in women), should not take biguanides. Caution should be taken when metformin is used in the elderly. A creatinine clearance test should be done on all individuals over the age of 80 years. The common side effect seen with biguanides are gastro-intestinal complaints, especially if the dosage is quickly advanced when initiated or initiated at too high a dose. This side effect is lessened when the medication is taken with food and/or gradually titrated or when an extended-release formulation is used. Many patients report a decrease in appetite and subsequent modest weight loss when taking biguanides (7).

Thiazolidinediones decrease insulin resistance primarily in muscle and adipose cells. Their glucose-lowering effect is not based on stimulating insulin production; thus these agents do not produce hypoglycemia when used as monotherapy. Thia-zolidinediones have also been shown to have both lipid-lowering and antihyper-tensive effects (6). The main side effects associated with thiazolidinediones are weight gain and edema. Patients should be observed for signs and symptoms of heart failure. Thiazolidinediones are not recommended for use in patients with New York Heart Association (NYHA) Class III and IV heart failure (7). Liver tox-icity was a concern with an earlier medication in this class. The newer thiazo-lidinediones do not seem to produce this side effect, but, as a precaution, should be used with caution in liver disease. Liver function tests should be done before initiating therapy and according to the prescriber's discretion. If any elevation is present at baseline, more frequent testing is prudent.

SLOWING GLUCOSE ABSORPTION

Unlike the other medications used to treat type 2 diabetes that increase insulin production or decrease insulin resistance, α-glucosidase inhibitors work on the intestinal tract by slowing glucose absorption (Table 5.3). These medications are usually most effective in the early stages of type 2 diabetes, where postprandial excursions of glucose seem to be the primary issue involved in controlling glu-cose (6,16), and in patients who ingest large amounts of carbohydrates (6). The most common side effects seen in this class of medication are flatulence and, occa-sionally, diarrhea. These side effects seem to subside after 3–4 weeks of use (6,7). α-Glucosidase inhibitors do not cause hypoglycemia when used as monotherapy (16). Hypoglycemia can occur when these agents are used in combination with other diabetes medications that can cause hypoglycemia, such as insulin secreta-gogues or insulin. Because α-glucosidase inhibitors slow down the digestion of carbohydrates into glucose, a monosaccharide such as glucose tablets or lactose (milk) must be used to effectively treat hypoglycemia (16).

ENCOURAGING WEIGHT LOSS

It is no coincidence that both diabetes and obesity are on the rise in the U.S. According to a study published in the *Journal of the American Medical Association*

Table 5.3 Medications that Reduce Glucose Absorption

α-Glucosidase inhibitors decrease carbohydrate absorption in the gastrointestinal tract.

Acarbose/Precose (25–100 mg), Miglitol/Glyset (25–100 mg); 3 times/day

Notes:
- Taken with the first bite of each main meal
- Flatulence and gastrointestinal complaints are the most common side effects
- Contraindicated
  - during pregnancy
  - during breast-feeding
  - for children
  - in cirrhosis of the liver
- Not recommended in patients with creatinine clearance of <25 ml/min (23) or inflammatory bowel disease

See also "Oral Agents" in RESOURCES.

---

(17), obesity rose from 19.8 to 20.9% of adults in the U.S. in the same year (2000–2001) that diagnosed diabetes rose from 7.3 to 7.9%. A strong correlation was found between being overweight and obesity and diabetes in all races, ages, educational levels, and smoking levels and in both sexes (17). Although being overweight is associated with insulin resistance, not all overweight people develop type 2 diabetes. Therefore, other factors besides obesity must be present to facilitate the onset of diabetes (18).

On a more positive note, even a modest weight loss in overweight adults significantly reduces the risk of developing diabetes. In one study, there was a 33% lower risk of developing diabetes in individuals for every kilogram lost per year over a 10-year period (18). In addition, in three randomized control trials in China, Finland, and the U.S., the incidence of type 2 diabetes in people who were at high risk for developing diabetes was reduced by up to 58% with lifestyle interventions that included modest weight loss (19–21).

Weight loss and regular physical activity are primary treatment strategies in type 2 diabetes. Over time, they can lead to a reduced need for medication as well as improved glycemic control. It is important for nurses to place the same emphasis on meal planning and physical activity as pharmacological interventions.

A simple strategy that can be used to promote weight loss is to assist individuals in recognizing the antecedents and consequences to overeating and their actual eating behaviors. An example would be asking a patient to examine how skipping a meal could promote overeating at the end of the day and then asking them to evaluate how they feel when they overeat (take note that this cannot be done if the patient is taking certain medications). Providers should tailor behavior changes accordingly (22). These lifestyle changes can help patients achieve the glycemic targets that will reduce their risk of serious complications. Sensible weight loss

> **PRACTICAL POINT**
>
> When addressing weight loss, work closely with a dietitian to set mutually acceptable and attainable goals. A possible first goal can be to not gain any weight between visits.

> **PRACTICAL POINT**
>
> As medications are being added or changed, remember to reinforce treatment goals with patients, stressing their relationship to avoiding diabetes-related complications.

takes time and perseverance. Many patients get frustrated and need ongoing guidance and support. Emphasizing even the smallest improvement in weight, especially if it correlates with a decrease in A1C level, helps keep patients encouraged and motivated. Referral to a dietitian and/or certified diabetes educator for medical nutrition therapy will be beneficial for the individual with type 2 diabetes.

TREATING TYPE 2 DIABETES

As type 2 diabetes progresses and β-cell function decreases or insulin resistance increases, medical treatment must be adapted (23). This often involves using more than one agent, with each targeting a different organ and defect. Coupled with the comorbidities associated with increased insulin resistance, such as hypertension and dyslipidemia (15), this often translates into an individual with type 2 diabetes taking a large number of medications daily (i.e., polypharmacy, see CHAPTER 23).

The use of polypharmacy in patients with type 2 diabetes creates several challenges for the nurse. First, the nurse must be diligent in learning the action, side effects, and drug-to-drug interactions of each medication so that he or she can educate the patient. Second, the nurse must find creative ways such as the use of pillboxes or reminder cues to assist the patient in adhering to complex medication regimens. Nurses must also be cognizant of the overall cost of taking multiple medications daily and assist patients with social services and pharmaceutical indigent care program referrals when needed.

Effective communication between the patient and health care provider is crucial if patients are to execute complex treatment recommendations. At least 14% of the nation's population speaks a language other than English at home (24). Adhering to complex medication regimens may be especially difficult when a nurse attempts to assist a patient whose primary language is not English. Nurses must be proactive in developing strategies to deal with the needs of culturally diverse populations. The use of bicultural/bilingual staff, use of internal language banks, and language skills training may assist nurses in facilitating communication between themselves and diverse patients (24).

> **PRACTICAL POINT**
>
> To facilitate adherence to treatment recommendations, make sure patients can describe how they should be taking their medications and what they should do if they have questions about their medications before they leave your facility.

Nurses should offer additional emotional and practical support to the individual with type 2 diabetes who must begin insulin therapy. Many of these patients need assistance in accepting this inevitable step in the progression of their disease and the reality that it is not their fault. Individuals with type 2 diabetes need information about the targets for glycemic control and the relationship between control and risk of complications. Avoiding diabetes-related complications is an important goal for both the nurse and the patient.

SUMMARY

Type 2 diabetes is a complex, progressive disease associated with numerous comorbidities including hyperlipidemia, hypertension, obesity, and depression. Due to the progressive nature of the disease, not the failure of the patient or health care provider, most patients will need insulin in their lifetime. The nurse will play an important role in assisting the patient in understanding the nature of their disease, including the necessity of medications to treat both insulin resistance and insulin deficiency and importance of healthy lifestyle behaviors.

REFERENCES

1. American Diabetes Association: Clinical Practice Recommendations 2004. *Diabetes Care* 27 (Suppl. 1):S1–S150, 2004
2. Harris R, Donahue K, Rathore S, Frame P, Woolf S, Lohr KN: Screening adults for type 2 diabetes: a review of the evidence for the U.S. Preventive Services Task Force. *Ann Intern Med* 138:215–290, 2003
3. American Diabetes Association: Type 2 diabetes in children and adolescents. *Diabetes Care* 23:381–389, 2000
4. Kaufman FR: Type 2 diabetes in children and young adults: a "new epidemic." *Clinical Diabetes* 20:217–218, 2002
5. Parmet S, Lynm C, Glass RM: Insulin. *JAMA* 289:2314, 2003
6. Beaser RS: *Joslin Diabetes Deskbook for Primary Care Providers.* Boston, MA, Joslin Diabetes Center, 2001
7. *Physicians' Desk Reference.* 57th ed. Montvale, NJ, Medical Economics, 2003
8. UK Prospective Diabetes Study Group: Intensive blood-glucose control with sulfonylureas or insulin compared with conventional treatment and risk of complications in patients with type 2 diabetes (UKPDS 33). *Lancet* 352: 837–853, 1998
9. DeWitt DE, Dugale DC: Using new insulin strategies in the outpatient treatment of diabetes. *JAMA* 289:2265–2269, 2003
10. DeWitt DE, Hirsch IB: Outpatient insulin therapy in type 1 and type 2 diabetes mellitus. *JAMA* 289:2254–2264, 2003
11. Aviles-Santa L, Sindling J, Raskin P: Effects of metformin in patients with poorly controlled insulin treated type 2 diabetes mellitus: a randomized, double-blind, placebo-controlled trial. *Ann Intern Med* 131: 182–188, 1999
12. Bergenstal R, Johnson M, Whipple D: Advantages of adding metformin to multiple dose insulin therapy in type 2 diabetes (Abstract). *Diabetes* 47 (Suppl. 1): A47, 1999
13. White JR: Clarifying the role of insulin in type 2 diabetes management. *Clinical Diabetes* 21:14–21, 2003
14. Bohannon NJV: Insulin delivery using pen devices: simple-to-use tools may help young and old alike. *Postgrad Med* 106:57–68, 1999
15. Reaven G: Metabolic syndrome: pathophysiology and implications for management of cardiovascular disease. *Circulation* 106:286–288, 2002
16. Franz MJ, Kulkarni K, Polonsky WK, Yearbough P, Zamudio V (Eds.): *A Core Curriculum for Diabetes Educators.* 4th ed. Chicago, IL, American Association for Diabetes Educators, 2003
17. Mokdad AH, Ford ES, Bowman BA, Dietz WH, Vinicor F, Bales VS, Marks JS: Prevalence of obesity, diabetes, and obesity-related health risk factors, 2001. *JAMA* 289:76–79, 2003

18. Resnick H, Valsania P, Halter J, Lin X: Relation of weight gain and weight loss on subsequent diabetes risk in overweight adults. *J Epidemiol Community Health* 54:596–602, 2003
19. Diabetes Prevention Program Research Group: Reduction in the incidence of type 2 diabetes with lifestyle intervention or metformin. *N Engl J Med* 346:393–403, 2002
20. Tuomilehto J, Lindstrom J, Eriksson JG, Valle TT, Hamalainen H, Ilanne-Parikka P, Keinanen-Kiukaanniemi S, Laakso M, Louheranta A, Rastas M, Salminen V, Uusitupa M, Finnish Diabetes Prevention Study Group: Prevention of type 2 diabetes mellitus by changes in lifestyle among subjects with impaired glucose tolerance. *N Engl J Med* 344:1343–1350, 2001
21. Pan XR, Li GW, Hu YH, Wang JX, Yang WY, An ZX, Hu ZX, Lin J, Xiao JZ, Cao HB, Liu PA, Jiang XG, Jiang YY, Wang JP, Zheng H, Zhang H, Bennett PH, Howard BV: Effects of diet and exercise in preventing NIDDM in people with impaired glucose tolerance: the Da Qing IGT and Diabetes Study. *Diabetes Care* 20:537–544, 1997
22. Wylie-Rosett J, Swencionis C, Friedler A, Schaffer N: *The Complete Weight Loss Workbook: Proven Techniques for Controlling Weight-Related Problems.* Alexandria, VA, American Diabetes Association, 1997
23. Weyer C, Tataranni PA, Bogardus C, Pratley RE: Insulin resistance and insulin secretory dysfunction are independent predictors of worsening of glucose tolerance during each stage of type 2 diabetes development. *Diabetes Care* 24:89–94, 2001
24. National Alliance for Hispanic Health: *A Primer for Cultural Proficiency: Towards Quality Health for Hispanics.* Washington, DC, Estella Press, 2001

Ms. Zaldivar is the Clinical Director at Northern General Diagnostic and Treatment Center, New York, NY. Ms. Seley is a Diabetes Nurse Practitioner at New York Presbyterian/Weill Cornell Medical Center, New York, NY.

6. Self-Management Practices

Deborah Hinnen, ARNP, CDE, FAAN, and
Richard A. Guthrie, MD, FACE, CDE

Self-monitoring of blood glucose (SMBG) was introduced in the late 1970s, replacing the retrospective and distasteful urine glucose testing methods previously used. The Diabetes Control and Complications Trial verified that glucose control could be achieved with intensive management, which required frequent monitoring and multiple insulin injections. Both monitoring and insulin delivery have continued to improve with technological advances in the past several decades.

Continuous glucose monitoring is available but not yet widely used. To be able to continuously collect glucose data that feed into an insulin delivery system, creating a closed loop, is the ultimate goal of diabetes management for insulin-requiring people. Until closed-loop technology is perfected, the mundane process of analyzing logbooks, or downloading data by patients who use computer software analysis to crunch the numbers, is necessary to make sense of all those glucose measurements.

Problem solving, detecting patterns, and making proactive changes in the food plan, physical activity, or the medication protocol are the essence of diabetes self-management (1). These are advanced skills for people with diabetes. First, the basic self-care skills for diabetes management must be mastered, including glucose monitoring, insulin injection and/or oral medication dosing and timing, hypoglycemia prevention and treatment, daily schedule delineation, basic meal planning, and learning when to call the practitioner. As a facet of continuous, lifelong outpatient diabetes education, all nurses working with people with diabetes can teach, reinforce, and verify these daily care activities.

GLUCOSE MONITORING: THE SPEEDOMETER OF DIABETES MANAGEMENT

Would you drive your car in rush-hour traffic or on a long trip if the speedometer didn't work? Determining your speed on the interstate is an important safety issue when driving. Determining your blood glucose level is equally important in diabetes management. Adult learners need to be able to learn new skills and information based on what they already know.

<table>
<tr><td>

PRACTICAL POINT

Adult learners learn best by experiential learning. Learning a skill such as glucose monitoring is a hands-on activity that must include a return demonstration to verify the patient's ability to obtain accurate results.

</td></tr>
</table>

Matching Meter to Patient

Here are the facts on today's glucose meters:

- All meters are essentially accurate if the manufacturer's instructions are followed.
- All newer meters are plasma referenced, which makes them comparable to the hospital and practitioner's office results.
- Today's meters require a nominal amount of blood.
- Most meters have a capillary "sipping" action, therefore drawing in a precise amount of blood.
- Most meters range in size from a deck of cards to a Pop-Tart.
- Meters have varying degrees of memory (10–3,000 data points).
- Newer meters provide results in <30 seconds and many in as little as 5 seconds.
- Most meters have some internal technology or computer software to assist with analyzing and summarizing the data.
- All major manufacturers have comparably priced test strips.
- Sample meters for patients are less available than in the past.

Given these facts, consider the following when helping a patient choose a meter:

- Does the patient have good vision and dexterity? If not, consider a meter with strips in a drum or disc to reduce the need for patients to have to open cans or foil wrappers.
- Does the patient have insurance to obtain strips and supplies? If not, refer him or her to a social worker or local resources for strip purchase at a reduced rate or consider a generic-labeled meter and test strip usage *and* less frequent but carefully staggered testing times.
- Does the insurance company have a preferred meter on formulary? If yes, then that is the meter to recommend. If yes, but there are no meter formulary restrictions, consider employment, lifestyle, and patient preference. For instance, people who are frequent computer users, piano players, guitar players, etc., may prefer alternate site testing (forearm, abdomen, or thigh). Earlier data about inaccuracies with alternate site testing have been refuted (2). Techno-savvy people may want a meter with extended memory, data storage, and data management capabilities. Seniors may need a meter that has fewer steps and a larger screen.

Key Meter Skills to Teach

- Do a test with control solution on the patient's finger initially, so the patient can see how simple it is to do a test.
- Help the patient get an adequate-sized blood sample.
  - Have the patient wash his or her hands in warm soapy water. There is no need to use alcohol to clean the skin; alcohol only dries the skin.
  - If using an alternate site, it is necessary to rub the site.
  - Select a finger that does not have calluses.

– Hang the hand in a dependent position for 30–60 seconds.
– Pretend you are shaking down a thermometer.
– After the puncture, gently milk (rather than squeeze) the finger.
– Adjust the lancing device depth (bigger number = deeper penetration).
- Have the patient do a test from start to finish with the nurse saying nothing.
- Give the patient an assignment: to call the toll-free customer service number (normally found on the back of the meter or on the packaging) for assistance in something, e.g., setting the date and time, changing the code.
- If an inpatient, have the patient do a test with his or her meter when it is the routine testing time. Patients can measure their blood glucose level and compare that value with results obtained from the laboratory. The values should be within 10–15% of each other.
- Carefully dispose of test strips and lancets in a container, not the trash.

Common User Errors

- Not enough blood
- Blood not adequately/completely filling the test strip chamber
- Meter not calibrated to the current strips
- Ruined strips: out of date, mail-order strips got too hot or too cold
- Patient not familiar with control solution or opened for >90 days, but date on bottle still current (make sure that patients date control solutions upon opening)

Tips for Motivating Reluctant Testers

- Experiment with blood glucose testing before and after certain foods, e.g., orange juice for breakfast, a meal with dessert, a fast-food meal (hamburger, fries, and soft drink).
- Many patients have symptoms that are nonspecific and describe it as "feeling funny." Tell patients to test when they feel "funny" to rule out diabetes problems when considering chest/heart problems or hypertension. One cannot discern a myocardial infarction, but if chest pain is present and the blood glucose is low, and then the patient treats the low blood glucose and the chest pain is relieved, then it is likely a symptom of low blood glucose.
- Ask the person with longstanding diabetes to try out a new meter and give an experienced person's opinion.
- Ask the person to speak at a diabetes support group meeting and show new patients how to keep a logbook and do beginning pattern recognition and problem solving.
- Negotiate with someone else at home to do the testing for 1 week.
- Negotiate the testing frequency based on what the patient is willing/able to do.
- Negotiate weekly data review with the patient by fax, phone, or e-mail.

New Glucose Monitoring Technology

- Continuous glucose monitoring equipment is available in clinics and physician office settings:

- Minimed/Medtronic's continuous glucose monitoring is available for 72 h of continuous data obtained via subcutaneous interstitial extraction. The several thousand dollars it costs makes it impractical for home use. Current use is for trending data to evaluate diet, exercise, and medication and make appropriate adjustments.
- GlucoWatch (Cygnus) technology is available to assess 12 h of glucose data from iontophoresis. The device is worn on the arm and provides a constant glucose reading, albeit 20 min old. An alarm can be set to go off when glucose reaches high and low targets. This device is also valuable for determining trending data. Finger-stick glucose monitoring is still required for calibration. A new glucose-sensing pad is needed after every 12 h of use. Other companies are near releasing similar and, in some cases, improved devices.
- Glucose meters that communicate with insulin infusion pumps are now available. Therasense and BD have glucose meters that, via infrared technology, communicate blood glucose value to the Deltec Cozmo and Minimed Paradigm pumps, respectively. The pump software is now sophisticated enough to automatically calculate correction factors when glucose data are provided. The insulin pump has safety features that require manual initiation of the bolus of insulin, if the individual agrees with the data calculations from the pump program.

Glucose Monitoring Schedules

Patients who use insulin are often asked to test four times per day: fasting and 2 h after each meal. Recent studies and consensus conferences of major organizations support postprandial testing. This information most closely correlates to glycated hemoglobin A_{1c} (A1C) (3–5). When glycemic goals are reached in type 2 diabetes, testing may be less frequent (four times per day, 3–4 days per week). People who are carbohydrate counting and using insulin-to-carbohydrate ratios will test before meals to determine how much insulin to take for the meal. Women who are pregnant and people using insulin pumps are asked to test every day, four to six times per day.

People using oral agents test less often after reaching glycemic goals. Recommendations are not consistent in the literature. If the person is insured by Medicare, 100 test strips for a 3-month period are covered. This dictates testing frequency to a great degree. If people choose to test fasting daily or during fasting and at 4:00 P.M., they will miss postprandial glucose excursions. Therefore, alternating days and times during the day to provide a more complete glucose pattern would be a better use of testing supplies. Testing four times per day, 2 days per week is consequently the recommendation for many people on oral agents (1,6,7). Some practitioners recommend testing two times per day, 4 days per week. Individualization is the key to successful testing. For instance:

- All patients need more tests with illness, medication change, dietary changes, and stress (1).
- During acute illness, premeal or hourly testing is needed to determine the need for and dose of any supplemental insulin.
- Asymptomatic hypoglycemia, i.e., hypoglycemia unawareness, requires more frequent and regular testing on a daily basis, particularly at peak

insulin times and before driving, as a precaution for identifying low blood glucose levels.

- Pregnancy requires frequent SMBG, e.g., five to seven times per day, every day to make the adjustments needed to optimize blood glucose control.

LONGER-TERM MEASURES OF GLUCOSE CONTROL

A1C

The gold standard in overall diabetes control is A1C level. This measure of control provides an average (or weighted mean) of the glucose over the past 2–3 months. The glycation process, when glucose attaches to the hemoglobin molecule, is irreversible and linear, with higher glucose levels causing increased glycation, thus higher A1C values. Therefore, A1C measures the average blood glucose level seen during the 120-day lifespan of the hemoglobin molecule.

The American Diabetes Association (ADA) has effectively promoted a standardization process for this test (8). High-performance liquid chromatography and immunoassay methods are now commonly used to measure A1C. The normal range is 4–6%. With consistency from hospital, clinic, and physician laboratories, this test and the anticipated normal ranges allow practitioners to speak a common language in regard to diabetes control.

Many pharmaceutical companies provide teaching materials, charts, and graphs to explain the relationship of a normal A1C value of 6% to a correlated average glucose of 135 mg/dl (6.7 mmol/l) for the past 2–3 months. As the A1C value goes up 1 percentage point, the glucose averages go up ~35 mg/dl (1.7 mmol/l). Consequently, an A1C of 7% equals an average glucose of 170 mg/dl (9.4 mmol/l).

The ADA's standards of care recommend an A1C goal <7% (corresponding to average blood glucose values of 170 mg/dl [8.3 mmol/l]) and <6% in some populations (9). Testing should be done every 3 months until glycemic goals are reached and then every 6 months. The recommendation to take action if the value is >7% is critical to the prevention of long-term complications of diabetes.

Fructosamine: Glycated Albumin

The glycation of serum albumin is a process similar to glycation of hemoglobin. The result, however, provides a glucose average of the past 10 days. Conceptually, this would be valuable for medication adjustment. Fructosamine would be especially useful in situations when short-term measurements are needed, such as pregnancy, elderly patients, or patients unable to do SMBG. Fructosamine may also be very helpful in patients with hemoglobinopathies where the A1C may not be accurate.

Normal ranges vary with the different methods used. This test is not as standardized as the A1C. The lack of standardization of the testing procedure has limited the use of this measure.

Ketone Testing

Ketone testing provides an important indicator of fat metabolism and free fatty acid conversion in the liver. In the face of hyperglycemia, this is an indication of insulin insufficiency and alternate fuel availability. The ketone bodies are weak acids: acetone, acetoacetic acid, and β-hydroxybutyric acid. The accumulation of these acids decreases the pH and eventually leads to diabetic ketoacidosis (DKA). Therefore, it is important to test for ketones when glucose levels are elevated.

Ketones can be tested by a urine dipstick or plasma testing for β-hydroxybutyric acid with some of the newer glucose meters. Urine ketone testing is done by dipping a ketone test strip into a urine sample and comparing it with the color chart in the appropriate time period advised by the manufacturer.

Ketones are rarely present in patients with type 2 diabetes because they still have endogenous insulin production. However, on sick days, the counterregulatory hormones and catecholamines may trigger ketosis in patients with type 2 diabetes as well as in those with type 1 diabetes (see also "Be Prepared: Sick Day Management," a patient handout in RESOURCES). Therefore, all people with diabetes need to test for ketones when they are ill. The presence of ketones can also indicate inadequate calories. In pregnant women, ketones and hyperglycemia (DKA specifically) during the first trimester are incompatible with fetal viability. Later in the pregnancy, positive ketones are usually an indication of a hypocaloric situation called starvation ketosis.

Indications for ketone testing are

- when blood glucose levels exceed 250–300 mg/dl (13.9–16.6 mmol/l), especially in patients with type 1 diabetes
- during illness
- when fasting, during pregnancy
- if glucose levels exceed 150 mg/dl (8.3 mmol/l) during pregnancy
- during weight loss to verify fat metabolism.

PROBLEM SOLVING AND SELF-MANAGEMENT

Concepts of Pattern Management

Pattern management is a comprehensive approach to blood glucose management that includes all aspects of current diabetes therapy (1,10–12). Although this approach is typically identified with intensive or flexible insulin therapy, pattern management should also include changes in nonpharmacologic therapies, i.e., nutrition therapy and physical activity, and combinations of oral agents to improve glycemic control.

Elements of pattern management include:

- The motivation to be an active participant in care
- Individualized blood glucose goals negotiated by the person with diabetes and diabetes care team
- Frequent SMBG, recorded in a logbook or with software, to provide data for making adjustments
- A food plan to follow, starting with eating consistent amounts of calories/carbohydrates as a basic skill. An advanced skill would be to determine insulin-to-carbohydrate ratios (developed by measuring the usual amount of insulin needed to cover varying amounts of carbohydrate), which are used for adjusting insulin dose based on carbohydrate intake (13)
- Multiple injections of insulin, insulin pump therapy, or combinations of oral agent(s)/insulin

- Self-adjustments, based on blood glucose monitoring data, of food intake, physical activity, and medication(s) to achieve glycemic goals
- Frequent interaction between individuals with diabetes and the diabetes care team, using telephone, fax, and e-mail to discuss glucose values between visits
- Comprehensive self-management training, including:
  - Coverage of the education content areas identified by the National Standards for Diabetes Self-Management Education (14)
  - The relationship of glucose levels, food, activity, and medications
  - Prevention of hypoglycemia or hyperglycemia
  - Sick-day management
  - Purpose, strategies, and value of pattern management for intensive therapy to achieve blood glucose goals
  - Empowerment of the patient through education for decision making and problem solving, goal setting, and long-term motivation
  - An understanding of the personal belief systems related to the value of health and intensive diabetes management
  - Access to diabetes and health-related supplies
  - Support systems to provide emotional and clinical management support
  - Diabetes care team with on-call clinical support
  - Ongoing education such as support groups offered via the ADA, hospital, or education center (15,16)

Strategies for Pattern Management

Pattern management involves reviewing several days of glucose records and making adjustments in diabetes treatment based on trends, rather than reacting to a single high or low blood glucose reading. Adding supplemental or sliding-scale insulin at the time of the elevated glucose level solves the problem only for that particular point in time but does not prevent the problem from occurring again (17–19). Effective pattern management takes into account all variables that affect blood glucose levels—food, physical activity, stress, and illness—not just insulin or other medication adjustments (1).

The patient must have a food plan that he or she can consistently follow. The number of calories and/or carbohydrate servings is determined by the person with diabetes in consultation with a dietitian. To determine patterns, food intake, physical activity, and timing and doses of insulin or other medications must be as consistent as possible. This helps prevent blood glucose fluctuations that can mask true patterns.

In individuals using insulin, if blood glucose levels are out of goal range, consider whether

- the individual prefers to change calorie/carbohydrate intake, change physical activity, or make adjustments in insulin or other medications. Although it is easier to make insulin or other medication adjustments, weight management must be a consideration. Increasing insulin to cover extra food or carbohydrates will anabolically store total calories and potentially increase weight.
- the individual is on enough insulin, too much insulin, or on the wrong insulin regimen (20–22).

In individuals with type 2 diabetes, if blood glucose levels are out of goal range, consider whether the individual

- has a food plan that he or she is able to follow.
- requires a change in medication dose.
- requires the addition of a second or third oral medication (23).
- requires the addition of evening insulin.
- requires a change to a comprehensive insulin-only regimen.

The first step in pattern management is to identify blood glucose trends in relation to glucose goals. The individual with diabetes needs to provide multiple data points at critical times for evaluation and problem solving and to collect sufficient data to evaluate whether goals are being met. Ideally, this means monitoring four to six times a day, but adequate data can be obtained by testing four times a day, 2–3 days per week or testing two times per day, at alternating times, for 1 or 2 weeks. Food records with the number of calories and carbohydrate servings compared with blood glucose readings can then be analyzed once or twice a week.

When looking for patterns, read down the columns of blood glucose records to review all of the readings at the same time of day, e.g., fasting. A sample blood glucose record is provided in Table 6.1. Three high readings at the same time each day is a pattern of high blood glucose levels. Several low readings at the same time is a pattern of low blood glucose levels. If blood glucose readings are high for 3–5 days at a specific time, that is a pattern. Potential causes for the elevated levels should be examined so that the problem can be corrected. Causes of high blood glucose levels can be any of the following:

- Eating too much carbohydrate or more calories than usual
- Doing less physical activity than usual
- Taking too little insulin, missing an insulin dose, or having problems with the dose, type, or combination of oral medications
- Using expired or improperly stored insulin or not taking oral agents as prescribed
- Experiencing emotional or physical stress, including illness
- Rebound response from the liver releasing excessive amounts of glucose from glycogen as a result of hypoglycemia
- Overtreatment of hypoglycemia

If blood glucose levels are low for several days at the same time, potential causes should be examined. Low blood glucose levels are usually corrected before high levels. Untreated hypoglycemia can cause a rebound glucose response,

Table 6.1 Sample Blood Glucose Log

	Fasting blood glucose (mg/dl)	After breakfast (mg/dl)	After lunch (mg/dl)	After supper (mg/dl)
Monday	106	198	84	112
Tuesday	159	210	178	191
Wednesday	141	188	—	113
Thursday	139	222	132	233

induced by the counterregulatory hormone glucagon, with hyperglycemia to occur later. Causes of low blood glucose levels can be any of the following:

- Eating too little carbohydrate or less than usual, i.e., too few calories
- Doing more physical activity than usual
- Taking too much insulin or oral medication
- Taking a hot bath/shower for an extended period of time

Questions to Ask When Evaluating Blood Glucose Readings

- Is there a pattern when evaluating 3–5 days of blood glucose readings?
- Does something happen at the same time every day, such as an insulin reaction, high glucose after breakfast, etc.?
- Are there blood glucose readings representing all "times" of the day?
- Are there blood glucose readings reflecting the "peak" times of each medication (insulins and/or oral agents)?
- Are there readings to represent peak glucose readings after all meals?
- Are there "other notes" or "changes" to account for observed patterns, such as meal times, carbohydrate or calorie variances, exercise changes, unusual hours of work or school, stress, illness, etc.?
- Is prevention of weight gain or weight loss important for the patient? If so, consideration must be given to trying to reduce the use of hypoglycemic medications (i.e., insulin or insulin secretagogues), especially if low blood glucose levels are occurring routinely.
- Does the patient have a history of weight gain? Is the weight gain the result of overtreatment of frequent episodes of hypoglycemia?
- Does the patient have a history of weight loss? Is the weight loss caused by poor glycemic control (1)?

Interpreting Blood Glucose Readings

Knowing what the glucose level means based on when the test was performed is critical to effective decision making.

- Premeal glucose measurements are needed to monitor basal (or background) insulin dose(s) (e.g., NPH, glargine, or ultralente). If fasting or predinner readings are out of the target range, consider adjusting basal insulin doses. Premeal testing may also be used to determine a supplemental/correction insulin dose to add or subtract from the bolus dose.
- Two-hour postprandial glucose readings are needed to titrate rapid-acting insulin (e.g., lispro insulin or aspart insulin) for mealtime injections. If the difference in premeal and postprandial glucose readings is >20–40 mg/dl (1.1–2.2 mmol/l), consider adjusting the mealtime rapid-acting insulin by 10% (24).
- Two-hour postprandial readings are also used to evaluate the effectiveness of thiazolidinediones, glipizide, glyburide, repaglinide, nateglinide, α-glucosidase inhibitors, and other glucose-lowering agents. Two-hour postprandial glucose testing is helpful in patients with type 2 diabetes when evaluating the effect of meals and certain foods on blood glucose levels (23).

- Elevated fasting glucose levels require 3:00 A.M. testing and recording for at least once a week to determine the cause. High fasting glucose levels can be caused by any of the following:
  - Overnight lows that trigger the liver to release glucose (Somogyi or rebound effect)
  - Normal hormonal changes that trigger the liver to release excessive glucose in the early morning (dawn phenomenon)
  - Insufficient basal or background insulin
  - In youth, growth hormone secreted at night during growth spurts
  - Excessive hepatic glucose release in type 2 diabetes

A Case in Problem Solving: John

John is a 57-year-old man who has had type 2 diabetes for 5 years. He works as a manager at Wal-Mart and has no known complications. John is taking the following diabetes medications:

- Morning: 10 mg glipizide, 1,000 mg metformin
- Evening: 10 mg glipizide, 1,000 mg metformin

His food plan consists of 1,800 calories.

	Monday	Wednesday	Saturday
Glucose values (mg/dl)			
Fasting	187	199	203
2 h after breakfast	139	144	148
Before lunch			
2 h after lunch	152	133	121
Before dinner			
2 h after dinner	128	146	138

Changes in schedule/routine
Diet
Insulin/medication
Reactions
Activity

Problem: High fasting blood glucose levels

Possible cause: Inadequate medication in evening or at bedtime to prevent excessive hepatic glucose release

Options:

- Assure John that the high fasting glucose levels are likely not because he ate too much at dinner or during the evening. Explain that food that is eaten is used or stored in 4–5 h. Explain how the liver releases excessive glucose in the early morning hours if adequate insulin is not available.
- Consider adding bedtime NPH or a glargine insulin dose (initiate bedtime basal dose at 10% of total body weight).
- Consider adding a third oral agent.

A Case in Problem Solving: Mary Jane

Mary Jane is a 40-year-old woman who has had type 1 diabetes for 18 years. She works in a call center. Mary Jane has mild peripheral neuropathy in both feet, with no visual changes. Recently, she began a daily four-injection regimen to improve her glucose control.

- Breakfast: 12 units insulin lispro
- Lunch: 10 units insulin lispro
- Dinner: 14 units insulin lispro
- Bedtime: 40 units insulin glargine

Her food plan consists of 1,600 calories (three meals and one snack) with an additional 2 units insulin lispro for each additional carbohydrate choice (15 g) eaten (1:7 insulin-to-carbohydrate ratio).

	Wednesday	Friday	Sunday
Glucose values (mg/dl)			
Fasting	100	110	103
2 h after breakfast	315	292	248
Before lunch			
2 h after lunch	269	233	149
Before supper			
2 h after supper	144	136	137
Changes in schedule/routine			
Food	Donut	O.J., toast	Pancakes
Insulin/medication			
Reactions			
Activity			Walk after lunch

Problem: Pattern of high blood glucose levels after breakfast on 3 days and lunch on 2 days

Possible causes:
- Too much carbohydrate at breakfast/lunch for the current insulin dose
- Too many calories for breakfast
- Not enough insulin before breakfast/lunch
- Insulin-to-carbohydrate ratio is incorrect, needs to be recalculated
- Not counting carbohydrate correctly
- Not using insulin-to-carbohydrate ratio

Options: Consider changing something in routine *before* the high tests:
- Decrease total carbohydrate at breakfast/lunch.
- Change the composition of breakfast (i.e., add protein and fat to carbohydrate).
- Decrease total calories at breakfast/lunch.
- Increase the dose of insulin lispro before breakfast/lunch, e.g., by 10%.
- Increase the insulin-to-carbohydrate ratio at breakfast, e.g., 1:6 (2.5 units insulin lispro per carbohydrate serving).
- Include exercise after breakfast; it was effective on Sunday after lunch.

LIFESTYLE ISSUES

Self-management is central to integrating successful glycemic control with flexibility of lifestyle. Two common issues illustrate how this is done.

Traveling

Travel is not the cumbersome experience it once was for people with diabetes. However, security issues have changed in recent years. People with diabetes must familiarize themselves with the Federal Aviation Administration (FAA) guidelines. The information is summarized on the ADA web site at www.diabetes.org.

- All medications must have the pharmacy label. Insulin boxes are typically where the pharmacy label is applied, so advise individuals to save boxes, even from insulin pens.
- Meters, pumps, and supplies can go through the security check without damage to the equipment.
- Patients may order diabetic meals for their in-flight service, but airlines should be notified well in advance or during the purchase of tickets.
- All supplies (medication, testing supplies, items to treat hypoglycemia, and snacks) should be in a carry-on bag, not packed in checked luggage. Temperature-sensitive supplies are protected, and supplies are at hand.
- Documentation from a practitioner explaining that the person has diabetes and must carry various medications and supplies is not required by the FAA because of the increased risk of forgery. However, Canadian customs agents accept such letters.
- Education on travel outside of the country should include emergency medical contacts.
- Instructions on acquiring medication if the traveler has his or her carry-on bag stolen should include going to the emergency room or pharmacy in that country. Insulin may be a different concentration, i.e., U40 (40 units/cc) or U80 (80 units/cc) rather than U100 (100 units/cc). However, the person can obtain that country's "meal/bolus" insulin and "basal" insulin and syringes to match. A unit of insulin is an international measure. The dilution of the insulin will be variable. If the person needs 10 units of insulin lispro for lunch, he or she will need 10 units of regular (or other available rapid insulin) in U80 or U40 strength, drawn up in the appropriate U80 or U40 syringe. The amount will look different because of the dilution of the insulin.
- In the past, crossing time zones has been the greatest challenge for insulin users. The use of insulin glargine has made this much less difficult. Keep the injection time for glargine on the same schedule as in the patient's original time zone. Other meal insulins may change to match the meal times of the new destination. People using insulin pumps may need to adjust the timing of their nighttime basal rates based on when they sleep in the new time zone. However, flexibility in meal times continues to be a strength for those using pumps.
- Keeping supplies from getting too hot is another consideration whether flying or driving. Travel kits with cool gel packs are available from pharmacies for a reasonable cost. Insulated lunch bags are also useful for moderating temperatures.
- Traveling always requires that snacks and glucose for treating hypoglycemia be available and within reach at all times. Temperature

control for supplies is a concern. People should not leave their emergency snacks or medication in the car when they go into a restaurant for lunch.

- Traveling to high altitudes may affect meter readings and reduce appetite. If skiing or hiking, the insulin dose may need to be reduced because of increased activity and lower caloric intake. Snacks and glucose should be carried in a pocket or backpack.

Drinking Alcohol

The literature is confusing regarding the benefits and risks of alcohol intake. If the person with diabetes chooses to drink, the key is understanding the physiology and making informed decisions.

- Alcohol is detoxified in the liver, where the glycogen reserves are stored and normally released in case of hypoglycemia. At the time alcohol is consumed, glucose values will likely rise because of the carbohydrate in the beer, wine, or mixed drinks. However, the later and more dangerous effect of alcohol is a hypoglycemic effect. This hypoglycemic effect may take place anywhere from 10–20 h after drinking. If the person has had enough to drink and becomes hypoglycemic during the night while sleeping, the liver may not be able to release glycogen reserves to protect and correct the low blood glucose. This situation is potentially fatal.
- Drug interactions are known to occur with several oral agents.
  1. Secretagogues (especially the older Diabinese) may cause an Antabuse, or disulfiram, reaction when the person drinks. This will be evident by flushing and nausea.
  2. Binge drinking (defined by the ADA as five or more drinks on one occasion) while on metformin can increase lactate levels, potentially leading to lactic acidosis. Flu-like symptoms may be a confusing side effect that can also occur with intoxication.
- For the person who chooses to drink, the key is moderation.
  1. If the person is in optimal glycemic control, the ADA guidelines for alcohol intake suggest a maximum of one to two drinks per day.
  2. Alcohol should be consumed with food.
  3. Alcohol calories should be calculated into the total daily intake.
  4. Even if blood glucose values are elevated, the bedtime snack should not be skipped.

SUMMARY

Monitoring-based self-management has become the standard of diabetes care in the past decade. The technology, medications, and education of people with diabetes and providers have vastly improved. These pieces of the puzzle, when put together in an organized fashion, create a picture of flexibility and optimal glycemic control that is clearer now than ever before. The elusive nature of the "water color painting" of diabetes care and glycemic control has been replaced with a sharper image—a clearly focused, detailed picture of diabetes management that is patient driven. Nurses can help patients take ownership in this intensive management approach. Commitment to long-term self-care, together with education on diabetes care rationale and goals, empowers the patient to set personal short- and long-term goals and to seek help with obstacles, including the challenge of maintaining long-term motivation.

REFERENCES

1. Hinnen D, Guthrie D, Childs B, Friesen J, Rhiley D, Guthrie RA: Pattern management. In *A Core Curriculum for Diabetes Education.* 5th ed. Franz M, Ed. Chicago, IL, American Association of Diabetes Educators, 2003
2. Ellison JM, Stegmann JM, Colner SL, Michael RH, Sharma MK, Ervin KR, Horwitz DL: Rapid changes in postprandial blood glucose produce concentration differences at finger, forearm, and thigh sampling sites. *Diabetes Care* 25:961–964, 2002
3. Avignon A, Radauceanu A, Monnier L: Nonfasting plasma glucose is a better marker of diabetic control than fasting plasma glucose. *Diabetes Care* 20:1822–1826, 1997
4. Bell D, Ovalle F, Shadmany S: Postprandial rather than preprandial glucose levels should be used for adjustment of rapid-acting insulins. *Endocr Pract* 6:477–478, 2000
5. Brewer KW, Chase HP, Owen S, Garg SK: Slicing the pie: correlating HbA_{1c} values with average blood glucose values in a pie chart form. *Diabetes Care* 21:209–212, 1998
6. Guthrie DW, Guthrie RA (Eds.): *Nursing Management of Diabetes Mellitus.* 5th ed. New York, Springer, 2002
7. Guthrie DW, Guthrie RA: Approach to management. *Diabetes Educ* 16: 401–406, 1990
8. American Diabetes Association: Tests of glycemia in diabetes (Position Statement). *Diabetes Care* 27 (Suppl. 1):S91–S93, 2004
9. American Diabetes Association: Standards of medical care in diabetes (Position Statement). *Diabetes Care* 28 (Suppl. 1):S4–S36, 2005
10. Davidson J, Reader D, Rickheim O: *Blood Glucose Patterns: A Guide to Achieving Targets.* Minneapolis, MI, International Diabetes Center Park Nicollet Institute, 2003
11. Pearson J, Bergenstal R: Fine-tuning control: pattern management versus supplementation: pattern management: an essential component of effective insulin management. *Diabetes Spectrum* 14:75–78, 2001
12. Farkas-Hirsch R (Ed.): *Intensive Diabetes Management.* 2nd ed. Alexandria, VA, American Diabetes Association, 1998
13. American Dietetic Association, American Diabetes Association: *Advanced Carbohydrate Counting.* Chicago, IL, American Dietetic Association; Alexandria, VA, American Diabetes Association, 2003
14. American Diabetes Association: National standards for diabetes self-management education (Position Statement). *Diabetes Care* 27 (Suppl. 1): S143–S150, 2004
15. Norris S, Engelgau M, Narayan V: Effectiveness of self-management training in type 2 diabetes: a systematic review of randomized controlled trials. *Diabetes Care* 24:561–587, 2001
16. Pieber TR, Brunner GA, Schnedl WJ, Schattenberg S, Kaufmann P, Krejs GJ: Evaluation of a structured outpatient group education program for intensive insulin therapy. *Diabetes Care* 18:625–630, 1995
17. Hirsch IB, Farkas-Hirsch R: Sliding scale or sliding scare: it's all sliding nonsense. *Diabetes Spectrum* 14:79–81, 2001

18. Shagan BP: Does anyone here know how to make insulin work backwards? Why sliding-scale insulin coverage doesn't work. *Pract Diabetol* 9:1–4, 1990
19. Sawin CT: Action without benefit: the sliding scale of insulin use. *Arch Intern Med* 157:489–491, 1997
20. Guthrie RA, Childs B, Guthrie D: *Rapid and Long Acting Insulin Analogs: Strategies for Patient Use.* Monograph. 2nd Ed. Wichita, KS, Quontum Press, August 2004
21. Hirsch I: Implementation of intensive diabetes therapy for IDDM. *Diabetes Reviews* 3:288–307, 1995
22. Brunelle BL, Llewelyn J, Anderson JH, Gale EA: Meta-analysis of the effect of insulin lispro on severe hypoglycemia in patients with type 1 diabetes. *Diabetes Care* 21:1726–1731, 1998
23. Childs BP, Guthrie RA, Carr M, McDaniel J, Rhiley D: Incorporating new diabetes oral agents into clinical practice. *Diabetes Spectrum* 9:266–268, 1996
24. Bolli G: Clinical strategies for controlling peaks and valleys: type 1 diabetes. *Intern J Clin Pract* 120 (Suppl.):65–74, 2002

Ms. Hinnen is a Diabetes Clinical Nurse Specialist for the Department of Outreach and Prevention, Via Christi Regional Medical Center, Wichita, KS. She coordinates a multidisciplinary team that provides education and care through an American Diabetes Association–recognized program. Dr. Guthrie is the Medical Director at Mid-America Diabetes Associates, Wichita, KS.

COMPLICATIONS

7. Acute Complications of Diabetes

Irl B. Hirsch, MD

D iabetic ketoacidosis (DKA), hyperosmolar hyperglycemic syndrome (HHS), and hypoglycemia are the most common acute complications of diabetes. To prevent significant mortality and morbidity, it is important for the health care provider and the individual with diabetes to identify the symptoms and institute appropriate treatment promptly.

DKA AND HHS

Epidemiology

Despite the fact that insulin was first used clinically >80 years ago, hyperglycemic crisis continues to be a major public health problem. DKA has an incidence rate of four to eight cases per 1,000 patients with diabetes (1,2), and it appears that hospitalizations for DKA are increasing in the U.S. (3). Currently, DKA accounts for 4–9% of all hospitalizations for people with diabetes. HHS, on the other hand, is more difficult to quantify but is thought to comprise <1% of all hospitalizations for people with diabetes (4).

The cost of treating DKA is staggering. In the state of Rhode Island, it was estimated that the cost of DKA in 1983 was $225 million (2). More recently, the American Diabetes Association (ADA) estimated the cost of DKA to be approximately $1 billion each year (5). The mortality rates are <5% for DKA and ~15% for HHS, and the rates increase with age and comorbidities (5).

Pathophysiology

DKA consists of the triad of hyperglycemia, ketonemia, and acidemia. The ADA classifies DKA by level of acidemia and level of stupor. Although infection is usually thought of as the most likely precipitating factor, in both the U.S. and Europe, omission of insulin is actually the most common etiology. This omission may occur from the inability to obtain the insulin for financial reasons, as part of an eating disorder, or as part of some other type of psychological disease process.

Up to 20% of cases of DKA or HHS may present without a previous diagnosis of diabetes. HHS, more often a disease of the elderly, can be caused by acute illness or drug therapy. The former would most commonly include an infection such as pneumonia or sepsis, a vascular event such as a myocardial infarction or cerebrovascular accident, or acute pancreatitis. The latter includes agents such as glucocorticoids, diazoxide, diuretics, and β-blockers. In both DKA and HSS, the fundamental defect is a decrease in the net effective concentration of insulin coupled with a massive elevation of the counterregulatory hormones (glucagon, cortisol, growth hormone, and epinephrine). In DKA, the insulin deficiency is either absolute or relative in relation to the counterregulatory hormones that overwhelm the body's ability to suppress lipolysis. In HHS, there is a residual amount of insulin that suppresses ketosis but cannot control hyperglycemia. This leads to severe dehydration and impaired renal function that eventually leads to even more severe hyperglycemia. For this reason, hyperglycemia is more profound in HHS than in DKA.

At both the molecular and cellular levels, there has been a substantial improvement in our understanding of both of these conditions during the past 30 years. Despite this, what has not changed is that many of these hyperglycemic crises are preventable and that prevention is the fundamental goal.

Assessment and Clinical Presentation

DKA and HHS are both medical emergencies that require a brief but directed assessment. Key issues that require special assessment include *1*) airway patency, *2*) mental status, *3*) cardiovascular and renal status, *4*) possible source of infection, and *5*) state of hydration. Although there are many similarities in the presentation of DKA and HHS, there are some subtle differences. Table 7.1 presents the similarities and differences. DKA usually presents quickly, often over the span of 24 h, whereas HHS usually presents over several days because the level of consciousness often decreases in a less acute manner. DKA is also more often associated with nausea, vomiting, and abdominal pain. The classic rapid deep breaths observed with acidosis (Kussmaul breathing) is not generally seen with HHS. The fruity breath associated with DKA is a result of acetone loss through the lungs. Patients with HHS are more often hyperosmolar than those with DKA; thus, obtundation and coma are more common in this group. Another important detail for those with HHS is that even though infection is a common precipitating event, fever is rare, even with sepsis due to skin vasodilation related to the dehydration and volume depletion.

In a patient with known diabetes, a presumptive diagnosis can usually be made quickly by capillary glucose measurement and a urine dipstick. Because patients with DKA can present to the outpatient clinic, these tests are relatively easy to obtain, but for the obtunded individual in an emergency room, a urinary catheter is often required. Nevertheless, for definitive diagnosis, laboratory studies will be needed.

Labs and Tests

For either of the hyperglycemic emergencies, it is necessary to send *stat* labs for plasma glucose, electrolytes, urea nitrogen, creatinine, complete blood count (with differential), serum acetone, and arterial blood gas. The severity of the DKA is determined by the degree of acidemia and mental status: pH <7.24 and a stuporous level of consciousness is considered "moderate" DKA, whereas pH <7.00 with coma is considered "severe." Many mild cases of DKA, especially when there

Table 7.1 Comparison of DKA and HHS

	DKA	HHS
Features		
Age of patient	Usually <40 years	Usually >60 years
Duration of symptoms	Usually <2 days	Usually >5 days
Glucose level	Usually <600 mg/dl (<33 mmol/l)	Usually >800 mg/dl (>44 mmol/l)
Sodium concentration	Likely normal or low	Likely normal or high
Potassium concentration	High, normal, or low	High, normal, or low
Bicarbonate concentration	Low	Normal
Ketone bodies	Present	Usually absent
pH	Low, <7.3	Normal
Serum osmolality	Usually <350 mOsm/kg	Usually >350 mOsm/kg
Cerebral edema	Often subclinical	Rare
Assessment		
Skin	Flushed: dry, warm	Pallor: moist, cool
Breath	Fruity, acetone	Normal
Vital signs	Blood pressure decreased, pulse increased	Blood pressure decreased, pulse increased, afebrile
Gastrointestinal	Severe abdominal pain, nausea, vomiting	Mild abdominal pain, nausea, vomiting
Mental status	Lethargic	Lethargic
Prognosis	<5% mortality	15% mortality

are no abnormalities in mental status, can be managed in an outpatient setting or after volume repletion in an emergency room.

Note that a person can have DKA without substantial hyperglycemia. Euglycemic DKA is defined as DKA in an individual with plasma glucose level <300 mg/dl (<16.6 mmol/l). This condition most often occurs when volume depletion is not severe but there is absolute insulin deficiency, as in type 1 diabetes.

The initial urinalysis may need to be interpreted with caution. Urine (and for that matter, serum) ketones are evaluated by the nitroprusside reaction, which is a semiquantitative test for acetoacetate and acetone but not for β-hydroxybutyrate, the main keto acid of DKA (6). Therefore, laboratory assessment often underestimates the severity of the DKA.

PRACTICAL POINT

Euglycemic DKA can be seen in surgical patients with type 1 diabetes when adequate intravenous fluids are given to prevent dehydration but insulin is either withheld or administered in doses too low to prevent ketosis.

With the initial blood draw, if there is no obvious etiology, it is reasonable to draw blood for blood cultures. Obviously, if another etiology becomes apparent, the cultures can be cancelled. Similarly, a urine culture should be obtained with the initial laboratory assessment.

While waiting for the electrolytes to be analyzed, an electrocardiogram should be obtained, especially for adults. First, a myocardial infarction can precipitate DKA or HHS. In children, an electrocardiogram can give important clues to hypokalemia or hyperkalemia. Second, if there are abnormalities with the T-waves, suggesting abnormalities in potassium homeostasis, a telemetry device needs to be placed immediately because hypokalemia from the treatment of these emergencies is a common cause of mortality.

When evaluating laboratory data, it is important to understand two key formulas. Perhaps the most important is the anion gap, defined as the serum sodium – (chloride + bicarbonate). Often, the anion gap is calculated as part of the electrolyte measurement; if not, the clinician needs to perform the calculation. In modern assays, the normal anion gap is 7–9 mEq/l. An elevated anion gap confirms an unmeasured anion. Although this may include β-hydroxybutyrate (and acetoacetate), the differential diagnosis for an anion gap acidosis includes lactic acidosis, uremic acidosis, salicylate intoxication, rhabdomyolysis, and ethylene glycol intoxication. There are numerous different acid-base disturbances that need to be diagnosed because both metabolic alkalosis and primary respiratory diseases causing hypoventilation or hyperventilation may also present with DKA. Furthermore, a non–anion gap acidosis can be seen in DKA, as can a mixed–anion gap and hyperchloremic acidosis.

The other important formula that needs to be calculated is the total serum osmolality. This is calculated as:

$$2 \times [\text{serum sodium (mEq/l)}] + [\text{glucose (mg/dl)}/18]$$
$$+ [\text{blood urea nitrogen (mg/dl)}/2.8]$$

The normal range for this measurement is 290 ± 5 mOsm/kg. The diagnosis of HHS can be made with a serum osmolality >330 mOsm/kg, usually with a blood glucose level >600 mg/dl and the absence of significant ketonemia.

Several other issues related to laboratory assessment should be considered. The first is that serum creatinine may be falsely elevated because of acetoacetate interfering with the assay. After treatment, the creatinine level will usually return to normal or at least to the baseline level. Next, high amylase levels need to be interpreted cautiously in the initial evaluation of DKA because this may be the result of extrapancreatic secretion. A leukocytosis with very high white blood cell counts is common and does not necessarily reflect an infectious process. Again, with therapy for DKA, the white blood cell count will normalize, but if it remains high after successful treatment, investigation for an occult infection should be considered.

Hyperglycemia will result in a falsely low sodium level because of the movement of water from the intracellular to extracellular space in the presence of hyperglycemia. To calculate the corrected serum sodium level in the context of hyperglycemia, add 1.6 mEq/l to every 100 mg/dl above 180 mg/dl. If severe hyponatremia is still present after this calculation, other etiologies of hyponatremia need to be considered. Most patients with HHS present with profound hypernatremia, indicative of a severe free-water deficit. When the serum sodium is corrected for the hyperglycemia in these patients, the corrected sodium level is often >170 mEq/l.

Special attention needs to be paid to serum potassium levels. First, despite massive kaliuresis from hyperglycemia and often further potassium losses from vomiting, serum potassium levels are usually normal or even high. The reason for this is that insulin deficiency, acidemia, and hyperosmolarity all result in potassium moving from the cell into the blood. Clinicians should not be misled; potassium levels can drop quickly, leading to life-threatening arrhythmias as fluids and insulin are replaced. For this reason, potassium replacement is a key component of the therapy of DKA and HHS and is the reason many of these patients, especially older patients with possible coronary artery disease, need to be monitored with telemetry.

Treatments

Nursing plays a vital role in the therapy for acute hyperglycemic episodes. Appropriate monitoring is the first important component of therapy. This is best addressed with a complete flow sheet, which includes both physical examination findings (e.g., blood pressure, heart rate) and laboratory results (e.g., glucose, bicarbonate, potassium, phosphate). The flow sheet should also include aspects of therapy, e.g., rate and type of fluid, insulin and potassium rates, bicarbonate and phosphate rates. Table 7.2 presents an example of a flow sheet for tracking DKA therapy. Table 7.3 presents key treatment tips.

One of the most controversial areas in the treatment of hyperglycemic crisis has been the rate and type of fluids that should be infused. Initially, this should be determined by the volume status of the patient. Supine hypotension signifies an ~20% decrease in extracellular fluid, whereas orthostatic hypotension confirms a 15–20% reduction in extracellular volume. An orthostatic increase in pulse without a change in blood pressure suggests a 10% reduction in extracellular volume. For all of these situations, there is now agreement that the first fluid infused should be 0.9% normal saline, administered as quickly as possible over the first hour, followed by 500–1,000 ml/h for the next 2 h of either 0.9% normal saline or 0.45% normal saline, depending on the degree of hydration and serum sodium level. Even with severe dehydration and hypernatremia, 0.9% normal saline is hypotonic compared with the extracellular fluid. Some authors advocate hypotonic saline (0.45% normal saline) from the outset if the effective serum osmolality [calculated as 2 × measured sodium (mEq/l) + glucose (mg/dl)/18] is >320. Others, including this author, prefer the initial use of 0.9% saline for the first hour followed by 0.45% saline unless volume losses are severe and hypotension is not corrected after the first liter of fluid.

Dextrose (5%) should be added to the solution when blood glucose reaches 250 mg/dl (13.9 mmol/l) in DKA or 300 mg/dl (16.6 mmol/l) in HHS. There are two main reasons for this. First, it allows continued insulin administration to control ketogenesis in DKA. Furthermore, particularly in children, too rapid a decrease in blood glucose can result in cerebral edema. Another important point is that once blood pressure is stabilized and glucose levels decrease to the point that osmotic diuresis is not leading to further water and electrolyte losses, urine volumes will also decrease, allowing a decrease in intravenous fluids. This is critical in young children and older adults who are at a greater risk of overhydration. The excess of free water from overhydration can also result in cerebral edema. The exact fluid rate will vary depending on the clinical situation, but will generally range from 4–14 ml/kg/h. Although there are large variations, the average duration of time that intravenous hydration will be required is ~48 h.

Perhaps the most important point about the use of insulin therapy in either DKA or HHS is that electrolyte levels need to be confirmed before starting an intravenous insulin infusion. In the rare patient who presents with hypokalemia, insulin therapy needs to be postponed until the potassium levels are corrected. Although controversial, most authorities begin the insulin infusion (all human regular insulin) with an intravenous bolus of 0.1–0.15 units/kg, followed by 0.1 units/kg/h. Some endocrinologists will use intramuscular insulin at 7–10 units, except when hypotension is present, in which case only the intravenous route can ensure appropri-

Table 7.2 Suggested DKA/HHS Flowsheet

DATE: HOUR:	ER															
Weight (daily)																
Mental Status*																
Temperature																
Pulse																
Respiration/Depth**																
Blood Pressure																
Serum Glucose (mg/dl)																
Serum Ketones																
Urine Ketones																
ELECTROLYTES																
Serum Na^+ (mEq/L)																
Serum K^+ (mEq/L)																
Serum Cl^- (mEq/L)																
Serum HCO_3^- (mEq/L)																
Serum BUN (mg/dl)																
Effective Osmolality																
2[measured Na(mEq/L)]																
+ Glucose (mg/dl)/18																
Anion Gap																
A.B.G.																
pH Venous(V) Arterial(A)																
pO_2																
pCO_2																
O_2 SAT																
INSULIN																
Units Past Hour																
Route																
INTAKE FLUID/METABOLITES																
0.45% NaCl(ml) past hour																
0.9% NaCl(ml) past hour																
5% Dextrose(ml) past hour																
KCL (mEq) past hour																
PO_4 (mmol/l) past hour																
Other (e.g., HCO_3^-)																
OUTPUT																
Urine (ml)																
Other																

*A-ALERT D-DROWSY   S-STUPOROUS   C-COMATOSE
**D-DEEP S-SHALLOW   N-NORMAL

From ADA (7).

Table 7.3 Acute Complication Treatment Tips and Precautions

Establish diagnosis; if known to have diabetes and unable to test glucose, assume hypoglycemia and give intravenous glucose or glucagon.

If triage call, vomiting present, or hyperglycemia, request urine ketone measurement.

Treat the volume depletion first.

Insulin should not be replaced until the potassium level is known.

HHS/DKA usually requires intensive care monitoring for at least 12 h.

Monitor and replace potassium to prevent life-threatening arrhythmias.

Cerebral edema is a risk with too rapid correction of blood glucose.

Consider a major vascular incident in the elderly as etiology for hyperglycemic crisis.

---

ate absorption. Occasionally, insulin resistance will require much larger doses of insulin than the starting rates noted above. However, even very low doses of insulin will inhibit lipolysis and ketogenesis. When the blood glucose level reaches 250–300 mg/dl (13.3–16.3 mmol/l), the insulin infusion rate can be decreased and the intravenous dextrose added. In general, it is appropriate to measure blood glucose every hour in these patients. The electrolytes can be measured less frequently. The blood glucose should decrease at 50–70 mg/dl/h. If blood glucose is not improving, other etiologies should be investigated, such as patient's volume status not being corrected or an error in the insulin infusion mixture.

In general, these patients may have a 500- to 700-mEq/l potassium deficit when they present. Intravenous fluids will increase renal plasma flow, whereas intravenous insulin will result in a movement of potassium from extracellular to intracellular areas. These two events will lead to a profound decrease in serum potassium levels shortly after the treatment of a hyperglycemic emergency. When hypokalemia is present at the onset, potassium levels should be replaced at least to a level of 3.3 mEq/l before insulin is started. These patients should also be monitored with telemetry. In general, potassium replacement should not exceed 40 mEq the first hour and then 20–30 mEq/h after that. Because potassium chloride in addition to the saline used will usually result in hyperchloremia, many authors recommend replacing some of the potassium as either potassium phosphate or potassium acetate. However, there are no studies examining a change of outcomes with these alternate potassium solutions.

Bicarbonate use is also a controversial topic in the treatment of DKA. There is little reason to consider adding bicarbonate for most of those with DKA because acidemia will improve as bicarbonate is generated by the liver while the ketogenesis is reversed by insulin therapy. In children, it is suggested that bicarbonate will result in more profound altered consciousness and headache. Clearly, the addition of bicarbonate will lead to more profound hypokalemia. It is for this reason that some authors feel the only indication for the use of bicarbonate therapy is for life-threatening hyperkalemia. However, there are now controlled trials examining the use of bicarbonate therapy with severe acidemia (pH <7.0). It is for this reason that the ADA suggests bicarbonate therapy for those patients who present with this degree of severe acidemia (5). The solution should never be given as a bolus, but rather infused as 1 ampule (50 mmol) to another solution such as a liter of 0.45% normal saline.

As with potassium, initial levels of serum phosphate are often normal or increased despite a total-body deficit. Insulin therapy will result in a shift of phosphate into the cell, often resulting in hypophosphatemia during the treatment of DKA and HHS. However, in the rare situation of the serum phosphate dropping below 1 mg/dl, complications from hypophosphatemia are unusual. Furthermore, controlled trials have not demonstrated a benefit from routine use of phosphate therapy in the treatment of DKA. Current recommendations are to replace phosphate if levels drop below 1.0 mg/dl (5). This can be accomplished by adding 20–30 mEq/l of potassium phosphate to the intravenous solution over 2–3 h. The most important complication of phosphate replacement is hypocalcemia, so serum calcium levels need to be monitored during the time period.

Protocols for management of DKA and HHS are presented in Figs. 7.1 and 7.2. These protocols are taken from the ADA position statement on hyperglycemic crisis in patients with diabetes (7).

Unlike HHS, mild DKA can be managed on an outpatient basis. Patients are encouraged to call their providers when moderate or large urine ketones or unmanageable high blood glucose levels are noted. Early replacement of insulin using frequent doses of insulin lispro, insulin aspart, or intramuscular regular insulin (0.1 units/kg) every 2–3 h plus good hydration will allow the individual to decrease the blood glucose levels and restore hydration. Using sports drinks will assist in correcting the electrolyte imbalance. Sugared liquids will be required to prevent a rapid glucose drop from the supplemental insulin. Management principles follow the guidelines for hospital care. If the blood glucose does not decrease within 3–5 h or vomiting occurs, then the individual needs to be treated at the hospital. Antiemetics are not recommended because vomiting may be the symptom that guides whether the metabolic acidosis is being corrected.

Educational/Behavioral Considerations

The most important area for educational consideration is determining how DKA and HHS can be prevented. Because a large percentage of these patients develop these life-threatening emergencies because of insulin omission, factors leading to this need to be explored and attempts need to be made to correct the situation. The patient who returns with a hyperglycemic crisis on a frequent basis must be assessed for underlying causes. These patients (previously termed *brittle*) often return in crisis because of some other major problem that could be related to a severe psychological stress, an eating disorder, or even major financial troubles that make obtaining insulin difficult. Alternatively, some patients with frequent hospitalizations have waited too long to ask for assistance during a pump malfunction or systemic infection. If the etiology is related to a psychological problem, the patient will require special attention. A referral to a mental health specialist would be appropriate for the vast majority of these patients.

Education of the individual with diabetes and family is essential. See

> **PRACTICAL POINT**
>
> Education is the key to the prevention of the acute complications of diabetes: hypoglycemia and hyperglycemia. Nurses should review with patients their strategies for treating high and low blood glucose levels and potential precipitating causes. Reinforce good practices.

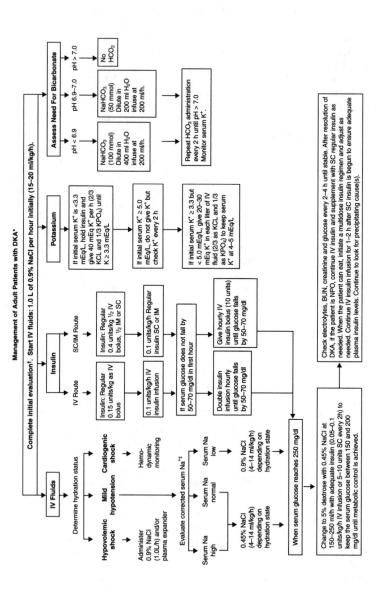

Figure 7.1 Protocol for the management of adult patients with DKA. *DKA diagnostic criteria: blood glucose >250 mg/dl, arterial pH <7.3, bicarbonate <15 mEq/l, and moderate ketonuria or ketonemia. Normal ranges vary by lab; check local lab normal ranges for all electrolytes. †After history and physical examination, obtain arterial blood gases, complete blood count with differential, urinalysis, blood glucose, blood urea nitrogen (BUN), electrolytes, chemistry profile, and creatinine levels *stat* as well as an electrocardiogram. Obtain chest X-ray and cultures as needed. ‡Serum Na should be corrected for hyperglycemia (for each 100 mg/dl glucose >100 mg/dl, add 1.6 mEq to sodium value for corrected serum sodium value). IM, intramuscular; IV, intravenous; SC, subcutaneous. *From* American Diabetes Association: Hyperglycemic crises in diabetes (Position Statement). *Diabetes Care* 27 (Suppl. 1):S94–S102, 2004.

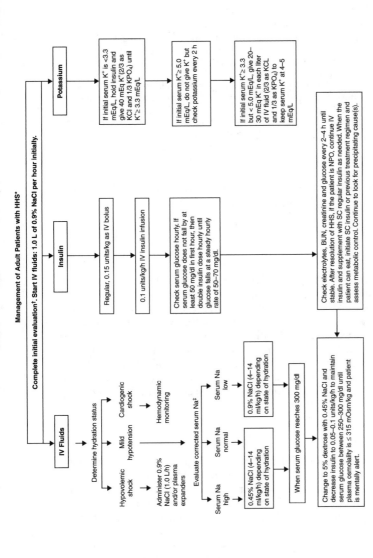

Management of Adult Patients with HHS*

Potassium

If initial serum K⁺ is <3.3 mEq/L, hold insulin and give 40 mEq K⁺ (2/3 as KCl and 1/3 KPO₄) until K⁺ ≥ 3.3 mEq/L.

If initial serum K⁺ ≥ 5.0 mEq/L, do not give K⁺ but check potassium every 2 h

If initial serum K⁺ ≥ 3.3 but < 5.0 mEq/L, give 20–30 mEq K⁺ in each liter of IV fluid (2/3 as KCL and 1/3 as KPO₄) to keep serum K⁺ at 4–5 mEq/L

Insulin

Regular, 0.15 units/kg as IV bolus

0.1 units/kg/h IV insulin infusion

Check serum glucose hourly. If serum glucose does not fall by at least 50 mg/dl in first hour, then double insulin dose hourly until glucose falls at a steady hourly rate of 50–70 mg/dl.

IV Fluids

Determine hydration status

Hypovolemic shock

Administer 0.9% NaCl (1.0 L/h) and/or plasma expanders

Mild hypotension

Cardiogenic shock

Hemodynamic monitoring

Evaluate corrected serum Na‡

Serum Na high

0.45% NaCl (4–14 ml/kg/h) depending on state of hydration

Serum Na normal

Serum Na low

0.9% NaCl (4–14 ml/kg/h) depending on state of hydration

When serum glucose reaches 300 mg/dl

Change to 5% dextrose with 0.45% NaCl and decrease insulin to 0.05–0.1 units/kg/h to maintain serum glucose between 250–300 mg/dl until plasma osmolality is ≤ 315 mOsm/kg and patient is mentally alert.

Check electrolytes, BUN, creatinine and glucose every 2–4 h until stable. After resolution of HHS, if the patient is NPO, continue IV insulin and supplement with SC regular insulin as needed. When the patient can eat, initiate SC insulin or previous treatment regimen and assess metabolic control. Continue to look for precipitating cause(s).

Complete initial evaluation†. Start IV fluids: 1.0 L of 0.9% NaCl per hour initially.

Figure 7.2 Protocol for the management of adult patients with HHS. *Diagnostic criteria: blood glucose >600 mg/dl, arterial pH <7.3, bicarbonate <15 mEq/l, mild ketonuria or ketonemia and effective serum osmolality >320 mOsm/kg H₂O. This protocol is for patients admitted with mental status change or severe dehydration who require admission to an intensive care unit. For less severe cases, see text for management guidelines. Normal lab ranges vary by lab; check local lab normal ranges for all electrolytes. Effective serum osmolality calculation: 2[measured Na (mEq/l)] + glucose (mg/dl)/18. †After history and physical examination, obtain arterial blood gases, complete blood count with differential, urinalysis, plasma glucose, blood urea nitrogen (BUN), electrolytes, chemistry profile, and creatinine levels stat as well as an electrocardiogram. Obtain chest X-ray and cultures as needed. ‡Serum Na should be corrected for hyperglycemia (for each 100 mg/dl glucose >100 mg/dl, add 1.6 mEq to sodium value for corrected serum value). IV, intravenous; SC, subcutaneous. *From* American Diabetes Association: Hyperglycemic crises in diabetes (Position Statement). *Diabetes Care* 27 (Suppl. 1):S94–S102, 2004.

Table 7.4 Patient Education Tips

Problem	Key Education Points
Insulin omission	Access to care, including insulin supply Poor storage of insulin, old insulin
Failed sick-day management	Access to ketone monitoring supplies Recognition of symptoms of DKA, HHS, and hypoglycemia Understanding of action needed if ketones present Access to glucose-containing fluids Understanding of when to treat Importance of continuing insulin, even with illness Guidelines for when to call the health care provider/emergency medical services Guidelines, if appropriate, for insulin supplementation during illness
Frequent DKA	Referral to mental health professional

Table 7.4 for educational tips. Referral to appropriate resources should occur to prevent the next episode.

HYPOGLYCEMIA

Epidemiology

Hypoglycemia, defined as a blood glucose level <50–60 mg/dl (<2.8–3.3 mmol/l) is common in type 1 diabetes. It is estimated that most people with type 1 diabetes have at least two symptomatic episodes each week, meaning that they may have thousands of episodes over the course of a lifetime (8). Severe hypoglycemia, defined as requiring the assistance of another person, may occur in many at least once yearly. It is estimated that 2–4% of deaths in patients with type 1 diabetes occur because of hypoglycemia (9). Iatrogenic (as a result of treatment) hypoglycemia is much less common in type 2 diabetes. Estimates vary, but severe hypoglycemia appears to occur at a fraction of the rate seen in type 1 diabetes (5). Hypoglycemic death from sulfonylureas has been documented.

Pathophysiology

Normally, as glucose levels decline, both glucagon and epinephrine levels respond as a protective mechanism against hypoglycemia. In nondiabetic individuals, the glycemic threshold for this counterregulatory response is between 65 and 70 mg/dl (3.6 and 3.9 mmol/l), but this shifts to higher levels in individuals with suboptimally controlled diabetes and lower levels in individuals with near-normal A1C levels. The glucagon and epinephrine response will result in an increase of hepatic glucose output in addition to a suppression of glycogenesis. Furthermore, the elevated epinephrine levels will result in the autonomic symptoms frequently seen with hypoglycemia: tremor, palpitations, and anxiety. Common signs include an elevated heart rate, pallor, and an elevated systolic blood pressure. A cold sweat and hunger appear to be cholinergic (not related to epinephrine). Eventually, if oral or parenteral glucose is not provided, neuroglycopenic symptoms will occur, e.g., nausea, diplopia, confusion, seizures, and even coma may result from profound hypoglycemia. These neuroglycopenic symptoms occur after the autonomic symptoms.

The mechanisms for hypoglycemia and hypoglycemia unawareness are better understood in type 1 than in type 2 diabetes. In the former, as endogenous insulin secretion declines, the normal glucagon response to hypoglycemia diminishes to the point that the patient's only initial response is epinephrine secretion. Furthermore, the brain adapts to antecedent hypoglycemia so that the epinephrine response to hypoglycemia is shifted to a lower plasma glucose level. A severely reduced epinephrine response can be seen in the absence of classic autonomic dysfunction, leading to hypoglycemia unawareness. However, the presence of autonomic neuropathy typically diminishes the epinephrine response, leading to an even higher risk of severe hypoglycemia.

For individuals with type 2 diabetes, the frequency of severe hypoglycemia is similar to that in individuals with type 1 diabetes when matched for duration of insulin therapy. Given the progressive nature of insulin deficiency in type 2 diabetes, clinical hypoglycemia becomes a greater problem as endogenous insulin secretion declines. Table 7.5 lists risk factors for the development of hypoglycemia.

Alcohol is a common etiology of hypoglycemia. Alcohol can inhibit gluconeogenesis, especially in a starved state, placing an insulin-requiring patient at high risk for iatrogenic hypoglycemia. Indeed, even individuals without diabetes can develop hypoglycemia from alcohol. In the fed state, alcohol may actually increase hepatic glucose production, thus making alcohol ingestion quite risky because it may be quite difficult to predict the glycemic effects at any given time. To further complicate matters, the type of alcohol ingested may alter the glucose. For example, a sweet liqueur may raise the glucose, whereas a dry wine may lower it depending on the fed state of the individual. Given this wide variability, alcohol can be dangerous and should be ingested in moderation. Furthermore, frequent blood glucose testing should be performed to help guide treatment, espe-

---

Table 7.5 Risk Factors for Hypoglycemia

Risk Factors	Possible Causes
Insulin excess	Too much insulin, insulin secretagogue, or insulin sensitizer, taken at the wrong time or wrong type
Decreased exogenous glucose	Missed meal or snack, not enough food Overnight fast
Decrease in endogenous glucose production	Alcohol
Increased glucose utilization	Too much exercise or activity without enough food
Increased insulin sensitivity	Late after exercise Improved fitness Weight loss Use of an insulin sensitizer Middle of the night
Decreased insulin clearance	Renal failure
Compromised glucose counterregulation	Insulin deficiency, history of severe hypoglycemia, aggressive therapy and glucose goals, lower A1C

cially as it relates to the prevention of hypoglycemia because typical symptoms may be altered.

Labs and Test

Usually, very little needs to be done for the diagnosis of insulin or sulfonylurea-induced hypoglycemia. In a symptomatic patient, a capillary blood glucose level will confirm the diagnosis. Those with hypoglycemia unawareness need more frequent self-monitoring of blood glucose in an attempt to avoid severe hypoglycemia. Often, these patients are found to be hypoglycemic on routine blood checks even though they may not have any symptoms.

Treatment

Most episodes of symptomatic and asymptomatic (found by checking blood glucose) hypoglycemia can be treated with the ingestion of oral carbohydrate. This carbohydrate may be in the form of glucose tablets, juice, milk, or crackers. The vast majority of these cases can be treated with 15–20 g carbohydrate. This step can be repeated in 15–20 min if the symptoms have not improved or the blood glucose level has not increased. The most common mistake by patients is to overtreat the hypoglycemic episode because of insatiable hunger, failure of the symptoms to resolve immediately, and/or fear of a continuing drop in glucose levels. All too often this results in posthypoglycemic hyperglycemia because additional insulin is not injected for the extra food ingested.

Treating Severe Hypoglycemia

Parenteral therapy is required when the patient is unable to take carbohydrate orally. Crushed glucose tablets or gel should not be placed in the mouth or rubbed onto the buccal mucosa of a person who is not able to swallow. Glucagon or intravenous glucose is the only remedy. Subcutaneous or intramuscular glucagon is often used by family members in patients with type 1 diabetes. Glucagon is less helpful for individuals with type 2 diabetes because it stimulates insulin secretion as well as glycogenolysis. After glucagon administration, the patient will often experience nausea, vomiting, and headache.

When possible, intravenous glucose is the preferred treatment for severe hypoglycemia. The usual treatment is 10–25 g of 50% dextrose administered over 1–3 min. A blood glucose level should be checked after completion of the administration. Doses are variable, based on the weight of the individual, the type of diabetes, and the cause of the hypoglycemia. A continuous glucose infusion of 10% dextrose may be needed because the glucose bolus is transient. In patients who are unable to ingest oral carbohydrates or those with sulfonylurea-induced hypoglycemia, the hypoglycemia may be prolonged.

A patient who has been treated for hypoglycemia with glucagon or intravenous glucose should be provided oral carbohydrates as soon as he or she is able to eat.

Hypoglycemia Unawareness

Hypoglycemia unawareness is defined as the loss of the epinephrine-mediated warning symptoms of hypoglycemia. Hypoglycemia unawareness is associated with hypoglycemia frequency. The more hypoglycemia a patient experiences, the lower the threshold for symptoms. Fortunately, clinical trials have shown that this type of hypoglycemia unawareness may be reversed by strict avoidance of hypoglycemia. Most clinicians advise individuals with hypoglycemia unawareness to measure their glucose before driving. Until the technology for glucose sensors improves, it would seem prudent for these individuals to measure their blood glucose when driving—more frequently if the trip is during a time of suspected glycemic reduction, e.g., after exercise, 1–2 h after injecting a rapid-acting analog (Table 7.6).

Educational/Behavioral Considerations

All patients at risk for iatrogenic hypoglycemia need to learn typical symptoms and treatment. These patients would include individuals prescribed sulfonylureas, insulin secretagogues, and insulin. Treatments that require review include strategies for prompt oral treatment and avoidance of overtreatment. Family members of individuals with type 1 diabetes need training in the use of subcutaneous/intramuscular glucagon.

Patients who develop a severe fear of hypoglycemia (usually after one or more episodes of severe hypoglycemia) require special attention. Families can also become extremely fearful. The provider needs to appreciate that this fear can be overwhelming and that individuals may intentionally maintain extremely high blood glucose levels because of this fear. Often, they require psychological counseling. Slowly lowering glycemic targets over time can be an effective method to address this fear and return to glycemic goals.

SUMMARY

Prevention is the key to effective management of the acute complications of diabetes. These complications are costly, not only in the expenditure of health care dollars, but also in the decrease in the quality of life for people with diabetes.

Table 7.6 Reduction and Treatment of Hypoglycemia Unawareness

Goal	Actions
Increase symptoms of hypoglycemia	Rigorous avoidance of hypoglycemia Increased glucose monitoring Increase glucose targets for at least 3 weeks
Assist patient in identifying nonclassic symptoms	Possible: Blurred vision, numbness in limbs or lips, nausea, many others Encourage documentation in symptom log Log should include exercise, food, insulin timing Use log to identify atypical symptoms and patterns
Secure assistance at work, school, and home	Identification and training of family, friends, and coworkers to give glucagon and/or know when to call emergency medical services

Specific protocols, order sets, treatment algorithms, and clinical pathways should be developed and implemented to guide the best practices in the hospital (see CHAPTER 31). Nurses should take a leadership role in developing and implementing these clinical pathways. Monitoring of the patient with DKA and HHS by the nurse will be crucial. Preventing future episodes of DKA or HHS will depend on patient and family/caregiver education. Managing mild DKA and hypoglycemia at home will require a patient and family who are well educated. The nurse should take every opportunity to assess the patient and family's knowledge level and ability to prevent and treat hyperglycemia and hypoglycemia.

REFERENCES

1. Johnson DD, Palumbo PJ, Chu C: Diabetic ketoacidosis in a community-based population. *Mayo Clin Proc* 55:83–88, 1980
2. Faich GA, Fishbein HA, Ellis SE: The epidemiology of diabetic acidosis: a population-based study. *Am J Epidemiol* 117:551–558, 1983
3. Centers for Disease Control and Prevention, Division of Diabetes Translation: *Diabetes Surveillance, 1001.* Washington, DC, U.S. Govt. Printing Office, 1992, p. 635–1150
4. Fishbein HA, Palmubo PJ: Acute metabolic complications in diabetes. In *Diabetes in America.* 2nd ed. Harris MI, Cowie CC, Stern MP, Boyko EJ, Reiber GE, Bennett PH, Eds. Washington, DC, U.S. Govt. Printing Office, 1995, p. 283–291 (NIH publ. no. 95-1468)
5. Kitabchi AE, Umpierrez GE, Murphy MB, Barrett EJ, Kreisberg RA, Malone JI, Wall BM: Management of hyperglycemic crisis in patients with diabetes (Technical Review). *Diabetes Care* 24:131–153, 2001
6. Stephens JM, Sulway MJ, Watkins PJ: Relationship of blood acetoacetate and β-hydroxybutyrate in diabetes. *Diabetes* 20:485–489, 1971
7. American Diabetes Association: Hyperglycemic crises in diabetes (Position Statement). *Diabetes Care* 27 (Suppl. 1):S94–S102, 2004
8. Cryer PE: Hypoglycemia: the limiting factor in the glycaemic management of type I and type II diabetes. *Diabetologia* 45:937–948, 2002
9. Laing SP, Swerdlow AJ, Slater SD, Botha JL, Burden AC, Waugh NR, Smith AW, Hill RD, Bingley PJ, Patterson CC, Qiao Z, Keen H: The British Diabetic Association Cohort Study. II. Cause-specific mortality in patients with insulin-treated diabetes mellitus. *Diabet Med* 26:466–471, 1999
10. Kitabchi AE, Fisher JN, Murphy MB, Rumbak MJ: Diabetic ketoacidosis and the hyperglycemic hyperosmolar nonketotic state. In *Joslin's Diabetes Mellitus.* 13th ed. Kahn CR, Weir GC, Eds. Philadelphia, Lea & Febiger, 1994, p. 738–770

Dr. Hirsch is a Medical Doctor, Diabetes Care Center, at the University of Washington Medical Center, Seattle, WA.

8. Cardiovascular Complications

DEBORAH A. CHYUN, RN, MSN, PHD, FAHA, AND
LAWRENCE H. YOUNG, MD, FACC, FAHA

PATHOPHYSIOLOGY

Cardiovascular disease (CVD), which includes stroke, peripheral vascular disease, hypertension, angina, myocardial infarction (MI), heart failure, and sudden cardiac death, is the leading cause of death in patients with type 1 or type 2 diabetes. Patients with diabetes are two to three times more likely to develop CVD than people without diabetes, and women with diabetes are at especially high risk (1). Hypertension, which is present in ~40–60% of patients with type 2 diabetes, plays a major role in the development of stroke, MI, and heart failure.

The pathophysiology of CVD in individuals with diabetes is complex, and the development of atherosclerotic coronary artery disease (CAD), the focus of this chapter, involves the interaction of many factors, including hypertension, hyperlipidemia, impaired endothelial function, inflammation, central adiposity, and hemostatic abnormalities involving platelet function, thrombosis, and fibrinolysis. Although the direct role of hyperglycemia remains controversial, hyperglycemia has an important role in the development of microvascular complications that contribute to adverse outcomes, as well as to lipid and coagulation abnormalities that directly influence the development and progression of CAD. In patients with diabetes, CAD is generally more widespread, with stenosis in a greater number of vessels, along with more obstructive lesions within each vessel. Diffuse disease involving long segments and/or the distal aspects of the artery may be present, thereby limiting the usefulness of either percutaneous or surgical revascularization. Therefore, multiple risk factors must be controlled for successful prevention and management of CAD.

CLINICAL PRESENTATION

In the early stages, minor atherosclerosis may lead to plaque buildup. Plaque rupture may subsequently lead to acute coronary syndromes such as unstable angina and acute MI. More advanced atherosclerosis significantly narrows the vessel lumen and restricts blood flow, leading to myocardial ischemia during exercise or emotional stress. Myocardial ischemia sometimes results in angina or dyspnea, but some patients with diabetes may be asymptomatic. The first manifestation of CVD in these individuals may be acute MI, heart failure, or sudden cardiac death. Although as many as one in five individuals with type 2 diabetes may have completely asymptomatic or "silent" ischemia (2), CVD also occurs in patients who have symptomatic ischemia with angina. The mechanisms responsible for asymptomatic CAD in patients with diabetes may include cardiac autonomic neuropathy (3,4), and abnormalities in cardiac autonomic function may also serve as a risk marker in individuals with underlying asymptomatic myocardial ischemia (2). The clinical presentation of CVD is outlined in Table 8.1.

Table 8.1 Clinical Presentation of CVD

Stable angina

- Transient symptoms usually brought on by activity and relieved by rest or nitroglycerin: pressure, squeezing, fullness, or pain in center of chest lasting more than a few minutes; pain or discomfort in one or both arms, back, neck, jaw, or stomach; feeling out of breath with or before the chest discomfort
- In absence of anginal symptoms, "anginal equivalents": excessive fatigue, dyspnea, breaking out into a cold sweat, nausea, or lightheadedness
- Diagnostic: transient ST-segment depression on exercise electrocardiogram, regional contractile abnormalities on exercise echocardiogram, or stress-induced myocardial perfusion imaging

Acute coronary syndromes

- Symptoms: as with stable angina, but change in pattern with increased frequency, severity, and duration, lasting more than a few minutes and not relieved by rest or nitroglycerin
- Signs: cool, clammy skin; increased or irregular heart rate; decreased blood pressure; restlessness; altered mental status
- Diagnostic: ST-segment elevation or depression, significant Q-waves, deep T-wave inversions, left bundle branch block, ventricular arrhythmias or heart block on electrocardiogram; elevation of serum cardiac markers; echocardiogram, myocardial perfusion imaging, and angiogram may be ordered

Heart failure

- Symptoms: swelling in feet, ankles, and legs (edema); difficulty breathing, shortness of breath, dyspnea on exertion, orthopnea paroxysmal nocturnal dyspnea; weight gain; weakness or dizziness
- Signs: elevated heart rate and blood pressure; S3, S4, cardiac murmurs; crackles on lung examination; jugular venous distention and abdominojugular reflux
- Diagnostic: chest x-ray consistent with heart failure or pulmonary edema; echocardiogram, myocardial perfusion imaging, and angiogram may be ordered

Stroke

- Symptoms: sudden numbness or weakness in face, arm, hand, or leg, especially on one side of body; sudden inability to see out of one eye or to one side; sudden confusion, trouble understanding or speaking; sudden trouble walking, dizziness, or loss of balance or coordination; sudden, severe headache without known cause
- Signs: depends on site involved but may include restlessness, lethargy, altered mental status, hemiplegia, or hemiparesis
- Diagnostic: computed tomographic scans, magnetic resonance imaging, carotid or transcranial ultrasound, cerebral angiography, lumbar puncture

PREVENTION

As the understanding of the pathophysiological mechanisms responsible for CVD in individuals with diabetes continues to evolve, it has become apparent that the development of both diabetes and CVD share many common antecedents. The most effective way of preventing CVD in patients is to prevent diabetes in the first place. Although it is critical that the primary prevention of CVD in all patients with diabetes become a top priority, because CVD may already be established when the person is diagnosed with diabetes, identification of underlying CVD and limiting its progression are additional goals. There is some discrepancy in treatment goals among published clinical practice guidelines, particularly for blood pressure and lipids, as well as for levels at which medications should be started. Yet, no matter how lenient the goal, it is clear that the goals for cardiac risk factors or for blood glucose are not being achieved in most patients with diabetes. Goals and strategies for multifactorial risk reduction are presented in Table 8.2 (5–13).

The importance of blood pressure control was demonstrated in the U.K. Prospective Diabetes Study (14). American Diabetes Association (ADA) goals call for reduction of blood pressure to <130/80 mmHg (8), whereas more recent guidelines call for the need to reduce blood pressure even further (13). Therapeutic lifestyle approaches should be initiated when blood pressure levels are between 130/80 and 139/89 mmHg (8,15). For blood pressure >140/90 mmHg, antihypertensive medications are usually instituted immediately, in addition to therapeutic lifestyle interventions (Table 8.3). The major lipid abnormalities associated with insulin resistance and type 2 diabetes include reduced HDL cholesterol and increased triglyceride levels (16). Increased atherogenicity may be related to the presence of oxidized, small, dense LDL cholesterol particles, even though overall elevations in LDL cholesterol are not specifically related to diabetes (17). Although the ADA recommends LDL cholesterol levels <100 mg/dl, the current guidelines do not call for the initiation of pharmacological therapy for levels between 100 and 129 mg/dl unless macrovascular disease is present (6). Goals for HDL and triglyceride levels also vary and are secondary to LDL lowering (6,12,15). Recently, further LDL lowering to <70 mg/dl, along with a lowering of the threshold for drug treatment to 100 mg/dl, have been recommended for very-high-risk patients, such as those with established CVD and diabetes (18).

Physical inactivity and obesity play major roles in the development of type 2 diabetes and CVD. Regular physical activity, structured exercise, and dietary modifications have beneficial effects on glycemic control, lipids, weight, and blood pressure. Table 8.4 illustrates the approximate and cumulative effect on LDL cholesterol reduction achieved by dietary modification (13).

> ### PRACTICAL POINT
>
> Lowering LDL to <70 mg/dl, along with a lowering of the threshold for drug treatment to 100 mg/dl, have been recommended for very-high-risk patients, such as those with established CVD and diabetes.

Individualized exercise recommendations are required in patients with peripheral vascular disease or cardiac autonomic neuropathy, severe retinopathy, or known CAD (9). Because of the possibility of unrecognized CAD, particularly in individuals with type 2 diabetes, these patients should generally engage in moderate-intensity exercise regimens. Sedentary individuals should always initiate exercise programs at a low level and gradually

Table 8.2 Goals and Strategies for Prevention of CVD in Patients with Diabetes

Blood pressure <130/80 mmHg (8,13,15)

- Measure at each visit; if ≥130/80 mmHg, confirm on second day
- Lifestyle modification (weight control, physical activity, limit sodium and alcohol intake) before initiation of medication if blood pressure <140/90 mmHg
- Angiotensin-converting enzyme (ACE) inhibitor or angiotensin receptor blocker considered first-line therapy for renal-protective effect

LDL cholesterol <100 mg/dl (5,6,11,12,15,18)

- Tested annually or every 2 years if low risk
- Suggested daily intake: carbohydrates, 50–70%; protein, 15–20%; total fat, 25–35%; saturated fat <7–10%; up to 10% polyunsaturated and 20% monounsaturated; cholesterol <200–300 mg; fiber 20–30 g/day
- Regular physical activity
- Weight and glycemic control
- Medication if LDL ≥135 mg/dl; optional (fibric acid derivative or niacin) if HDL is <40 mg/dl and LDL is 100–129 mg/dl (unless known CAD)
- HMG-CoA reductase inhibitors (statins) preferred as first-line therapy; fibrate with statin if triglycerides elevated

Regular physical activity three to four times per week for 30 min (9,15)

- Routinely assess physical activity and exercise status
- Encourage increase in daily activities and moderate aerobic regimen such as brisk walking

- With multiple CAD risk factors, diabetes complications, or long duration of diabetes, consider screening for CAD
- Individualization of exercise prescription and caution with peripheral or cardiac autonomic neuropathy or proliferative retinopathy
- Patient education regarding symptoms of angina and MI

Maintain BMI 21–25 kg/m² and waist circumference <102 cm (40.2 in) in men and <88 cm (34.7 in) in women (15)

- Measured at each visit
- Weight control
- Regular physical activity

Complete smoking cessation (10,15)

- Assess smoking status
- Provide counseling, problem solving, or coping skills training and pharmacotherapy

Aspirin therapy (7,15)

- Consider enteric-coated aspirin, 75–162 mg/day, if age >30 years with one or more additional CAD risk factors
- Initiate in presence of CAD

A1C <7% (11)

- Tested two to three times annually if meeting goal; four times annually if above goal or therapy changed
- Medical nutrition therapy
- Weight control
- Regular physical activity
- Self-monitoring of blood glucose
- Education in self-management and problem solving

---

increase the intensity of exercise. All patients should be educated about the typical and atypical symptoms of myocardial ischemia and instructed to report these symptoms to their care provider if they occur. When patients want to engage in high-intensity exercise, those with a long duration of diabetes, multiple CAD risk factors, or known diabetes-related complications should undergo screening for underlying CAD (21). Exercise stress testing with myocardial perfusion imaging or echocardiography is recommended for risk stratification in the patient with cardiac symptoms or evidence of ischemia or MI on electrocardiogram. In the asymptomatic patient with diabetes, screening may be considered in patients with peripheral or carotid occlusive disease, cardiac autonomic neuropathy, or multiple (two or more, including microalbuminuria) cardiac risk factors in addition to diabetes.

Table 8.3 Lifestyle Modifications to Manage Hypertension

Modification	Recommendation	Approximate Systolic Blood Pressure Reduction
Weight reduction	Maintain normal body weight	5–20 mmHg/10 kg weight loss
Adopt DASH eating plan	Consume a diet rich in fruits and vegetables and low-fat dairy products with a reduced content of saturated and total fat	8–14 mmHg
Dietary sodium restriction	No more than 2,400 mg/day	2–8 mmHg
Physical activity	Regular aerobic activity such as brisk walking at least 30 min/day most days of the week	4–9 mmHg
Moderation of alcohol consumption	Limit to no more than two drinks per day for men, one for women	2–4 mmHg

From Hinnen et al. (19). DASH, National Heart, Lung, and Blood Institute's dietary approaches to stop hypertension.

Current recommendations for the use of aspirin call for initiation of low-dose therapy in the presence of known CVD, and aspirin therapy should be considered in individuals with diabetes who are at high risk (7). These individuals include people over the age of 30 years; current smokers; individuals with a family history of CVD; or those with hypertension, obesity, micro- or macroalbuminuria, or elevated lipid levels. Many individuals with diabetes continue to smoke, and complete smoking cessation should be the goal (10). Although glucose control is more strongly linked with microvascular complications of diabetes than with macrovascular disease, optimal glucose control is important to the control of lipid levels and hemostatic function and may have an impact on cardiac events. Recent studies have shown an improved outcome in both mortality and morbidity with optimal

Table 8.4 Approximate and Cumulative LDL Cholesterol Reduction Achievable by Dietary Modification

Dietary Component	Dietary Change	Approximate LDL Cholesterol Reduction
Major		
Saturated fat	<7% of calories	8–10%
Dietary cholesterol	<200 mg/day	3–5%
Weight reduction	Lose 10 lb	5–8%
Other LDL-lowering options		
Soluble fiber	5–10 g/day	3–5%
Plant sterol/stanol esters	2 g/day	6–15%
Cumulative estimate 20–30%		

From Kruger et al. (20).

glucose control during acute treatment of MI. As shown in the Diabetes Mellitus, Insulin Glucose Infusion in Acute Myocardial Infarction (DIGAMI) study, intensive insulin treatment produced improved survival at 1 year and at the follow-up at 3.4 years (22). The intensive treatment of diabetes with patient self-monitoring of blood glucose levels and target glycated hemoglobin A_{1c} (A1C) concentrations <7% is supported by both the ADA and the American Heart Association (15).

TREATMENT

Nonsurgical Intervention

Once the diagnosis of CAD is made, aggressive treatment of dyslipidemia and hypertension, prevention of thrombosis with aspirin, and medications to reduce the occurrence of myocardial ischemia become even more essential, following the same principles outlined above (Table 8.2). Specific medication therapies for CVD management in patients with diabetes, along with precautions to observe in this population, are outlined in Table 8.5.

The diagnosis of heart failure presents additional challenges. Treatment of heart failure in patients with diabetes should focus not only on the management of heart failure, but on coexistent hypertension, CAD, and renal disease, as well as management of glucose control. Guidelines for the overall management of heart failure, based on Class I evidence (evidence and/or general agreement that the procedure or treatment is useful and effective) and the four stages of heart failure, are shown in Table 8.6 (23). Stage A includes individuals at high risk of developing heart failure, stage B includes individuals with left ventricular dysfunction but without symptoms, and stage C includes individuals with left ventricular dysfunction with either current or prior symptoms. Refractory, end-stage heart failure is considered stage D.

Blood pressure should be lowered to <130/80 mmHg, and in most patients, even more aggressive lowering of blood pressure is indicated in an attempt to reduce afterload and reverse left ventricular hypertrophy when present (14). Treatment of heart failure in patients with diabetes with ACE inhibitors improves clinical outcome, with less frequent hospitalizations for heart failure and fewer deaths (24). ACE inhibitors have an additional benefit in diabetes because of their proven renal protective effect (25,26), even in high-risk patients without heart fail-

---

PRACTICAL POINTS

Aspirin should be considered in individuals with diabetes who are at high risk (7). These individuals include people aged >30 years; current smokers; individuals with a family history of CVD; or those with hypertension, obesity, micro- or macroalbuminuria, or abnormal lipid levels.

Smoking cessation assistance is available online at the American Cancer Society's web site at http://www.cancer.org/docroot/PED/PED_10_3x_Find_Support.asp (accessed 19 November 2004).

Table 8.5 Cardiac Medications in Patients with Diabetes

Angiotensin-Converting Enzyme (ACE) Inhibitors

- Contraindications: angioedema, severe cough, bilateral renal artery stenosis, anuric renal failure, significant hyperkalemia, hypotension, shock
- Monitor renal function and potassium levels

β-Blockers

- Caution: assess for worsening of glycemic and lipid control
- Contraindications: bradycardia, second- or third-degree arteriovenous block, hypotension, moderate or severe heart failure, active wheezing
- Assess risk of masking hypoglycemia in patients requiring insulin
- If used in the presence of bronchospastic disease, active heart failure, and conduction system disease, assess for deterioration
- Initiate slowly and avoid abrupt withdrawal

Calcium Channel Blockers

- Diltiazem and verapamil are contraindicated in patients who have heart failure with systolic dysfunction; amlodipine and felodipine may be used to treat angina in patients with heart failure
- Caution: heart failure, left ventricular dysfunction, arteriovenous block, sinus node dysfunction

Digoxin

- Contraindications: sinus node dysfunction or arteriovenous block
- Potential interactions with many medications
- Monitor renal function and electrolytes (hypokalemia and hypomagnesia)

Diuretics

- Aldosterone antagonist; spironolactone useful, particularly in patients with heart failure, but caution in patients with renal insufficiency because of possible hyperkalemia

Lipid-Lowering Agents

- HMG-CoA reductase inhibitors (statins) contraindicated with acute liver disease, heavy alcohol intake, or significant elevations in liver function tests (LFTs); monitor LFTs and closely monitor patients with hepatic dysfunction; assess for myalgias and potential myopathy with creatine phosphokinase (CPK) measurement, especially when used in combination with fibrates

Nitrates

- Use with caution in patients with autonomic neuropathy
- Avoid nitrate tolerance by dosing with 8- to 12-h nitrate-free period
- Caution in setting of acute MI with presence of hypotension or right ventricular infarction

Platelet Inhibitors and Anticoagulants

- Monitor for bleeding with anticoagulants
- Maintain partial thromboplastin time (aPTT) (heparin) and prothrombin time/International Normalized Ratio (PT/INR) (warfarin)
- Provide patient education regarding possible medication and dietary interactions with warfarin
- In patients allergic to or unable to take aspirin, use clopidrel

---

See also "Antihypertensive Medications" and "Lipid-Lowering Medications" in RESOURCES.

Table 8.6 Recommendations for Treating Heart Failure

■ Achieve adequate blood pressure and lipid control
■ Avoid smoking, alcohol, and illicit drugs
■ Use ACE inhibitors
  – Add β-blockers in stage B and prior MI and in all of stage C, once compensated, unless contraindicated
■ Control ventricular rate in atrial fibrillation
■ Treat thyroid disorders
■ Evaluation and treatment for signs and symptoms
  – Periodic if stage A and regularly if in other stages
  – In stage B and higher, consider valve replacement or repair for hemodynamically significant stenoses/regurgitation
  – In stage C and higher
    □ diuretics if evidence of fluid retention
    □ digitalis unless contraindicated
    □ withdrawal of drugs known to adversely affect clinical status
  – In stage D
    □ meticulous treatment of fluid retention
    □ referral for heart failure program and cardiac transplantation

---

ure or known low ejection fractions (27,28). Although there is often reluctance to treat diabetes patients with β-blockers, they clearly benefit from such treatment after MI (29,30). The β-blocker carvedilol has been shown to improve ventricular function and survival in patients with chronic heart failure and depressed left ventricular function (31). Diuretics also may have an important role in the treatment of advanced symptomatic heart failure (stage C) (32). Generally, calcium channel blockers should not be used in the treatment of heart failure in individuals with diabetes. Although metformin and thiazolidinediones (TZDs) are not recommended in patients with moderate to severe heart failure because of the risk of lactic acidosis (metformin) and worsening of heart failure (TZDs), these medications are still used in patients with diabetes and heart failure. Careful monitoring for the development of these complications is therefore necessary. In addition, with TZDs, careful assessment of valve status prior to initiation of therapy, lower doses in the presence of known heart disease, and slow increases in dosage are advocated (33).

Increasing evidence suggests that individuals with diabetes have an increased risk for cardiomyopathy that is independent of the atherosclerosis. In patients with diabetes who are unresponsive to medical therapy, consideration should be given to cardiac transplantation. Transplant rejection is a relatively rare occurrence in the current era of immunosuppressive therapy (34). However, patients requiring insulin are at higher risk for poor outcomes at transplantation. Higher doses of insulin and other adjuvant hypoglycemic agents are usually required during the early posttransplantation phase, when high doses of corticosteroids are used.

In the setting of acute coronary syndromes, which include unstable angina and acute MI, early and appropriate management is critical to limit myocardial damage and prevent complications. MI may occur without the warning of prior angina, and patients may have atypical symptoms that delay them in seeking medical attention and the benefits of timely reperfusion. Although early coronary reperfusion, aspirin, β-blockers, ACE inhibitors, lipid-lowering agents, and coronary revascularization have dramatically improved the survival of patients with diabetes and MI, those patients with known CVD and diabetes-related micro-vascular complications still have a higher risk of complications than nondiabetic patients, both during and after hospitalization (Table 8.7) (35–39).

Patients with diabetes presenting with ST-segment elevation, indicative of MI, who are within 12 h of the onset of symptoms, should be considered for primary angioplasty with stent placement, particularly when there is evidence of heart failure or hemodynamic stability, where the establishment of secure vessel patency may be critical. At times, however, surgical revascularization is necessary, particularly when significant residual CAD is present with recurrent angina or inducible ischemia (40). After thrombolytic therapy or percutaneous coronary intervention (PCI), hemostatic abnormalities in individuals with diabetes remain problematic. Therefore, subsequent antithrombotic treatment to prevent reocclusion is an important part of follow-up care. Placement of intracoronary stents with adjuvant antithrombotic treatment with glycoprotein IIb/IIIa inhibitors is a common approach to treating ST-segment elevation MI in patients with diabetes. In addition, during the acute MI period, aggressive control of blood glucose may improve both short- and long-term outcomes (41,42). After MI, aggressive management of cardiac risk factors is warranted (Table 8.2).

Unstable angina and non–ST-segment MI are also considered part of a spectrum of acute coronary syndromes that leaves the individual with diabetes at an increased risk for adverse outcomes (43), including death, progression to ST-segment elevation MI, and subsequent readmission for unstable angina (44). Patients with unstable angina and diabetes have more extensive CAD, involving a greater number and longer segments of vessels, often including the left main coronary artery. Some of these patients may have had prior coronary artery bypass graft (CABG), and patients presenting with imminent closure of a heavily diseased saphenous vein graft pose particular challenges. Symptoms often persist despite medical therapy, and revascularization strategies may be limited.

Cardiac autonomic neuropathy may further complicate management because of the associated increased heart rate and a decreased awareness of ischemic symptoms. The initial therapy of acute coronary syndromes includes the administration

---

Table 8.7 Complications to Assess and Prevent in Patients with Diabetes and CAD

After acute MI ■ Heart failure ■ Cardiogenic shock ■ Postinfarction angina ■ Heart block ■ Atrial arrhythmias ■ Renal insufficiency ■ Recurrent MI and heart failure after discharge **After percutaneous interventions** ■ MI ■ Renal failure ■ Stroke	■ Retroperitoneal bleeding, femoral hematoma, femoral or iliac artery dissection or occlusion, pseudoaneurysm formation ■ Restenosis, MI, and need for repeat revascularization **After coronary artery bypass surgery** ■ MI ■ Renal failure ■ Stroke ■ Sternal wound infection ■ Recurrent angina and heart failure

of β-blockers, aspirin, heparin, clopidrel or glycoprotein IIb/IIIa inhibitors, and nitrates. Those patients at significant risk for subsequent cardiac events, such as those with marked or widespread resting ST-segment depression, prior MI, decreased left ventricular function, or heart failure, may undergo early coronary angiography and revascularization. A noninvasive approach with further risk stratification based on stress echocardiography or myocardial perfusion imaging may be preferable in lower-risk patients and those with major comorbidity who are at high risk for the invasive approach.

Percutaneous or Surgical Revascularization

The decision to use PCI or surgical revascularization depends on a number of factors, including the suitability of the target vessels as well as overall risk status of the patient. PCI is usually reserved for single-vessel disease, and the use of drug-eluting intracoronary stents has improved PCI outcomes. Multivessel disease, frequently seen in patients with diabetes, often requires CABG. Although many patients with diabetes safely undergo CABG, older age and the presence of other diabetes-related complications (particularly nephropathy), place the individual at higher risk of poorer operative outcomes. Complications associated with both procedures, which should be assessed, are outlined in Table 8.7.

A major concern about the use of multivessel percutaneous transluminal coronary angioplasty (PTCA) in patients with diabetes was raised by the Bypass Angioplasty Revascularization (BARI) trial, which randomized patients to either PTCA or CABG in the late 1980s (45). The findings led to an alert, cautioning against the use of multivessel angioplasty in patients with diabetes (46) and to the suggestion that multivessel PTCA be abandoned in these patients (47). Although CABG is currently the preferred means of revascularization for multivessel disease in patients with diabetes, revascularization with PCI may be warranted in the future, along with the use of drug-eluting coronary stents, more effective platelet inhibitors, and careful observation after the initial procedure. Strategies for optimizing risk factor control after either PCI or surgical revascularization should be intensified in the population with type 2 diabetes. As with primary prevention in individuals free of CVD and secondary prevention in those with established CVD, there is a critical need for ongoing, intensive, multifactorial risk factor management after PCI or surgical revascularization (Table 8.2).

SUMMARY

Nurses need an understanding of the pathophysiology of CVD in individuals with diabetes, along with the clinical presentation of the various manifestations of CVD. Nurses should take an active role in coaching those with diabetes regarding the prevention and treatment of CVD. Nurses need to provide education regarding the goals of treatment.

REFERENCES

1. Kannel WB, McGee DL: Diabetes and cardiovascular risk factors: The Framingham Study. *Circulation* 59:8–13, 1979
2. Wackers FJT, Young LH, Inzucchi SE, Chyun DA, Davey JA, Barrett EJ, Taillefer R, Wittlin SD Heller GV, Filipchuk N, Engel S, Ratner RE, Iskandrian AE, DIAD Study Investigators: Detection of silent myocardial ischemia

in asymptomatic diabetic subjects: the DIAD study. *Diabetes Care* 27:1954–1961, 2004

3. Vinik AI, Mitchell BD, Maser RE, Freeman R: Diabetic autonomic neuropathy. *Diabetes Care* 26:1553–1579, 2003

4. Maser RE, Vinik AI, Mitchell BD, Freeman R: The association between cardiovascular autonomic neuropathy and mortality in individuals with diabetes. *Diabetes Care* 26:1895–1901, 2003

5. American Diabetes Association: Nutrition principles and recommendations in diabetes (Position Statement). *Diabetes Care* 27 (Suppl. 1):S36–S46, 2004

6. American Diabetes Association: Dyslipidemia management in adults with diabetes (Position Statement). *Diabetes Care* 27 (Suppl. 1):S68–S71, 2004

7. American Diabetes Association: Aspirin therapy in diabetes (Position Statement). *Diabetes Care* 27 (Suppl. 1):S72–S73, 2004

8. American Diabetes Association: Hypertension management in adults with diabetes (Position Statement). *Diabetes Care* 27 (Suppl. 1):S65–S67, 2004

9. American Diabetes Association: Physical activity/exercise and diabetes (Position Statement). *Diabetes Care* 27 (Suppl. 1):S58–S62, 2004

10. American Diabetes Association: Smoking and diabetes (Position Statement). *Diabetes Care* 27 (Suppl. 1):S74–S75, 2004

11. American Diabetes Association: Standards of medical care in diabetes (Position Statement). *Diabetes Care* 28 (Suppl. 1):S4–S36, 2005

12. National Cholesterol Education Program (NCEP): *Third Report of the NCEP Expert Panel on Detection, Evaluation and Treatment of High Blood Cholesterol in Adults (Adult Treatment Panel III)*. Bethesda, MD, National Heart, Lung, and Blood Institute, National Institutes of Health, 2001, p. 1–28

13. Chobanian AV, Bakris GL, Black HR, Cushman WC, Green LA, Izzo JL Jr, Jones DW, Materson BJ, Oparil S, Wright JT Jr, Roccella EJ: The seventh report of the Joint National Committee on Prevention, Detection, Evaluation and Treatment of High Blood Pressure. *JAMA* 289:1560–1572, 2003

14. UK Prospective Diabetes Study Group: Tight blood pressure control and risk of macrovascular and microvascular complications in type 2 diabetes: UKPDS 38. *Br Med J* 317:703–713, 1998

15. Grundy SM, Benjamin IJ, Burke GL, Chait A, Eckel RH, Howard BV, Mitch W, Smith SC Jr, Sowers JR: Diabetes and cardiovascular disease: a statement for healthcare professionals from the American Heart Association. *Circulation* 100:1134–1146, 1999

16. Stern MP, Haffner SM: Dyslipidemia in type 2 diabetes. *Diabetes Care* 14:1144–1159, 1991

17. Reaven GM, Chen YD, Jeppesen J, Maheux P, Krauss RM: Insulin resistance and hyperinsulinemia in individuals with small, dense low density lipoprotein particles. *J Clin Invest* 92:141–146, 1993

18. American Diabetes Association: Consensus development conference on the diagnosis of coronary heart disease in people with diabetes. *Diabetes Care* 21:1551–1559, 1998

19. Hinnen D, Childs BP, Maryniuk M, Vu J: Pharmaceutical treatment of hypertension and dyslipidemia in people with diabetes: an educator's perspective. Part 1: Hypertension. *Diabetes Spectrum* 17:60–64, 2004

20. Kruger DF, Cypress M, Maryniuk, Childs BP, Tieking J: Pharmaceutical treatment of hyperglycemia and dyslipidemia in people with diabetes: an educator's perspective. Part 2: dyslipidemia. *Diabetes Spectrum* 17:73–77, 2004

21. Malmberg K: Prospective randomised study on intensive insulin treatment on long term survival after acute myocardial infarction in patients with diabetes

mellitus. DIGAMI (Diabetes Mellitus, Insulin Glucose Infusion in Acute Myocardial Infarction) Study Group. *Br Med J* 314:1512–1515, 1997

22. American College of Cardiology/American Heart Association Task Force on Practice Guidelines: ACC/AHA guidelines for the evaluation and management of chronic heart failure in the adult: executive summary. *Circulation* 104: 2996–3007, 2001

23. Shekelle PG, Rich MW, Morton SC, Atkinson CS, Tu W, Maglione M, Rhodes S, Barrett M, Fonarow GC, Greenberg B, Heidenreich PA, Knabel T, Konstam MA, Steimle A, Warner Stevenson L: Efficacy of angiotensin-converting enzyme inhibitors and beta-blockers in the management of left ventricular systolic dysfunction according to race, gender, and diabetic status: a meta-analysis of major clinical trials. *J Am Coll Cardiol* 41:1529–1538, 2003

24. Lewis EJ, Hunsicker LG, Bain RP, Rohde RD: The effect of angiotensin-converting-enzyme inhibition on diabetic nephropathy: the Collaborative Study Group. *N Engl J Med* 329:1456–1462, 1993

25. Maschio G, Alberti D, Janin G, Locatelli F, Mann JF, Motolese M, Ponticelli C, Ritz E, Zucchelli P: Effect of the angiotensin-converting-enzyme inhibitor benazepril on the progression of chronic renal insufficiency: the Angiotensin-Converting-Enzyme Inhibition in Progressive Renal Insufficiency Study Group. *N Engl J Med* 334:939–945, 1996

26. Heart Outcomes Prevention Evaluation Study Investigators: Effects of an angiotensin-converting enzyme inhibitor, ramipril, on cardiovascular events in high-risk patients. *N Engl J Med* 342:145–153, 2000

27. Heart Outcomes Prevention Evaluation (HOPE) Study Investigators: Effects of ramipril on cardiovascular and microvascular outcomes in people with diabetes mellitus: results of the HOPE study and MICRO-HOPE substudy. *Lancet* 355:253–259, 2000

28. Kjekshus J, Gilpin E, Blackey A, Henning H, Ross J Jr: Diabetic patients and beta-blockers after acute myocardial infarction. *Eur Heart J* 11:43–50, 1990

29. Viscoli CM, Horwitz RI, Singer BH: Beta-blockers after myocardial infarction: influence of first-year clinical course on long-term effectiveness. *Ann Intern Med* 118:99–105, 1993

30. Bristow MR, Gilbert EM, Abraham WT, Adams KF, Fowler MB, Hershberger RE, Kubo SH, Narahara KA, Ingersoll H, Krueger S, Young S, Shusterman N: Carvedilol produces dose-related improvements in left ventricular function and survival in subjects with chronic heart failure: MOCHA Investigators. *Circulation* 94:2807–2816, 1996

31. Pitt B, Perez A: Spironolactone in patients with heart failure. *N Engl J Med* 342:132–136, 2000

32. Masoudi FA, Wang Y, Inzucchi SE, Setaro JF, Havranek EP, Foody JM, Krumholz HM: Metformin and thiazolidinedione use in Medicare patients with heart failure. *JAMA* 290:81–85, 2003

33. Grundy SM, Cleeman JI, Merz CN, Brewer HB Jr, Clark LT, Hunninghake DB, Pasternak RC, Smith SC Jr, Stone NJ, National Heart, Lung, and Blood Institute, American College of Cardiology Foundation, American Heart Association: Implications of recent clinical trials for the National Cholesterol Education Program Adult Treatment Panel III guidelines. *Circulation* 110:227–239, 2004

34. Nesto RW, LeWinter M, Bell D, Bonow RO, Semenkovich CF, Fonseca V, Smith SJ, Grundy SM, Young LH, Horton ES Kahn R: Thiazolidinedione

use, fluid retention, and congestive heart failure. *Diabetes Care* 27:256–623, 2004
35. Behar S, Boyko V, Reicher-Reiss H, Goldbourt U: Ten-year survival after acute myocardial infarction: comparison of patients with and without diabetes. *Am Heart J* 133:290–296, 1997
36. Granger CB, Califf RM, Young S, Candela R, Samaha J, Worley S, Kereiakes DJ, Topol EJ: Outcome of patients with diabetes mellitus and acute myocardial infarction treated with thrombolytic agents. *J Am Coll Cardiol* 21:920–925, 1993
37. Barbash GI, White HD, Modan M, Van de Werf F: Significance of diabetes mellitus in patients with acute myocardial infarction receiving thrombolytic therapy. *J Am Coll Cardiol* 22:707–713, 1993
38. Chyun DA, Vaccarino V, Murillo J, Young LH, Krumholz HM: Acute myocardial infarction mortality in the elderly with diabetes. *Heart Lung* 31:327–339, 2002
39. Chyun D, Vaccarino V, Murillo J, Young L, Krumholz H: Mortality, heart failure and recurrent myocardial infarction in the elderly with diabetes. *Am J Crit Care* 11:504–519, 2002
40. Hasdai D, Granger CB, Srivatsa SS, Criger DA, Ellis SG, Califf RM, Topol EJ, Holmes DR Jr: Diabetes mellitus and outcome after primary coronary angioplasty for acute myocardial infarction: lessons from the GUSTO-IIb Angioplasty Substudy: Global Use of Strategies to Open Occluded Arteries in Acute Coronary Syndromes. *J Am Coll Cardiol* 1502–1512, 2000
41. Malmberg K, Ryden L, Efendic S, Herlitz J, Nicol P, Waldenstrom A, Wedel H, Welin L: Randomized trial of insulin-glucose infusion followed by subcutaneous insulin treatment in diabetic patients with acute myocardial infarction (DIGAMI Study): effects on mortality at 1 year. *J Am Coll Cardiol* 26:57–65, 1995
42. Malmberg K, Norhammar A, Wedel H, Ryden L: Glycometabolic state at admission: important risk marker of mortality in conventionally treated patients with diabetes mellitus and acute myocardial infarction. *Circulation* 138:2626–2632, 1999
43. Braunwald E, Antman EM, Beasley JW, Califf RM, Cheitlin MD, Hochman JS, Jones RH, Kereiakes D, Kupersmith J, Levin TN, Pepine CJ, Schaeffer JW, Smith EE 3rd, Steward DE, Theroux P, Gibbons RJ, Alpert JS, Eagle KA, Faxon DP, Fuster V, Gardner TJ, Gregoratos G, Russell RO, Smith SC Jr: ACC/AHA guidelines for the management of patients with unstable angina and non-ST-segment elevation myocardial infarction: executive summary and recommendations: a report of the American College of Cardiology/American Heart Association Task Force on Practice Guidelines (committee on the management of patients with unstable angina). *Circulation* 102:1193–1209, 2000
44. Malmberg K, Yusuf S, Gerstein HC, Brown J, Zhao F, Hunt D, Piegas L, Calvin J, Keltai M, Budaj A: Impact of diabetes on long-term prognosis in patients with unstable angina and non-Q-wave myocardial infarction: results of the OASIS (Organization to Assess Strategies for Ischemic Syndromes) Registry. *Circulation* 102:1014–1019, 2000
45. BARI Investigators: Influence of diabetes on 5-year mortality and morbidity in a randomized trial comparing CABG and PTCA in patients with multivessel disease: the Bypass Angioplasty Revascularization Investigation (BARI). *Circulation* 96:1761–1769, 1997

46. Ferguson JJ: NHLBI BARI clinical alert on diabetics treated with angioplasty. *Circulation* 92:3371, 1995
47. O'Neill WW: Multivessel balloon angioplasty should be abandoned in diabetic patients. *J Am Coll Cardiol* 31:20–22, 1998

Dr. Chyun is an Associate Professor and Director of the Adult Advanced Practice Nursing Specialty Program at Yale University School of Nursing, New Haven, CT. Dr. Young is a Professor of Medicine, Section of Cardiovascular Medicine, at Yale University School of Medicine, New Haven, CT.

9. Peripheral Vascular Disease

LINDA HAAS, PHC, RN, CDE

Peripheral vascular disease is an inclusive term referring to peripheral arterial disease (PAD), vasculitis, venous thrombosis, venous insufficiency, and disorders of the lymphatic system (1). However, because PAD is more common in individuals wih diabetes (2), this disorder is the focus of this chapter, with some reference to venous disease. The critical importance of PAD in diabetes is evidenced by this disorder being a marker for atherosclerotic disease of other blood vessels, including the coronary arteries (2), and a major risk factor for lower-extremity amputation (3).

EPIDEMIOLOGY

PAD affects ~12 million people in the U.S. (2). Although there are no hard data on the incidence and prevalence of PAD in diabetes, the Framingham Heart Study showed that 20% of people with symptomatic PAD had diabetes (4). Thus, there may be ~2.5 million people with diabetes and PAD in the U.S. This figure may underestimate the prevalence of PAD in people with diabetes because these individuals may have asymptomatic PAD due to sensory peripheral neuropathy.

Risk factors for PAD are cigarette smoking, diabetes, older age, hypertension, and dyslipidemia (5). In addition to these general PAD risk factors, risk factors in diabetes patients are diabetes duration, African-American or Hispanic ethnicity, and peripheral neuropathy (2). Risk factors for venous disease are age, immobility, recent surgery, living in a residential care facility, previous hospitalization for deep or superficial vein thrombosis, obesity, and trauma (6).

PATHOPHYSIOLOGY

PAD is an atherosclerotic disease of the lower extremities, with vascular inflammation, altered cellular contents of the vasculature and blood cells, and abnormal hemostatic factors. There are abnormalities of endothelial function and regulation of the vasculature, including loss of normal nitrous oxide function, increased atherosclerotic activity in the smooth muscle cells lining blood vessel walls (7), increased oxidative stress, platelet aggregation, and hypercoagulation (8).

PAD in individuals with diabetes is increased because of vascular inflammation and derangement in cellular components. Elevated levels of C-reactive protein (CRP) are strongly associated with the development of PAD (9). In diabetes and impaired glucose tolerance, CRP levels are abnormally elevated. Not only is CRP a marker for the disease process, it may also play a causative role in the impairment of fibrinolysis and the regulation of vascular tone (2). Vascular abnormalities may present before diagnosis of diabetes and increase with duration of disease and worsening of glucose control.

Venous disease includes varicose veins, caused by incompetency of venous valves, superficial or deep vein thrombosis, or chronic venous insufficiency. The latter is caused by chronic incompetence of the deep veins (6).

ASSESSMENT AND CLINICAL PRESENTATION

Intermittent claudication is the most common manifestation of PAD. Patients should be asked about cramping pain in their calves, thighs, or buttocks that occurs with activity and is relieved by rest. If venous disease is suspected, patients should be asked about feelings of fullness in their legs, a "bursting" sensation, dull aching, and pruritus. These symptoms are usually worse at the end of the day. Table 9.1 provides guidance for forming assessment questions for peripheral vascular disease.

The feet and lower legs should be examined. The lower extremities in PAD can demonstrate dependent rubor, with pallor on elevation. Presence or absence of hair should be assessed, as well as the condition of the nails, which may be dystrophic in PAD. The area between the toes (interdigital spaces) should be carefully inspected for cracks, fissures, and infection. Debris between the toes may indicate that patients cannot reach their feet to clean between their toes or are not aware of the importance of this hygienic measure. Table 9.1 delineates assessment and intervention strategies for patients with PAD or venous disease.

TESTS AND VALUES

Pedal pulses may be difficult to feel in many patients, particularly for an inexperienced examiner. In addition, the process of locating them can have many false-positive and false-negative results. Thus, the ankle-brachial index (ABI) is a preferred measure for screening for PAD in the legs and should be measured for all patients with diabetes over age 50 years who have other risk factors for PAD (2). This test involves measuring the systolic blood pressure just above the ankle and over the brachial artery in the arm with a handheld Doppler device. A ratio is calculated from these measures, with the radial blood pressure as the denominator and the ankle value as the numerator. See Table 9.2 for interpretation of the ABI.

If PAD is diagnosed, or strongly suspected, patients should have segmental pressures and pulse volume recordings in a vascular laboratory. Some patients may require treadmill testing, for which a >20-mmHg decrease in ankle pressure usually indicates PAD (2). To confirm the diagnosis of venous disease, continuous-wave Doppler, plethysmography, bidirectional ultrasound, duplex ultrasound, or venography are used in the vascular laboratory (6).

TREATMENTS AND INTERVENTIONS

Treatment of PAD has several aspects. All the conventional risk factors for cardiovascular disease should be addressed, including cigarette smoking cessa-

Table 9.1 Nursing Assessment and Interventions and Patient Self-Management Education for Diabetes Patients with Peripheral Arterial and Venous Disease

PAD	Venous Disease
Ask patient about:	**Ask patient about:**
■ Intermittent claudication (pain in calves when walking, especially uphill, relieved by rest) ■ Pain at rest *Gradual onset,* narrowing of vessels *Sudden onset,* complete occlusion ■ May complain of feet feeling cold	■ May have no symptoms ■ Aching discomfort ■ "Bursting" feeling ■ Tenderness ■ Pruritus ■ Footwear too small ■ Feet too swollen for usual shoes
Examination	**Examination**
Color	**Color**
■ Pale or blue, purple ■ Dependent rubor (redness) ■ Blanching when elevated to 45°	■ Brownish, reddish ■ Mottled
Skin	**Skin**
■ Cool to touch ■ Shiny, thin ■ Loss of hair on toes, lower legs ■ Thickened ridged toenails ■ Nonhealing, distal wounds or ulcers ■ Gangrenous	■ Warm to touch ■ Dry and scaly ■ Edematous (except for toes) ■ Stasis ulcers on malleolus, lower leg
Pulses	**Pulses**
■ Diminished or absent dorsalis and posterior tibialis	■ Peripheral pulses may be difficult to locate related to edema
Interventions	**Interventions**
■ Encourage and support efforts at smoking cessation ■ Encourage and support efforts toward increasing walking	■ Encourage and support efforts at smoking cessation
Instruct patients to:	**Instruct patients to:**
■ Inspect daily for cracks and sores ■ Prevent/protect from trauma ■ If interdigital spaces macerated, wind lamb's wool loosely between toes ■ Sit with feet supported below heart to reduce pain ■ Do not use circular bandages or ace wraps on legs ■ Avoid constriction (tight sock band, garters, rubber bands/garters to hold up socks)	■ Inspect daily for cracks and sores ■ Prevent/protect from trauma ■ Use support hose ■ Elevate feet above heart for 20 min three times a day ■ Avoid constriction (tight sock band, garters, rubber bands/garters to hold up socks) ■ Elevate feet when sitting. Use recliners, foot stools, boxes ■ Tie shoes loosely or wear shoes with an adjustable toebox, e.g., post-op shoes with Velcro closures

Table 9.2 Interpretation of ABI

Ratio	Interpretation
0.91–1.3	Normal
0.7–0.9	Mild obstruction
0.4–0.69	Moderate obstruction
<0.4	Severe obstruction
>1.3	Poorly compressible*

*May indicate medial arterial calcification; ABI is less reliable in this situation.

tion (10,11) and hypertension and dyslipidemia treatment (2). Antiplatelet therapy is indicated, and clopidogrel may be beneficial in patients with diabetes and PAD (12).

Cigarette smoking is the single most important modifiable risk factor for the development and exacerbation of PAD (2). Tobacco use is associated with increased risk of amputation.

Hypertension is associated with a two- to threefold increase in claudication and contributes to the development of atherosclerosis. Aggressive blood pressure control, achieving a level of <130/80 mmHg in patients with PAD and diabetes, will help reduce cardiovascular risk.

Although no studies have directly examined the effects of lipid lowering in individuals with diabetes and PAD, there is evidence that lipid-lowering therapies decrease the severity of claudication. In the Scandinavian Simvastatin Survival Study (4S), the reduction of cholesterol level by simvastatin reduced the risk of new or worsening symptoms of intermittent claudication by 38% (13).

A very important PAD treatment modality is a walking program, which has been shown to increase blood flow, improve collateral circulation, lengthen walking distance capability, decrease the oxygen cost of exercise and the heart rate, and improve functional well-being (14,15). Walking programs are usually carried out in the home setting but may be part of a structured program conducted through a cardiac rehabilitation or physical therapy department. Before starting a walking program, the health care provider or cardiac rehabilitation or physical therapy department should determine if such a program will be safe for the patient.

Walking programs must be maintained to be effective, and dropout rates are high. Strategies to assist patients in maintaining a walking regimen include doing some of the cardiac rehab program at home (16), semi-weekly phone calls from health care providers, and daily self-monitoring of progress (17). In addition, a computerized feedback system, which tracked progress and set goals, decreased and delayed dropout rates in a walking program (17).

A major intervention for venous disorders is use of compression stockings, which should have at least 30–40 mmHg of compression and extend to the knee, or higher if feasible (6). Patients should avoid long periods where their legs are dependent, prolonged travel without getting up and walking, and hot weather as much as is feasible. In addition, patients should follow a low-sodium diet to decrease fluid retention. Anticoagulation is usually implemented for superficial or deep vein thrombosis.

> ### PRACTICAL POINT
>
> The use of compression stockings can be difficult for patients who live alone and cannot put on the stockings without help. Silk inner toe liners, stockings with zippered sides, and other devices to help put on the elastic stockings are especially helpful for these patients.

INFECTIONS

Patients with diabetes and PAD are more likely to develop severe foot infections. When both neuropathy and PAD are present, the foot is at much greater risk for traumatic ulceration, infection, and gangrene. Patient education in preventive foot

Education/Behavioral Considerations for Peripheral Vascular Disease

Problem	Considerations
Patients with PAD have pain associated with walking	■ Encourage and assist to implement a walking program ■ Identify barriers to program (external barriers are more easily overcome than internal) ■ Problem solve ways to overcome these barriers ■ Identify or assist patients to identify community resources, such as cardiac rehabilitation, YMCA, senior centers, and shopping mall walking programs, because people are more apt to stay with exercise programs if they have social support
Many people cannot adequately examine their feet because of obesity, decreased vision, and/or decreased flexibility	■ Mirrors on handles may facilitate visual inspection of the plantar surfaces of their feet ■ Problem solve methods to raise the feet so patients can reach their feet to wash and dry them appropriately ■ Long-handled sponges can enable people to clean their feet and long-handled pointed sponges enable cleaning of the interdigital spaces

care measures becomes critically important in reducing amputation risk. Ischemic ulcers typically form at the edges of the foot, including the tips of the toes and the back of the heels. Footwear for the neuroischemic foot must fit well to avoid the creation of pressure points or shearing force.

In individuals with diabetes and foot infection, the presenting signs and symptoms are often diminished. An impairment of the neuroinflammatory response reduces the early warning signs of infection. Differentiating between the erythema of cellulitis and the rubor of ischemia may be difficult. The redness of ischemia will disappear on elevation, but in cellulitis, the redness remains, irrespective of positioning.

In cases of severe infection, broad-spectrum intravenous antibiotics will be necessary because the infections are frequently polymicrobial. However, antibiotic treatment alone is not enough to treat most infections. Surgical assessment for debridement and drainage, offloading the ulcer, and appropriate dressings plays a vital role in the treatment process.

FUTURE NURSING RESEARCH

What strategies will facilitate continuance of walking programs and in which populations? What strategies assist patients to wear appropriate footwear?

SUMMARY

PAD is significantly underdiagnosed and undertreated (18,19). A careful nursing assessment, particularly about exercise patterns and barriers, may identify clues, such as leg pain, that indicate PAD. In addition, careful examination of the lower extremities can also suggest PAD. The nursing assessment can also generate ideas for strategies to assist patients to implement and maintain an exercise program. These clues include, but are not limited to, previous activity/exercise patterns, occasions when walking was pleasurable, and support systems such as family, friends, pets, a senior group, and interest in walking groups that might give support for initiation and maintenance of a walking program. Because use of support hose is critical in the treatment of venous insufficiency, the patients' ability to put these on should be assessed. If patients have difficulty putting compression stockings on, a family member can help; if that is not feasible, a sock assister is very helpful.

PAD is a serious complication associated with diabetes and is often asymptomatic. The clinical presentation varies greatly. Some patients will maintain activity while others will have difficulty performing daily activities. Since patients with diabetes can present with symptoms that can be confused with neuropathy, PAD can be missed. Clinical evaluation that includes diagnostic vascular testing is important to establish the diagnosis. Vascular consultation followed by appropriate treatment is necessary to preserve and protect the affected limb. Foot care education is a main component in the prevention of foot ulcers and infections. Surgery to restore circulation may be necessary to avoid loss of the limb.

REFERENCES

1. Creager MA, Libby P: Peripheral arterial diseases. In *Heart Disease: A Textbook of Cardiovascular Medicine*. Braunwald E, Zipes DP, Libby P, Eds. Philadelphia, W. B. Saunders, 2001, p. 1457–1484
2. American Diabetes Association: Peripheral arterial disease in people with diabetes (Consensus Statement). *Diabetes Care* 26:3333–3341, 2003
3. Pecoraro RE, Reiber GE, Burgess EM: Pathways to diabetic limb amputation: basis for prevention. *Diabetes Care* 13:513–521, 1990
4. Murabito JM, D'Agostino RB, Silbershatz H, Wilson WF: Intermittent claudication: a risk profile from the Framingham Heart Study. *Circulation* 96:44–49, 1997
5. Criqui MH: Peripheral arterial disease: epidemiological aspects. *Vasc Med* 6 (Suppl. 1):3–7, 2001
6. Wennberg PW, Rooke TW: Diagnosis and management of diseases of the peripheral arteries and veins. In *Hurst's The Heart*. Fuster V, Alexander RW, O'Rourke RA, Eds. New York, McGraw-Hill, 2001, p. 2427–2440
7. Veves A, Akbari CM, Primavera J, Donaghue VM, Zacharoulis D, Chrzan JS, DeGirolami U, LoGerfo FW, Freeman R: Endothelial dysfunction and the expression of endothelial nitric oxide synthetase in diabetic neuropathy, vascular disease, and foot ulceration. *Diabetes* 47:457–463, 1998
8. Schneider D, Sobel B: Diabetes and thrombosis. In *Diabetes in Cardiovascular Disease*. Johnstone M, Veves A, Eds. Totawa, NJ, Humana Press, 2001
9. Ridker PM, Cushman M, Stampfer MJ, Tracy RP, Hennekens CH: Plasma concentration of C-reactive protein and risk development of peripheral vascular disease. *Circulation* 97:425–428, 1998
10. Haire-Joshu D, Glasgow R: Smoking and diabetes (Technical Review). *Diabetes Care* 22:1887–1898, 1999
11. Lassila R, Lepantalo M: Cigarette smoking and the outcome after lower limb surgery. *Acta Chir Scand* 154:635–640, 1988
12. Mehler PS, Coll JR, Estacio R, Esler A, Schrier RW, Hiatt WR: Intensive blood pressure control reduces the risk of cardiovascular events in patients with peripheral arterial disease and type 2 diabetes. *Circulation* 107:753–756, 2003
13. Scandinavian Simvastatin Survival Study Group: Randomised trial of cholesterol lowering in 4444 patients with coronary artery disease: the Scandinavian Simvastatin Survival Study (4S). *Lancet* 444:1383–1389, 1994
14. Hiatt WR: Medical treatment of peripheral arterial disease and claudication. *N Engl J Med* 344:1608–1621, 2001
15. Tan KH, De Cossart L, Edwards P: Exercise training and peripheral vascular disease. *Br J Surg* 87:553–562, 2000
16. Carlson JJ, Johnson JA, Franklin BA, VanderLaan RL: Program participation, exercise adherence, cardiovascular outcomes, and program cost of traditional versus modified cardiac rehabilitation. *Am J Cardiol* 86:17–23, 2000
17. King A, Taylor C: Strategies for increasing early adherence to and long-term maintenance of home-based exercise training in healthy middle-aged men and women. *Am J Cardiol* 61:628–632, 1988
18. McDermott MM, Mehta S, Ahn H, Greenland P: Atherosclerotic risk factors are less intensively treated in patients with peripheral arterial disease than in patients with coronary artery disease. *J Gen Intern Med* 12:209–215, 1997

19. Mukherjee D, Lingam P, Chetcuti S, Grossman PM, Moscucci M, Luciano AE, Eagle KA: Missed opportunities to treat atherosclerosis in patients undergoing peripheral vascular interventions: insights from the University of Michigan Peripheral Vascular Disease Quality Improvement Initiative (PVD-Q12). *Circulation* 106:1909–1912, 2002

Ms. Haas is the Endocrinology Clinical Nurse Specialist at the VA Puget Sound Health Care System, Seattle, WA.

10. Ocular Changes with Diabetes

ROGER H. PHELPS, OD, FAAO, CDE

D iabetic retinopathy is the leading cause of new blindness in Americans aged 20–74 years, and up to 90% of diabetes-related blindness is preventable (1–3). Nurses can participate in this prevention by

- knowing the range of effects that diabetes has on the eyes
- assessing the patient's glycated hemoglobin A_{1c} (A1C) history and level of retinopathy (if any) and when the last dilated eye examination was done
- encouraging diabetes self-management knowledge and skills to promote glycemic and blood pressure control

For every 1% lowering of A1C, there is an ~35% risk reduction in the development or progression of retinopathy. Timely detection and treatment of proliferative diabetic retinopathy can reduce the risk of severe visual loss by 50% (4,5).

The American Diabetes Association (1) recommendations on diabetic retinopathy state that

- an ophthalmologist or optometrist who is knowledgeable and experienced in diagnosing the presence of diabetic retinopathy and is aware of its management perform annual dilated eye examinations of patients with diabetes
- patients who have been identified with a specific risk of visual loss be promptly referred to an ophthalmologist who is knowledgeable and experienced in the management and treatment of diabetic retinopathy, i.e., an ophthalmologist who is experienced in fluorescein angiography and panretinal photocoagulation

Herein, the term *retinal specialists* will refer to ophthalmologists who have had specific retinal fellowship training beyond their general ophthalmological training. All eye doctors are licensed to do comprehensive dilated eye examinations and are responsible for detecting diabetic retinopathy (6). Nurses working with diabetes patients should know which practitioners on referral lists have specific experience with diabetic eye diseases.

Ophthalmologic Examination Schedule

Patient group	Recommendation for exam	Minimum routine follow-up
Type 1 diabetes	Within 3–5 years after diagnosis of diabetes once the patient is aged ≥10 years	Yearly
Type 2 diabetes	At time of diagnosis of diabetes	Yearly
Pregnancy with preexisting diabetes	Prior to conception and during first trimester	Physician discretion, pending results of first trimester exam

From ADA (1).

TEMPORARY REFRACTIVE CHANGES

Temporary blurry vision can occur any time individuals with diabetes have a major change in their average glycemic control. Either a major increase or decrease in A1C can change the osmotic balance between the aqueous and the crystalline lens in the eye. This is usually a temporary change that is reversible with glycemic stabilization. However, it remains important that the patient have a dilated eye examination any time there is a complaint of blurry vision to rule out any serious cause for blurry vision. Most eye doctors will discuss the costs versus benefits of purchasing a pair of glasses for temporary use while driving or reading before the refractive error stabilizes.

LEVELS OF DIABETIC RETINOPATHY

Microvascular disease of the retina is best predicted by the A1C history and duration of diabetes in a patient (5). The continued hyperglycemia of inadequately controlled diabetes can lead to blindness by the following process. First, high glucose levels damage the capillary walls of the retina, leading to leakage and small blot hemorrhages and microaneurysms. Continued glycemic insult leads to more capillary non-

---

PRACTICAL POINT

The nurse should encourage all patients with diabetes to learn how to establish and maintain glycemic control. When working with individuals who are experiencing significant changes in glycemic control, inform the eye doctor of these changes and send a copy of the most recent A1C value. There appears to be no long-term effect of this temporary refractive change.

Eye Anatomical Terms (see Fig. 10.1)

- **Aqueous:** The clear fluid that is constantly produced by the eye. It drains out of the eye in a circular canal near the iris root.
- **Iris:** The diaphragm that forms the pupil, located in the front portion of the eye. The color of the iris is considered the "eye color."
- **Lens:** The crystalline lens is just behind the iris and is responsible for about one-third of the optical power of the eye. It can change focus until about the age of 40 years.
- **Vitreous:** The vitreous body is the clear gel-like body that fills the large posterior portion of the eye. It is bathed in aqueous fluid, as is the entire inside of the eye, and tends to liquefy with increasing age.
- **Retina:** The photosensitive membrane that lines the inside back of the eye and acts like the film in a camera. It is connected to the brain's seeing mechanism through the optic nerve. It is nourished by its own capillary bed as well as from vessels that underlie it.
- **Optic disk:** The opening in the retina where the optic nerves and major retinal vessels enter and exit the back of the eye.
- **Macula:** This small area of the retina is the most sensitive and central part of our vision.

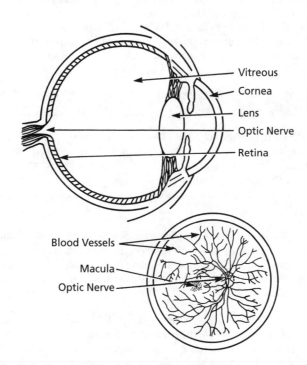

Figure 10.1 Illustration of a normal eye. *From* American Diabetes Association: *Type 2 Diabetes: A Curriculum for Patients and Health Professionals.* Funnell MM, Arnold MS, Lasichack AJ, Barr PA, Eds. Alexandria, VA, American Diabetes Association, 2002, p. 347

perfusion and the development of intraretinal microvascular abnormalities, venous beading, and the stimulation of chemical factors such as vascular endothelial growth factor. New fragile vessels then grow out from the retina into the vitreous. These leak and bleed easily, forming adhesions between the retina and vitreous, which then lead to traction retinal detachment, vitreous bleeding, and blindness (7).

There are surgical interventions available to stop or slow this process (4), but the best intervention is to optimize glycemic control to keep the retinal capillaries healthy. Often, if the retinopathy is severe, improving glycemic control too quickly can lead to increased retinopathy at first, but after 2–3 years, the benefit of the maintained glycemic control will be realized.

No Diabetic Retinopathy

This level indicates that no disease is visible on the retina. Although this has been historically uncommon after a long duration of diabetes, it is now becoming more probable with ongoing, consistent glycemic control combined with a timely diagnosis of diabetes.

Nonproliferative Diabetic Retinopathy

This level, also called *background retinopathy*, indicates that there has been some damage to the retinal capillary bed but not to the point that new vessel growth has been stimulated into the vitreous body, which signifies proliferative diabetic retinopathy. These background changes are usually put into three categories: mild, moderate, and severe (or preproliferative) (8).

PRACTICAL POINT

The health of the retinal capillary bed can be best diagnosed by fluorescein angiography. A dye is given through an intravenous line, and then carefully timed photographs are taken of the retina to show areas of capillary nonperfusion and leakage.

Mild nonproliferative diabetic retinopathy. Some scattered small blot hemorrhages and microaneurysms begin to appear on the retina. These can be difficult to see and are easily missed during a nondilated eye examination. There are documented incidences of patients at this mild stage improving their glycemic control and reversing these changes.

Moderate nonproliferative diabetic retinopathy. There is a significant increase in the number of small blot hemorrhages and microaneurysms, with the additional findings of intraretinal microvascular abnormalities or venous beading. This is the point at which the experienced eye doctor will consider a consultation with a retinal specialist.

Severe nonproliferative (preproliferative) diabetic retinopathy. Retinal changes are now becoming a real threat to vision. The retina capillary bed is severely compromised, and more of the retinal findings of the previous moderate stage are present. The chemical mediators are now strongly calling out for new vessel growth. The patient should immediately see a retinal specialist for fluorescein angiography and probable treatment.

Proliferative Diabetic Retinopathy

Proliferative diabetic retinopathy indicates that there has been sufficient insult to the vessels and the body has started to try to fix the problem by growing new vessels. However, this "fix" results in more problems for the eye. The new vessels most commonly grow from the optic nerve head, but can also grow elsewhere in the retina and on the iris of the eye (called *rubeosis iridis*). Rubeosis iridis can lead to neovascular glaucoma. A retinal specialist needs to be immediately involved at this stage to minimize the high probability of blindness.

Retinal Detachment

The proliferative new vessels are leaky and cause adhesions and tractions that can then pull apart the two layers of the retina, in turn detaching them from the eye wall. If the retina is not surgically reattached, it will deteriorate quickly. Many times, this finding is the first indication of an eye problem in a patient with suboptimally controlled diabetes who has not had an eye examination or routine annual screening. It is not always possible to reattach the retina, resulting in permanent blindness.

Vitreous Hemorrhage

A vitreous hemorrhage occurs when the fragile new vessels growing in proliferative diabetic retinopathy break and bleed into the vitreous body. This can be seen as an oily, pink haze or sometimes as a total blockage of vision. Again, this may be the first indication of a diabetes-related eye problem. A retinal specialist usually does a vitrectomy at this point. This surgical procedure removes the jelly-like vitreous material, allowing clear aqueous fluid to fill the eye.

Clinically Significant Macular Edema

Retinal edema can appear at almost any level of retinopathy and is usually accompanied with some hard exudates. Sometimes these changes can be very subtle and missed by an inexperienced examiner who fails to dilate the pupil. Grid laser treatment, guided by fluorescein angiography, needs to be done as soon as possible to minimize the damage caused by the edema to the sensitive macular area.

OTHER RETINAL CHANGES IN THE EYE SOMETIMES ASSOCIATED WITH DIABETES

Hypertensive Retinopathy

High blood pressure combined with weakened retinal capillary beds in suboptimally controlled diabetes can cause a rapid progression in diabetic retinopathy. Hypertensive effects include infarcts in the retinal nerve fiber layer evidenced by cotton wool spots and flame-shaped retinal hemorrhages. These can resolve with

Interventions for Diabetic Ocular Complications

- Glycemic control
- Blood pressure control
- Panretinal photocoagulation. A retinal specialist will use a laser to carefully place hundreds of microburns to the peripheral retina. This will decrease the peripheral vision somewhat, but will reduce the demand for new blood vessel growth. This usually dries up the neo-vascular growth in proliferative diabetic retinopathy, thus preserving the central vision.
- Grid laser treatment. If a fluorescein angiography determines areas of leakages around the macula, a small-grid pattern of microburns will be placed, usually drying up the clinically significant macular edema to prevent further permanent loss to the macular function.
- Vitrectomy. A retinal specialist, in microsurgery, will remove the vitreous body while carefully protecting the retina from detachment, removing traction membranes.
- Follow-up. Most retinal specialists do not do routine eye care or pre-scribe low-vision aids, so the optometrist or general ophthalmologist will continue to monitor the patient's visual needs and, if necessary, refer him or her to a low-vision specialist for visual rehabilitation.
- Visual rehabilitation. Similar to physical therapy after a stroke, many patients can learn to adapt to their reduced vision with various new low-vision aids and techniques.
- Many new pharmacological interventions are being studied and show some promise in turning off the chemical mediators in the eye that call out for new blood vessel growth.

better control of blood pressure; however, continued hypertension, even without diabetes, can lead to sight-threatening retinal changes.

Central Retinal Vein Occlusion

Central retinal vein occlusion (CRVO) appears as a hemorrhagic stroke resulting from an occlusion in the central vein of the eye or a branch of it (BRVO). This problem threatens sight and is more related to the macrovascular changes in diabetes. Cholesterol management together with blood pressure control best prevent it (see ABCs of diabetes, CHAPTER 2). Some of the branch occlusions can resolve, and others need laser treatment similar to that in proliferative diabetic retinopathy. Central retinal artery occlusions can happen as well.

Age-Related Macular Degeneration

Although not specifically associated with diabetes, age-related macular degeneration is the leading cause of legal blindness in senior adults. When a patient with diabetes has this problem, special devices, low-vision aids, and proper training can greatly assist the patient in his or her self-management needs, such as in reading blood glucose meters and drawing up insulin.

NONRETINAL CHANGES IN THE EYE SOMETIMES ASSOCIATED WITH DIABETES

Diplopia

A sudden onset of double vision in a patient with diabetes is commonly associated with a complete or partial paresis of cranial nerves III, IV, and VI, which affect the extraocular muscles controlling eye position and movement. Most of these patients can be followed conservatively for 2–3 months, and many times, there is a dramatic recovery. The important exception is when either a third nerve palsy affects the pupil or if any palsy lasts >3 months. This situation requires an extensive neuroradiological workup to rule out the possibility of a brain aneurysm or other serious cranial problems.

Cataracts

Most people who live long enough will benefit from cataract extraction because the lens of their eye becomes less clear in the natural aging process. When the crystalline lens is removed, an artificial lens (intraocular lens) is usually put behind the iris to keep it in proper focus. Although cataracts are more common in individuals with suboptimally controlled diabetes, they are easily detected in routine eye examinations and easily treated when they sufficiently interfere with vision. However, no surgery is without risk, and individuals with diabetes who have a significant amount of retinopathy are at a higher risk of complications during and after the surgery. Many cataract surgeons will request a consultation from a retinal specialist to determine the best time for surgery in these cases.

Glaucoma

There are basically three types of glaucoma: primary open-angle glaucoma, primary angle-closure glaucoma, and neovascular glaucoma. All three types are associated with an intraocular pressure that is too high for the health of the optic nerve fibers.

Primary open-angle glaucoma (also known as chronic open-angle glaucoma). It is uncertain whether the diabetic population is at higher risk of developing this most common type of glaucoma. However, the potential for loss of vision is higher in individuals with suboptimally controlled diabetes because of compromised microvascular circulation. Detection and continuous treatment of this condition are important to minimize or prevent vision loss. Almost all routine eye examinations check for glaucoma. Because it is usually asymptomatic, patients are unaware of its presence until much of their peripheral vision is lost. Most patients can be successfully controlled with daily eye drops that lower their eye pressure.

Primary angle-closure glaucoma. Primary angle-closure glaucoma is an ocular emergency and is usually very painful. The cause is an anatomical closure of the drainage canal by the iris. It is also called narrow angle glaucoma. Quick treatment usually prevents any visual loss. Prevention of this condition begins when a narrow drainage angle is discovered during a routine eye examination. The patient would then be referred to an ophthalmologist, who has a special laser to open a drainage hole in the iris. This procedure (called *YAG iridotomy* [neodymium:yttrium aluminum garnet pulsed laser]) can be performed during an office visit, usually permanently prevents closure, and requires no ongoing medication.

Neovascular glaucoma. Neovascular glaucoma is a very serious condition and is associated with suboptimally controlled diabetes. This is a form of proliferative diabetic retinopathy in which new blood vessels form and proliferate along the iris (rubeosis iridis) and into the normal drainage canal of the eye, blocking the normal outflow of the aqueous, causing a painful increase in eye pressure. It is treated in the same way as other proliferative diabetic retinopathy, with panretinal laser photocoagulation and other medical and surgical interventions. Treatment, however, is not always successful in saving vision.

SUMMARY

The nurse can play an important role in reducing the incidence of diabetic retinopathy through education in maintaining blood glucose control, helping ensure timely eye examinations, and assisting individuals to achieve better control of blood pressure and lipids. Optimal diabetes control may prevent or delay the onset of diabetic retinopathy. Early detection and treatment also decreases

Abbreviations Commonly Used in Ocular Charts and Reports

A1C:	Glycated hemoglobin A_{1c}
AMD:	Age-related macular degeneration (sometimes ARMD)
BDR:	Background diabetic retinopathy (same as NPDR)
CRVO:	Central retinal vein occlusion
CSME:	Clinically significant (diabetic) macular edema
CW:	Cotton wool spots (on retina)
DME:	Diabetic macular edema
DR:	Diabetic retinopathy
FA:	Fluorescein angiography
H/ma:	Small-blot hemorrhages and/or microaneurysms
IRMA:	Intraretinal microvascular abnormalities
NPDR:	Nonproliferative diabetic retinopathy (same as BDR)
NVD:	New vessels on the optic disk (this is PDR)
NVE:	New vessels elsewhere in the retina (this is PDR)
NVG:	Neovascular glaucoma
OD:	Oculus dexter (right eye)
OS:	Oculus sinister (left eye)
OU:	Oculus uterque (both eyes)
PACG:	Primary angle closure glaucoma
PDR:	Proliferative diabetic retinopathy
POAG:	Primary (or chronic) open-angle glaucoma
PRP:	Panretinal laser photocoagulation
RD:	Retinal detachment
RI:	Rubeosis iridis (this is PDR)
VB:	Venous beading (with retinal veins)
VH:	Vitreous hemorrhage

the incidence of blindness. Encouragement by the nurse to achieve optimal control and to have annual dilated eye exams is important.

REFERENCES

1. American Diabetes Association: Retinopathy in diabetes (Position Statement). *Diabetes Care* 27 (Suppl. 1):S84–S87, 2004
2. Chous AP: *Diabetic Eye Disease: Lessons from a Diabetic Eye Doctor: How to Avoid Blindness and Get Great Eye Care.* Auburn, WA, Fairwood Press, 2003
3. National Diabetes Education Program web site. Available from http://www.cdc.gov/diabetes/ndep/index.htm. Accessed 30 December 2004
4. American Academy of Ophthalmology (AAO) web site. Available from http://www.aao.org. Accessed 17 November 2004
5. Diabetes Control and Complications Trial Research Group: The relationship of glycemic exposure (HbA$_{1c}$) to the risk of development and progression of retinopathy in the Diabetes Control and Complications Trial. *Diabetes* 44:968–983, 1995
6. American Optometric Association (AOA) web site. Available from http://www.aoanet.org. Accessed 17 November 2004
7. Aiello LP, Aiello LM, Cavallerano JD: Visual loss. In *Therapy for Diabetes Mellitus and Related Disorders.* 4th ed. Lebovitz HE, Ed. Alexandria, VA, American Diabetes Association, 2004, p. 340–343
8. Aiello LP, Aiello LM, Cavallerano JD: Ocular complications: In *Therapy for Diabetes Mellitus and Related Disorders.* 4th ed. Lebovitz HE, Ed. Alexandria, VA, American Diabetes Association, 2004, p. 344–357

Dr. Phelps is an Adjunct Assistant Clinical Professor at the School of Optometry, Pacific University, Forest Grove, OR, and practices at Ojai Eyes Optometry, Ojai, CA.

11. Diabetic Nephropathy and End-Stage Renal Disease

BELINDA P. CHILDS, ARNP, MN, CDE, BC-ADM, AND
KRIS ERNST, RN, CDE, BSN

EPIDEMIOLOGY OF DIABETIC NEPHROPATHY

Approximately 20 million Americans have kidney disease. Of these, >8 million Americans have seriously reduced kidney function, and another 11 million have protein in their urine, a sign of early kidney disease. In 2000, there were nearly 400,000 people who had kidney failure that required dialysis or a kidney transplant. This figure is expected to double by the year 2010 (1). Diabetes accounts for as much as 40% of all new cases of kidney failure (2). This is partly because type 2 diabetes is increasing in prevalence and because people with diabetes now live longer. Minorities are disproportionately affected by kidney disease. African Americans are four times more likely and American Indians six times more likely than white Americans to develop end-stage renal disease (ESRD) (3). In all, 70–80% of people with diabetes never develop ESRD and may live without significant renal complications throughout their lives (4).

PATHOGENESIS OF DIABETIC NEPHROPATHY

Studies have suggested that diabetic nephropathy is primarily related to the metabolic changes associated with diabetes.

- Renal changes are initially absent in people with diabetes who have kidney biopsies at diagnosis.
- Renal changes occur in all types of diabetes.
- Renal damage occurs in animal models regardless of whether they have spontaneous or induced diabetes.
- In animal models, reversal of diabetes through intensive insulin therapy or transplantation prevents the renal disease and may reverse early histological changes (5).

The onset of diabetes seems to lead to hemodynamic changes in the renal circulation that leads to an increase in renal plasma flow, glomerular capillary hyperperfusion, and an increased glomerular pressure gradient. These hemodynamic changes are hypothesized to cause functional and structural damage to the glomeruli, which results in defects in glomerular capillary permeability, proteinuria, mesangium changes, and glomerulosclerosis (6). The natural progression of diabetic nephropathy and some of the contributing factors are shown in Fig. 11.1.

RISK FACTORS FOR DIABETIC NEPHROPATHY

Risk factors that contribute to the development of renal disease include duration of diabetes, familial and genetic factors, hypertension, hyperglycemia, plasma prorenin activity, and lipid levels (6). One of the most important risk factors for the development of diabetic nephropathy is duration of diabetes; however, with type 1 diabetes, only 30–50% of patients develop diabetic nephropathy. Therefore, factors other than diabetes itself appear to affect the development of diabetic nephropathy.

Familial and Genetic Factors

In patients with type 1 diabetes, if one sibling has diabetes and nephropathy, then it is more likely that another sibling will also have nephropathy. In addition, some studies have found a difference in the distribution of HLA (human leukocyte antigen) markers between those with and without nephropathy in type 1 diabetes. There appears to be familial clustering in patients with type 2 diabetes as well (6).

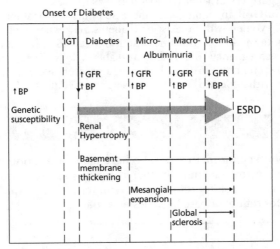

BP, blood pressure; IGT, impaired glucose tolerance; GFR, glomerular filtration rate; ESRD, end-stage renal disease.

Figure 11.1 Natural course of renal disease in diabetes. *Adapted from* Nelson et al. (6).

Hypertension

Hypertension may be a result of nephropathy but is also associated with progression and pathogenesis. Both systolic and diastolic hypertension accelerate the progression of diabetic kidney disease. Aggressive management of blood pressure can decrease the rate of fall of the glomerular filtration rate (GFR) (4).

Hyperglycemia

In the Diabetes Control and Complications Trial (DCCT), intensive therapy focused on attaining a hemoglobin A_{1c} (A1C) level as close to normal range (~7%) as possible reduced the occurrence of microalbuminuria (urinary albumin excretion ≥40 mg/24 h) by 39% and albuminuria (urinary albumin excretion ≥300 mg/24 h) by 54% in the combined cohort (7). Optimal diabetes control in the primary prevention group (those with retinopathy at baseline) in the U.K. Prospective Diabetes Study (UKPDS) demonstrated a reduction in the rate of progression of renal function end points (8).

Prorenin and Hyperlipidemia

Less clear is the role of prorenin and lipids in the development and progression of retinopathy. Prorenin is the precursor to renin, and an increase in plasma prorenin has been associated with the microvascular complications of diabetes. There are several small studies that have suggested that higher cholesterol level promotes the progression of renal disease.

Pregnancy

Pregnancy, regardless of whether a woman has diabetes, is associated with a transient rise in GFR and a moderate increase in urinary protein excretion (see CHAPTER 25). Women with preexisting diabetes may experience an increase in proteinuria from the first to third trimester, but this usually returns to normal after delivery. A pregnancy complicated by diabetes does not appear to adversely affect early diabetic renal disease; however, a greater risk of progression may occur in those with hypertension or more severe renal disease (6).

PRACTICAL POINT

A patient with nephropathy may also have diabetic eye disease. The presence of microalbuminuria in all age-groups has been associated with an increased risk for retinopathy. With renal disease, yearly screening for retinal disease becomes essential.

TREATMENT MODALITIES

Preventing and delaying the progression of diabetic nephropathy can be achieved with management of the known factors that influence the development and progression of the disease. Table 11.1 contains an outline of treatment approaches, divided into primary, secondary, and tertiary prevention strategies. Hypertension

Table 11.1 Strategies to Prevent or Delay the Progression of Diabetic Nephropathy

Primary prevention	*Goal:* Prevent diabetic nephropathy.
	Optimize glycemic control: A1C <7% *Blood pressure control:* <130/80 mmHg
Secondary prevention	*Goal:* Prevent or delay the progression from microalbuminuria to overt proteinuria.
	Aggressive control of blood pressure: <120/70 mmHg *Limit dietary protein:* ≤0.8 g/kg body wt/day (~10 of daily calories) *Medical intervention:* initiate ACE inhibitor or ARB treatment
Tertiary prevention	*Goal:* Prevent or delay the progression of overt diabetic nephropathy and improve clinical outcomes (tertiary care reduces morbidity and mortality by delaying time to dialysis or transplantation).
	Strategies as above for secondary prevention

Adapted from ADA (4,10) and DeFronzo (9).

is known to be the single most important factor in the progression of established renal disease. Both systolic and diastolic hypertension accelerate the progression of the disease (5).

According to the American Diabetes Association's (ADA's) Standards of Medical Care in Diabetes, blood pressure should be evaluated at each medical visit (10). If it is >130/80 mmHg, a second evaluation should be obtained in the near future. The primary goal is to lower blood pressure with lifestyle modifications, such as weight loss (if appropriate), reduction in salt and alcohol intake, and exercise. In 4–6 weeks, if blood pressure has not reached this goal and there are no contraindications for use, then an angiotensin-converting enzyme (ACE) inhibitor or angiotensin receptor blocker (ARB) should be initiated. If initial goals are met and well tolerated, decreasing the blood pressure further may be appropriate. The UKPDS indicated that continuing to lower blood pressure reduced the risk of microvascular complications (8).

EDUCATION AND SELF-MANAGEMENT

The patient with hypertension should self-monitor their blood pressure. Self-monitoring of blood pressure enhances educational efforts and allows the patient and health care team to work together in detecting, treating, and evaluating the risk for renal complications. Reviewing patients' technique and regularly checking blood pressure monitoring devices can help ensure accurate readings.

Dietary Protein Restriction

Animal studies have shown that reducing dietary protein intake reduces hyperfiltration and intraglomerular pressure and retards the progression of renal disease. Several small human studies have shown a modest reduction in the progression of renal disease using a restriction of 0.8 g/kg body wt/day. The current ADA recommendation is to prescribe the adult Recommended Daily Allowance (RDA) of 0.8 g/kg body wt/day (~10% of total calories) in the patient with overt nephropathy. Because most Americans eat in excess of the recommended amount of protein, portion control that includes weighing and measuring is necessary. It has been suggested that once the GFR begins to fall, it may be helpful to restrict protein intake to 0.6 g/kg/day (4).

Patients using protein-restricted meal plans must be continuously monitored for signs of malnutrition, including weight, muscle wasting, weakness, and hypoalbuminemia. In order to consume an adequate number of calories, other macronutrients may need to be increased. The additional amount of carbohydrate in this diet can cause blood glucose levels to rise, and insulin and/or oral medications may need to be adjusted. As the renal disease progresses, appetite frequently diminishes, and patients may have to be encouraged to eat adequate calories with enough protein. A dietitian should be consulted for any patient with moderate to severe nephropathy.

DIAGNOSIS AND RENAL FUNCTION TESTS

Diagnostic tests focus on early detection of microalbuminuria. Annual screening for microalbuminuria in type 1 diabetes patients should begin in puberty and/or after a 5-year disease duration. Among people with type 2 diabetes, screening for microalbuminuria should begin at the time of diagnosis. Screening for microalbuminuria can be performed by three methods:

- Measurement of the albumin-to-creatinine ratio in a random spot urine collection
- 24-h urine collection for creatinine and serum creatinine to measure creatinine clearance (CrCl)
- Timed (e.g., 4-h or overnight) collection

Analysis of the measurement of the albumin-to-creatinine ratio is the more commonly recommended screening method (4). The other two alternatives (24-h collection and a timed specimen) are rarely used for screening. Normal albumin excretion by spot collection is defined as <30 µg/mg, microalbuminuria is 30–299 µg/mg, and clinical albuminuria is ≥300 µg/mg (Table 11.2). Because of variability in urinary albumin excretion, at least two of three tests measured within a 6-month period should show elevated levels before a patient is designated as

Table 11.2 Definitions in Abnormalities in Albumin Excretion

Category	4-h Collection (mg/24 h)	Timed Collection (µg/min)	Spot Collection (µg/mg creatinine)
Normal	<30	<20	<30
Microalbuminuria	30–299	20–199	<30–299
Clinical albuminuria (≥300 µg/mg)	≥200	≥300	—

From ADA (4).

having microalbuminuria. Exercise within the preceding 24 h, infection, fever, congestive heart failure, vasculitis, other inflammatory processes (such as acute rheumatoid arthritis), and marked hyperglycemia and hypertension may elevate urinary albumin levels above baseline levels. If any of these problems were present at the time the urine sample was collected, the test should be repeated. If the albumin screening values are ≥300 µg/mg, then a 24-h urine is ordered to quantify the protein excretion and establish the GFR. In addition, a serum creatinine must be drawn during this time period to determine CrCl, if needed. CrCl is calculated by comparing the serum creatinine level with the urine creatinine level.

CrCl is the most widely used direct method of estimating GFR. This value is measured based on a carefully timed urine collection, usually over 24 h. It is critical to note an accurate time frame even if a full 24 h has not passed. A complete sample is imperative. Partial loss of a urine sample or a discrepancy in actual time collected will make the test invalid (11). Serum creatinine is an indirect measure of GFR. Subtle changes in serum creatinine, e.g., 0.8–1.3 mg/dl, may in fact indicate major functional loss.

An estimated GFR (eGFR) can also be calculated using the Levey modification of the Cockcroft and Gault method, which uses serum creatinine, patient age, and weight. The eGFR can be calculated by going to the web site www.kidney.org/kls/professionals/gfr_calculator.cfm (4).

CHRONIC RENAL DISEASE

Chronic renal disease is defined in two ways (11):

1. Kidney damage for ≥3 months, as defined by structural or functional abnormalities of the kidney, with or without decreased GFR, manifested by either
   • pathological abnormalities, or
   • markers of kidney damage, including abnormalities in the composition of the blood or urine or abnormal imaging tests.
2. GFR <60 ml/min/1.73 m² for ≥3 months, with or without kidney damage (11,12).

The stages are shown in Table 11.3.

CLINICAL PRESENTATION AND ASSESSMENT

Individuals are asymptomatic throughout the early stages of diabetic nephropathy. Clinical manifestations of diabetic nephropathy are evident when GFR is 20–35% of normal, and patients become nephrotic with a urinary protein excre-

Table 11.3 Stages of Chronic Kidney Disease

Stage	Description	GFR (ml/min/1.73 m²)
1	Kidney damage with normal or increased GFR	≥90
2	Kidney damage with mild decrease in GFR	60–89
3	Moderate decrease in GFR	30–59
4	Severe decrease in GFR	15–29
5	Kidney failure	<15 or dialysis

From the National Kidney Foundation (12,13).

tion of >4 g/day (14). The clinical management of diabetes with nephrotic syndrome presents a great challenge. The management of glucose control becomes more difficult as loss of renal function diminishes renal catabolism of insulin. Proteinuria is generally 4–8 g/day, but urinary protein loss can reach 20–30 g/day. Fluid retention is often massive, resulting in weight gain, peripheral edema, congestive heart failure, and pulmonary edema as uremia progresses. Fatigue and shortness of breath result in a reduction of daily activities. Hypertension may become uncontrolled, secondary to fluid volume overload. Uremia becomes evident because of the accumulation of metabolic wastes and toxins.

At equivalent levels of renal failure, patients with diabetes may appear more ill than those without diabetes. Underlying diabetes-induced neurological abnormalities such as gastroparesis can exacerbate uremia-induced nausea and vomiting.

A nephrologist should be consulted when GFR is <60 ml/min/1.73 m² or if difficulty occurs in the management of hypertension or hyperkalemia (4). Nephrologists should be consulted early in the diagnosis to assure that the patient receives all available preventive measures.

OTHER CONSIDERATIONS IN NEPHROPATHY PROGRESSION

Hypoglycemia

Hypoglycemia is a risk factor for patients with renal disease because most diabetes medications are metabolized in the kidney. It may be necessary to reduce the dosages of some antihyperglycemic medications and avoid the use of others. Of the oral agents, the sulfonylureas have the greatest risk for inducing and prolonging hypoglycemia. Glimepiride and the meglitinides are least likely to lead to hypoglycemia. Even with these medications, lower dosages will likely be necessary.

The kidneys catabolize one-fourth to one-third of injected insulin. As kidney function declines, exogenous insulin acts longer and in an unpredictable manner (9). Studies have concluded that the kidney can make and release glucose. Based on recent evidence, it would seem that the release of glucose by the kidney might play a role in the regulation of glucose homeostasis. The lack of this production and release may also be a contributing factor to hypoglycemia associated with kidney disease (14,15). Use of insulin analogs, intensive insulin therapy, and hypoglycemia awareness training may all aid in the reduction of severe hypoglycemia in the patient with renal impairment.

PRACTICAL POINT

Patients who present with frequent and unexplained hypoglycemia should have their renal status assessed.

Additional Complications

Management and rehabilitation of patients with ESRD are further complicated by the fact that >95% of patients with diabetic nephropathy have some degree of retinopathy, with 50% being blind or having significant vision loss (renal-retinal syndrome).

If either renal or retinal disease has been diagnosed, it is important to screen for disease in the other system. Also, microalbuminuria and proteinuria are prognostic indicators of cardiovascular disease in type 2 diabetes.

Other Threats to the Kidney

Urinary tract infections (UTIs). These are more common in older adults and in those with autonomic neuropathy affecting the bladder. UTIs are often asymptomatic or the patient may complain of unexplained hyperglycemia, incontinence, and vague symptoms, such as fullness in the suprapubic area. It is therefore important that a urinalysis be performed at each clinic visit. If leukocytes or nitrites are present, a urine culture should be obtained. Positive cultures should be treated with an antibiotic. Chronic infections can lead to pyelonephritis. There is debate regarding the importance of asymptomatic bacteremia and the necessity of treatment. Patient education on the symptoms of UTI is important.

Neurogenic bladder. This condition is more common in patients with diabetes, one that may predispose patients to UTIs. Symptoms such as frequent voiding, nocturia, incontinence, and recurrent UTIs may occur sporadically or be considered a result of age or prostatic hypertrophy. If diagnosed, the nurse can teach the Credé's manual voiding maneuvers, which should be performed every 8 h. This is often sufficient to prevent the postvoid residual. If not, parasympathetic agents may be tried. If pharmacologic therapy proves unsuccessful, intermittent straight catheterization should be performed two to three times daily.

Dye studies. Intravenous pyelography and other dye studies can be a risk for patients with diabetes as they are at increased risk for acute renal failure after any radiocontrast. Many times, an alternative diagnostic study can be performed. If contrast media are necessary, a minimum amount of dye should be used and adequate hydration with half-normal or normal saline should be ensured prior to the dye study. Serum creatinine tests should be checked daily for 2–3 days after the contrast study (5).

Nephrotoxic drugs. If these drugs (e.g., amphotericin B; aminoglycosides, such as gentamicin; acyclovir; nonsteroidal anti-inflammatory drugs [NSAIDs]) must be used, monitor serum creatinine levels and drug levels and reduce the dosage of the drug administered to patients with impaired renal function. Recommend acetaminophen rather than NSAIDs because these agents reduce prostaglandins and can damage the kidney.

Medication dosages. Because the presence of renal disease can increase the half-life of most medications, new medications should be started at one-half the recommended dosage, and other current medications should be reviewed for possible changes in dosage.

PRACTICAL POINT

In caring for patients with renal disease, consider the following:
- Identify UTIs early and treat aggressively
- Avoid nephrotoxic medications
- Avoid NSAIDs
- Avoid contrast dyes

SPECIAL CONSIDERATIONS

Anemia

Anemia caused by ESRD is the result of a decrease in the production of erythropoietin. Because erythropoietin stimulates the production of red blood cells, the anemia often leads to fatigue and decreased activity. The anemia of kidney disease is often managed with regular injections of erythropoietin.

When assessing patients with renal disease and anemia, patient symptoms may not correlate with capillary blood glucose values or with the A1C. Thus, it is important to be aware of how anemia can affect tests for glycemic control. With low hemoglobin and low hematocrit levels, some of the commonly used tests are affected and may give inaccurate results. A1C can give a falsely low value. Sometimes, a fructosamine test can be used to assess glycemic control. However, because the fructosamine test is affected by low albumin/protein levels, which are often seen in patients with ESRD, this test may not give an accurate assessment of glycemic control.

Additionally, capillary blood glucose tests can be affected by a low hematocrit level and therefore may also be altered by anemia. Capillary blood glucose results are most accurate when the hematocrit level is between 30 and 50%. However, some glucose meters have a documented accuracy with hematocrit ranges of 25–60% (16). If the patient's symptoms do not correlate with their capillary blood glucose levels, the nurse should compare the glucose meter value with a laboratory reference value. When a patient's symptoms do not correlate with a blood glucose value, verification by a laboratory measurement should be obtained.

Provided the difficulties concomitant with ESRD and anemia in testing blood glucose values, thorough and careful testing is advised in these patients. Evaluating which meter is less dependent on hematocrit will be important in assisting these patients. If a renal patient is reporting symptoms of hypoglycemia but obtaining normal or high capillary blood glucose levels, it would be prudent to obtain a blood glucose level by the reference laboratory with a simultaneous glucose meter reading.

Fluid Volume Excess

Fluid volume excess can result from the oliguria or anuria. Because of the thirst associated with ESRD, the patient tends to drink in excess and crave sodium, further contributing to the volume excess. The variation in hydration can also affect blood glucose levels. Edema may be a problem associated with the decreased serum osmolality. The nurse needs to assist the patient in identifying ways to relieve this thirst, such as with ice chips, mouth swabs, and sugar-free hard candies as appropriate. These patients are often on fluid restrictions, especially if they have not begun dialysis or are on hemodialysis, so a registered dietitian (RD) should be consulted. The nurse should reinforce these fluid restrictions and make it clear that foods that are liquids when at room temperature (e.g., Jell-O, pudding) are also fluids and subject to restriction. In patients who crave sodium, identifying foods that have alternative flavors without sodium, such as lemon, is an option.

Symptoms of electrolyte imbalance include weakness, muscle twitching, nausea, fatigue, headache, and heart palpitations. Other symptoms may include edema, alterations in ECG and chemistry panels, and positional blood pressure changes. Patients need to be cautioned about standing too quickly. This will reduce the potential of falling due to orthostatic hypotension and muscle weakness. Family members may need to be encouraged to support the patient.

Dietary Changes Associated With ESRD

Protein restriction may be used to prevent the progression of renal disease. But as the disease progresses, patients often experience anorexia, nausea, and vomiting. In addition, foods containing potassium and sodium are often restricted on the renal diet. With the multiple comorbidities of diabetes, it is not uncommon to see a patient trying to manage a meal plan that is low in fat, has consistent carbohydrate content, and is low in potassium and sodium, which can lead to confusion, anger, and feelings of deprivation. Malnutrition can occur because of reduced appetite and diet restrictions. The nurse should encourage a consultation with a dietitian and make every effort to offer additional food choices if the patient does not eat while in the hospital or in the dialysis unit. During dialysis sessions, dietary restrictions are modified, allowing the patient to enjoy a wider range of foods.

COORDINATION OF CARE

The patient with diabetic nephropathy presents a challenge for nursing. Renal disease itself presents a complex medical program of care. However, when renal disease is coupled with diabetes, the interaction of medical and nursing management issues demands a high level of nursing care and expertise. Research has demonstrated that excellent diabetes management must be maintained to retard renal deterioration, but with renal disease, diabetes self-management and the patient's ability to achieve glucose goals become increasingly difficult.

Foremost, the role of the nurse is to assist the patient in dealing with the complexity of the renal care regimen. A nurse will encounter many of these intricate aspects, including dietary issues and their effects on glucose levels, prevention of and treatment for hypoglycemia (including the use of glucagon), issues regarding alterations in activity and increased fatigue associated with anemia and uremia, skin dryness and pruritus, and mental health conditions such as depression. The patient will be interacting at many levels with the health care system: dietitians, renal and dialysis specialists, diabetes specialists and nurse educators, mental health providers, pharmacists, social workers, etc. As is evident, these many levels of interaction only increase the potential for miscommunication and faulty care coordination. The nurse is the ideal patient advocate to coordinate and facilitate care.

The renal patient has increased physical care needs. Table 11.4 identifies these needs and suggests nursing actions to meet them.

CHOOSING A TREATMENT OPTION FOR ESRD

Treatments for ESRD are aimed at replacing the work of the kidneys. People with diabetes who receive transplants or dialysis experience higher morbidity and mortality than patients without diabetes because of coexisting complications such as coronary artery disease, retinopathy, and neuropathy. Providing education and information on each treatment option allows the patient and family to make an informed choice and enhances the chances of a positive outcome. Benefits and risks of each treatment option should be reviewed with patients and family members for a comparison of options in treating uremia. Direct contact with other patients who are receiving different forms of therapy for ESRD may be valuable for education, emotional support, and instilling hope. Providing a list of useful web sites may also be helpful (see RESOURCES).

Table 11.4 Physical Care Needs for the Renal Patient With Diabetes

Physical Needs	Nursing Actions
Monitor fluid and electrolyte balance	1. Weigh patient for fluid retention and measure urinary output/fluid intake 2. Assess for signs of fluid overload/congestive heart failure 3. Assess blood pressure and orthostatic changes
Maintain adequate nutrition status	1. Evaluate food intake and dietary adherence 2. Collaborate with the dietitian and provide reinforcement on education regarding potassium and protein restriction 3. Assess weight changes and alterations in lab values and notify a doctor, if necessary 4. Educate patient in eating smaller, more frequent meals to reduce nausea and maintain blood glucose level
Maintain skin integrity	1. Maintain hygiene to prevent infection 2. Relieve dryness and pruritus by choosing alcohol-free creams and nondrying soaps
Prevent constipation	1. Use stool softeners and fiber products 2. Fluid restrictions and phosphate binders may aggravate constipation 3. Discourage use of over-the-counter (OTC) remedies that may cause electrolyte imbalances
Maintain target glucose levels	1. Help patient to identify times of the day when hypoglycemia is most likely to occur 2. Discuss appropriate treatment for hypoglycemia: oral medications and glucagon by injection 3. Discuss changes in glucose levels with continuous ambulatory peritoneal dialysis fluid changes or before and after dialysis 4. Encourage patient to keep a glucose log to assist in insulin adjustment decisions
Encourage safe level of activity	1. Assess patient's gait, balance, range of motion, muscle strength, and condition of feet 2. As tolerated, encourage activity to prevent bone demineralization and assist with glucose control
Increase understanding of complex regimen of care	1. Help patient to express treatment concerns/fears; refer to mental health professionals as appropriate 2. Assess treatment schedule to avoid unnecessary fatigue and to better coordinate with diabetes management program 3. Review alterations in diabetes therapy caused by changes in kidney status

Adapted from Nettina (17).

Dialysis and/or renal transplantation usually occurs earlier in the diabetes patient than in one who does not have diabetes. Typically, renal replacement therapy will begin when serum creatinine is >6 mg/dl or CrCl <20 ml/min, but more importantly, it should begin before the development of severe uremic symptoms such as uremic pericarditis, unresponsive hypertension, muscle deterioration, worsening of lethargy, nausea, and vomiting (9).

CANDIDATE SELECTION

Circumstances may be present that limit the patient's choice of treatment. For example, individuals with cardiovascular disease or vascular access problems might be less suitable candidates for hemodialysis. Likewise, individuals unable to tolerate fluid in the peritoneal cavity or those prone to infections would not be appropriate candidates for peritoneal dialysis.

Planning for treatment should begin early, usually when the serum creatinine level reaches 3 mg/dl (265 μmol/l). Early involvement with a nephrologist, which is usually recommended when creatinine is 2 mg/dl or GFR is <60 ml/min/1.73 m², is also important to optimize medical therapy as well as help the patient begin the adjustment process. Patients with renal disease will often feel that they are participating in a program in which the goal is to preserve kidney function as long as possible. Late referrals for treatment, which will require hasty decisions regarding type of dialysis or being put on a list for kidney transplantation, frequently result in sentiments of anger and betrayal at the primary care provider for not conveying the seriousness of the kidney disease. If transplantation is under consideration, planning includes tissue typing of family members or other living unrelated donors for possible kidney donation, being placed on a cadaver waiting list, and/or creating vascular access for dialysis.

BEHAVIORAL CONSIDERATIONS

Rates of depression, anxiety, and stress may be higher among patients with ESRD than among the general population. These psychological reactions may occur in response to the losses associated with diabetes and renal disease (e.g., loss of physical capacities and loss of control from the complications associated with diabetes). A variety of health care professionals, including mental health professionals, need to be involved in helping patients and families adjust to their losses and to select treatment options. In addition, the involvement of these professionals will make the task of learning a new, often complex treatment regimen more successful (18).

Some patients blame themselves when they develop diabetes complications. Scare tactics (e.g., "If you don't control your blood glucose, you will go into kidney failure") are not an effective behavior-change strategy. The fear, anxiety, and stress associated with renal disease may be expressed as anger toward the health care team and a reluctance to follow the recommended regimen. Some patients may make comments such as "why bother" or "well, I'm going to have a transplant, so I won't worry about it." It is important for the health care team to recognize and validate the patient's feelings in order to ensure that the patient follows the treatment regimen. Avoid giving "pat" answers or responses that can sound patronizing. To assess what feelings and concerns the patient may be experiencing, state the following: "This can be a difficult process for some people, and sometimes they blame themselves. How are you feeling about having a problem with your kidneys?" Allowing the patient to express his or her fears and concerns is the most important intervention.

**BEHAVIORAL CONSIDERATIONS WITHIN
THE HEALTH CARE TEAM**

The health care team may experience a range of emotions and may need the
help of a team member in expressing and dealing with their own feelings
about what the patient and family are going through and how they are coping.

Support groups and discussion with other individuals and families who have
experienced dialysis or transplantation can be an effective intervention for some
patients with ESRD. Patients can learn new information, coping skills, and behaviors and adopt positive attitudes from these role models. Having patients and their
families available in the clinic setting to meet new patients who are facing a recent
diagnosis of renal disease can be very valuable.

TREATMENT OPTIONS FOR ESRD

If treatment is not initiated for ESRD, death ensues. Survival is reduced in patients
with diabetes compared with those without diabetes. Nearly one-half of all
patients with diabetes who begin dialysis die within 2 years. For renal transplant
patients with diabetes, the survival rate is much better than that for the dialysis-
treated patient, primarily because those patients who have kidney or kidney/
pancreas transplants have fewer comorbidities.

No Treatment

A patient has the right to choose not to begin dialysis. The patient and family
should consider the no-treatment option only after the patient is dialyzed and is
not uremic because uremia can affect the mental status. Some patients could be
considered incompetent because of uremia. The nurse should encourage the
patient and family to discuss the decision not only with their physician but with
clergy, a psychologist, social worker, health care team, and other family members.
It is important to evaluate the patient for potentially undiagnosed and/or untreated
depression. Planning supportive care (e.g., home care, hospice care) is necessary for
the patient who chooses to forgo or discontinue renal replacement therapy.

Hemodialysis

Hemodialysis is the most commonly used kidney-replacement therapy for people
with ESRD in the U.S. The use of maintenance hemodialysis requires vascular
access, which can be more difficult in the patient with diabetes because of systemic
atherosclerosis. A synthetic graft may be used in the patient with diabetes.

Nursing considerations. Factors that can alter glucose levels for the patient receiving hemodialysis treatment include the glucose concentration in the dialysate
bath, appetite alteration on days with dialysis and days without dialysis, decreased
activity on dialysis days, and emotional stress. The following questions are useful
in eliciting information regarding causes of blood glucose variability in patients
with diabetes who are receiving hemodialysis treatment:

- "Tell me about your glucose pattern on the days you are having dialysis?"
- "Tell me about your pattern on other days?"
- "Tell me when and how much you eat on days you are having dialysis?"
- "What about other days?"
- "Tell me about your activity pattern on days you are having dialysis?"
- "Tell me about your activity pattern on other days?"

Altered hematocrit levels can alter the accuracy of some glucose meters (see "Anemia" above). Sometimes a change in the type of glucose meter used may be warranted to avoid erroneous measurements of blood glucose values. Meter manufacturers provide specifications of hematocrit ranges for their meters. The health care provider should be aware of this potential cause of variability.

Peritoneal Dialysis

Peritoneal dialysis has rapidly grown in popularity because of its advantages of rapid patient training and reduced cardiovascular stress. The use of the mechanical cyclers, called continuous cyclic peritoneal dialysis (CCPD), has simplified the process. Both CCPD and continuous ambulatory peritoneal dialysis carry the risks of peritonitis and gradual decrease in peritoneal surface area. Insulin, antibiotics, and other medications can be added to the dialysate. The amount of insulin required may vary based on the glucose concentration of the dialysate. Typically, regular insulin is added to the dialysate.

Patients requiring insulin can administer regular insulin directly into the dialysate before it is instilled into the peritoneal cavity. The advantage of intraperitoneal insulin is that there is a reduced need for injections because the insulin can be added to the dialysate. This represents a more physiologic way to deliver insulin because it is continuously absorbed by the hepatic system, much like insulin produced by β-cells.

Factors that can affect glucose regulation for patients on peritoneal dialysis include the concentration of the dialysate solution, method(s) of insulin delivery (e.g., intraperitoneal, subcutaneous, or both), and infection (peritonitis). Carefully written instructions will need to be provided. Self-monitoring of blood glucose is essential. Adjustments in the amount of insulin added to the dialysate should be based on glucose monitoring. A pattern approach should be used. The patient should be encouraged to keep good records, noting the glucose concentration of dialysate, calories/carbohydrates eaten, insulin added to dialysate, and insulin injected. Fast-acting insulin can be supplemented for meals and as a correction dose.

Kidney Transplantation

After transplantation, most individuals with diabetes will require a higher insulin dose because the immunosuppressive medications (i.e., steroids) have a hyperglycemic effect, the newly functioning kidney catabolizes the insulin, and the patient's appetite is often increased with resolution of the uremia due to the effect of the steroids. Patients should be aware that an unexplained rise in blood glucose may signal a problem with the transplanted kidney. Infection would likely cause a rise in blood glucose. Prolonged hypoglycemia may signify a reduction in kidney function and a potential rejection episode. If a rejection episode does occur, the medication to prevent the rejection likely will substantially increase blood glucose levels and, consequently, the insulin dose.

Simultaneous Kidney-Pancreas Transplantation

Kidney-pancreas transplantation restores both glucose metabolism and kidney function. Criteria for patient selection vary at each transplant center but typically include the diagnosis of type 1 diabetes, evidence of secondary complications such as moderate or severe neuropathy, metabolic instability, and adequate financial resources/insurance coverage. The complications of kidney-pancreas transplantation are cardiac incompetence, arterial or venous thrombosis, anastomotic leaks and bleeding, and side effects, which include immunosuppression, pancreatitis, and metabolic acidosis related to exocrine pancreatic function.

Renal transplant function is easier to measure than pancreas function. A rise in serum creatinine is a primary indicator of kidney rejection. A decrease in serum amylase or urinary amylase production can signal a jeopardized pancreas. Hyperglycemia occurs late in pancreas rejection. Signs of rejection can be detected earlier in the kidney and treatment can be initiated, thus providing some protection for the pancreas.

SUMMARY

Optimal control of blood glucose and blood pressure are the keys to the prevention of nephropathy. Early detection using the annual albumin-to-creatinine ratio will identify those who are at risk, and aggressive treatment may delay the progression of the disease. The nurse plays a vital role in prevention and detection. If the patient has developed ESRD, it is imperative that the nurse provide support to the patient and family when they are making a decision regarding treatment options.

FUTURE NURSING RESEARCH

Qualitative research is needed to develop a better understanding of how the diagnosis of ESRD affects the individual with diabetes and his or her family. Additional research issues may lie in the area of behavior-changing requirements that are specifically related to the lifestyle modification necessary for adapting to a diagnosis of diabetic nephropathy.

REFERENCES

1. Coresh J, Astor BC, Greene T, Eknoyan G, Levey AS: Prevalence of chronic kidney disease and decreased kidney function in the adult US population: Third National Health and Nutrition Examination Survey. *Am J Kidney Dis* 41:1–12, 2003
2. U.S. Renal Data System: 2004 ADR/reference tables [Internet]. Available from http://www.usrds.org/reference.htm. Accessed 22 November 2004
3. National Diabetes Information Clearinghouse (NDIC): Complications of diabetes in the United States [Internet]. Available from http://diabetes. niddk.nih.gov/dm/pubs/statistics/index.htm#13. Accessed 1 January 2005
4. American Diabetes Association. Diabetic nephropathy (Position Statement). *Diabetes Care* 27 (Suppl. 1):S79–S83, 2004

5. Bode BW (Ed.): Nephropathy. In *Medical Management of Type 1 Diabetes.* 4th ed. Alexandria, VA, American Diabetes Association, 2004, p. 198–207
6. Nelson RG, Knowler WC, Pettitt DJ, Bennett PH: Kidney disease in diabetes. In *Diabetes in America.* 2nd ed. Bethesda, MD, National Diabetes Data Group, 1995, p. 349–370 (NIH publ. no. 95-1468)
7. Diabetes Control and Complications Trial Research Group: The effect of intensive treatment of diabetes on the development and progression of long-term complications in insulin-dependent diabetes. *N Engl J Med* 329:977–986, 1993
8. UK Prospective Diabetes Study Group: Intensive blood-glucose control with sulfonylureas or insulin compared with conventional treatment and risk of complications in patients with type 2 diabetes (UKPDS 33). *Lancet* 352: 837–853, 1998
9. DeFronzo RA: Diabetic nephropathy. In *Therapy for Diabetes Mellitus and Related Disorders.* 4th ed. Lebovitz HG, Ed. Alexandria, VA, American Diabetes Association, 2004, p. 369–397
10. American Diabetes Association: Standards of medical care in diabetes (Position Statement). *Diabetes Care* 28 (Suppl. 1):S4–S36, 2005
11. Pfeettscher SA: Chronic renal failure and renal transplantation. In *Critical Care Nursing.* Bucher L, Melander S, Eds. Philadelphia, W. B. Saunders, 1999, p. 569–599
12. National Kidney Foundation: K/DOQI clinical practice guidelines for chronic kidney disease: evaluation, classification, and stratification [Internet], 2002. Available from http://www.kidney.org/professionals/kdoqi/guidelines_ckd/toc.htm. Accessed 18 November 2004
13. Levey AS, Coresh J, Balk E, Kausz AT, Levin A, Steffes MW, Hogg RJ, Perrone RD, Lau J, Eknoyan G: National Kidney Foundation practice guidelines for chronic kidney disease: evaluation, classification, and stratification. *Ann Intern Med* 139:137–147, 2003
14. Gerich JE, Meyer C, Woerle HJ, Stumvoll M: Renal gluconeogenesis: its importance in human glucose homeostasis. *Diabetes Care* 26:382–391, 2001
15. Cryer PE: Hypoglycemic disorders. *Hypoglycemia: Pathophysiology, Diagnosis, and Treatment.* New York, Oxford, 1997, p. 127–168
16. Tang, Z, Lee TH, Louie RF, Kost GJ: Effects of different hematocrit levels on glucose measurements with handheld meters for point-of-care testing. *Arch Pathol Lab Med* 124:1135–1140, 2000
17. Nettina SM (Ed): Renal and urinary disorders: chronic renal failure. In *Lippincott Manual of Nursing Practice.* 6th ed. Philadelphia, Lippincott-Raven, 1996, p. 610–615
18. Kleinbeck C: Challenges of diabetes and dialysis. *Diabetes Spectrum* 10:135–141, 1997

ADDITIONAL READING

Conrod BA, Ernst KL: Nephropathy. In *A Core Curriculum for Diabetes Education: Diabetes and Complications.* 5th ed. Franz MJ, Ed. Chicago, IL, American Association of Diabetes Educators, 2003, p. 153–185

Ms. Childs is a Diabetes Nurse Specialist at Mid-America Diabetes Associates, Wichita, KS. Ms. Ernst is a Public Health Advisor at the Centers for Disease Control and Prevention, Atlanta, GA.

12. Dental Issues in Patients with Diabetes

Geralyn Spollett, MSN, C-ANP, CDE, and Charles A. Crape, DMD

Individuals with diabetes are two to three times more likely than those without the disease to develop dental problems such as caries, periodontal and oral mucosal diseases, and tooth loss. Inadequately controlled diabetes can complicate routine dental visits as well as oral surgery and dental implant procedures. Maintaining appropriate blood glucose levels and following guidelines for good oral hygiene, including regular checkups, can reduce the incidence of dental problems.

PROMOTING DENTAL CARE

Nursing care of patients with diabetes should promote oral hygiene and prevention of dental disease as standard components of continuing diabetes management. Nurses need to emphasize routine dental care not only as a deterrent to tooth loss but also as an important measure in maintaining glycemic control. Patients must understand the relationship between dental care and glycemic control, in which a deterioration of one leads to the deterioration of the other.

The Centers for Disease Control and Prevention recommend that patients with diabetes see a dentist every 6 months and more frequently if periodontal disease is present (1). The American Diabetes Association Standards of Medical Care in Diabetes includes an examination of the oral cavity in the initial visit but offers no guidelines for periodic dental examinations.

People with diabetes are less likely than those without diabetes to have had a recent dental examination. In a study by Tomar and Lester (2), subjects who had not seen a dentist in the preceding 12 months cited a lack of perceived need for dental care and an underappreciation of the relationship between oral health and general health. In fact, when compared with other preventive care services (a dilated eye examination and a podiatric examination), dental care visits were the least likely to have occurred.

Inadequate dental care has a strong socioeconomic basis. Patients pay a much larger portion of dental costs out of pocket than they do for most other health care services. Medicare has no provision for dental care, and Medicaid provides only limited coverage in some states. Tomar and Lester found that the disparity in frequency of dental visits among racial, ethnic, and socioeconomic groups was greater than that for any other type of health care visit for subjects with diabetes (2). Among subjects whose annual household income was more than $50,000, 81.6% had seen a dentist in the preceding 12 months, compared with only 41.2% of those who earned less than $10,000 a year. Similar disparities did not exist for physician visits or foot examinations (2).

COMMON DENTAL PROBLEMS OF INDIVIDUALS WITH DIABETES

Although nursing care for people with diabetes focuses on promoting oral hygiene, nurses must recognize and understand the various dental diseases and conditions commonly found in their patients.

Dental Caries and Gingivitis

Prevention of dental caries is important for people with diabetes. Tooth decay and loss can compromise nutrition, further affecting diabetes control. Topical treatments such as fluoride applications, fluoride mouth rinses, and salivary substitutes can help prevent caries and also reduce dry mouth symptoms associated with diabetes.

Gingivitis, or inflammation of the gum tissue, is more prevalent in children and adults with diabetes, despite similar levels of plaque control as the general population (3). Patients with diabetes have more decayed and filled tooth surfaces, as well as a higher incidence of root caries, which may be associated with more gingival recession. Often, gingivitis progresses to periodontal disease and subsequent tooth loss. Patients who have partial or total tooth loss (edentulism) tend to be older and to have longer duration of disease. They also have higher glycated hemoglobin A_{1c} (A1C) levels and higher rates of microvascular complications, i.e., retinopathy, nephropathy, neuropathy, peripheral arterial disease.

Patient Education Topics for Promoting Oral Health

- Influences of diabetes on oral health
- Achieving glycemic control goals
- Tobacco cessation counseling
- Healthy eating habits
- Oral hygiene measures: routine and between meal brushing, flossing, using a water pick device
- Topical fluoride applications and dental sealants
- Adjustments in daily diabetes regimen for dental appointments or procedures (e.g., fasting, changes in insulin or diet prior to oral surgery, soft or liquid diet after a procedure)

Salivary Dysfunction and Xerostomia

Patients with type 2 diabetes show reduced salivary uptake and excretion (4), and they lack the protective components of saliva that help reduce oral bacteria. During episodes of hyperglycemia, glucose levels in the saliva can increase, providing a medium for bacterial growth. The resulting infection further increases glucose levels, and a vicious cycle of infection and hyperglycemia may ensue.

Xerostomia, or dry mouth, may be related to salivary dysfunction, polydipsia, changes in the salivary basement membranes, or the dehydration associated with hyperglycemia. Diuretics, antihistamines, and antidepressants can also affect salivation and aggravate xerostomia.

Patients with xerostomia may experience difficulties in lubricating, masticating, tasting, and swallowing, which can impair nutritional intake and further affect glycemic control. Complications resulting from xerostomia include mucositis, ulcers, and desquamation, as well as opportunistic bacterial, viral, or fungal infections (5). Improvement in glycemic control may alleviate dry mouth and prevent further oral health problems.

Oral Mucosal Diseases

Oral mucosal diseases occur more frequently in patients with diabetes, perhaps as the result of chronic immunosuppression or acute hyperglycemia. Optimizing glycemic control is the key to prevention and treatment for each of these diseases.

Candidiasis. Fungal infections such as candidiasis are common in individuals with diabetes, particularly smokers with inadequately controlled glucose levels or patients who have dentures or other mouth appliances. Because candidiasis thrives in a warm, moist environment, denture wearers who have diabetes need to remove and clean their dentures daily to maintain healthy gums and oral membranes. Some indicated medications are fluconazole and nystatin.

Lichen planus. Lichen planus, a chronic mucocutaneous disease, appears to be an immunologically mediated process involving a hypersensitivity reaction at a microscopic level. The lesions associated with lichen planus can contain increased numbers of CD4, CD8, macrophages, dendritic cells, and other immune-regulating cells. Because the corticosteroids and immunomodulating drugs used to treat this condition can lead to hyperglycemia, diabetes therapy must be carefully regulated to reduce glucose levels that can inhibit the healing process.

Angular cheilitis. Angular cheilitis, a lesion that occurs at the outer corners of the mouth, is commonly associated with fungal infections. It is treated with an antifungal cream or an antifungal-steroid preparation applied to the area three to four times a day for 2 weeks. Again, improved glucose levels can help promote healing.

Burning mouth syndrome. Patients with burning mouth syndrome may complain of tongue or mucosal sensations when no lesion is present. Suboptimal glucose control, salivary dysfunction, candidiasis, and neurological abnormalities may all contribute to the syndrome. Treatment may include prescribing salivary substitutes or using benzodiazepine or tricyclic antidepressant therapy to reduce the burning sensation. Patients who decrease their alcohol and caffeine intake may also find relief. Interestingly, burning mouth syndrome has been found in patients with undiagnosed diabetes. When diabetes is diagnosed and glucose control achieved, the symptoms of burning mouth syndrome resolve.

Oral ulcers. Oral ulcers, whether the benign aphthous ulcers or the potentially fatal palatal ulcers, occur more frequently in the diabetic population and must be treated with care. Because individuals with diabetes tend to develop more severe infections, oral ulcers require aggressive management and evaluation by a dental professional.

Periodontal Disease

The prevalence of periodontitis in patients with diabetes is 17% compared with 9% in the nondiabetic population (6). The rate increases dramatically among smokers with diabetes, who are 20 times more likely to develop periodontitis with loss of supporting bone than individuals without diabetes (7). The incidence and severity of periodontal disease increase with inadequate glucose control, age, and duration of disease. Patients with inadequate glycemic control of either type 1 or type 2 diabetes have more interproximal loss of connective tissue attachment and alveolar bone loss than patients with well-controlled diabetes. Many factors contribute to the difficulty in preventing and treating periodontal disease in individuals with diabetes (Table 12.1).

Immune response. Although severe periodontal disease is related to increased plaque or calculus, other mechanisms may also play a role in the development of the disease (8). The presence of diabetes can activate a protective humoral immune response. Smoking and/or the presence of diabetes can alter neutrophil function, lowering the protective response and placing the patient at greater risk for infection. Impairment of the polymorphonuclear leukocyte also leaves the patient with a reduced defense against gram-negative microbial infection. Any defect in the function of the polymorphonuclear leukocyte may mean a shift in the balance between destruction and repair in the initiation or progression of periodontal disease (8).

Collagen formation. Hyperglycemia reduces the growth of the fibroblast, an essential element in the building of collagen for the peridontium. A fine balance

---

Table 12.1 Physiological Problems in the Patient with Diabetes that Make Treating Periodontal Disease Difficult

Increased susceptibility to infection
Impaired wound-healing ability
Magnified inflammatory response
Vascular changes
  Inhibition of vasodilation
  Vasoconstriction
  Accelerated atherosclerosis
  Focal thrombosis
Neuropathies from accelerated connective tissue damage
Gingival changes compromising periodontal integrity

From Hein (6).

between destruction and repair of the periodontal tissue already exists; therefore, any element that decreases collagen formation will result in a loss of tissue turnover and will ultimately affect periodontal integrity. Patients with diabetes have an alteration in collagen metabolism and suppressed white blood cell function. Together, these factors increase susceptibility to periodontal infection and reduce healing.

Patients with diabetes may also have an increased level of collagenase, an enzyme that, when activated, can lead to the loss of connective tissue attachment. The decreased formation of collagen and the increased production of collagenase alter the homeostasis within the periodontal tissues (9). This is commonly manifested by "loose teeth," which limits the patient's ability to properly chew food. Once this connective tissue attachment is lost, it cannot be regenerated and usually leads to multiple tooth extractions.

Wound healing and recovery time. Advanced glycosylation end products (AGEs), the result of prolonged hyperglycemia, may alter wound healing and contribute to the severity of periodontal disease. AGEs can change the solubility of collagen and alter its turnover rate. Not only do AGEs bind to phagocytes, initiating an inflammatory response to the bacteria present in the mouth, but they can also activate collagenase. AGEs may also cause a thickening of the basement membrane of blood vessels, which further compromises the wound healing process by inhibiting the activation or exchange of nutrition, oxygen, and various antibodies (9).

Glucose control affects recovery time after treatment of periodontal disease. In one study, patients with well-controlled diabetes had an uneventful recovery, whereas those with inadequately controlled diabetes did well initially but had a more rapid reoccurrence of pockets and a less favorable prognosis (10). Sustaining long-term metabolic control in patients with diabetes is necessary to ensure periodontal health (11). A collaborative effort between dental health providers and the diabetes care team is essential in achieving positive outcomes in periodontal care.

Treatment. In some patients, undiagnosed periodontal disease may disrupt glucose control and increase A1C values. Periodontitis-induced bacteremia may elevate serum proinflammatory cytokines, leading to hyperlipidemia and furthering insulin resistance. Treatment of the dental problem is important to improve glycemic control (12).

PRACTICAL POINT

Advanced periodontitis can present with diffuse gingival inflammation and generalized bleeding of the gum tissue on examination. Patients may complain of "tender gums" that bleed whenever they brush their teeth. This discomfort may lead to increased reluctance to pursue oral hygiene. During treatment for periodontitis, patients must follow specific hygienic measures: use of an automatic toothbrush, interdental cleaning, irrigation with a water pick, and mild abrasive dentifrices (6). Patients with periodontitis will also need more frequent checkups.

Antibiotics, particularly tetracycline and doxycycline, have been prescribed for periodontitis. These drugs seem to reduce the formation of collagenase and/or inhibit the degradation of collagen. They are used with mechanical therapy and may help reduce glucose levels by controlling the infection. Mechanical therapy alone does not completely eliminate periodontal disease when the organisms have invaded connective tissue (6). Chronic gram-negative periodontal infection triggers and sustains systemic inflammation (13).

DENTAL VISITS

To prevent hypoglycemic episodes during the dental examination, the patient must have proper food intake before the appointment. However, some procedures, such as conscious sedation, may require the patient to withhold food for a period of time before or after the procedure (14). In these cases, a reduction in the amount of medication or insulin may be necessary. To avoid hypoglycemia, patients should not schedule the dental appointment during the hours of peak insulin activity or at a usual mealtime. If a hypoglycemic event occurs, the dental procedure should be stopped and 15 g carbohydrate administered. Glucose tabs or gel are often the quickest and easiest form of treatment, and if they do not already do so, patients should be advised to carry emergency carbohydrate.

Certain dental surgeries should not be done during episodes of severe hyperglycemia because of the risk of infection and poor wound healing. One study showed that the risk of infection was linked to fasting glucose level (15). Patients with levels <206 mg/dl had no increased risk, whereas patients with glucose levels >230 mg/dl had an 80% risk of developing infection.

MANAGING DENTAL IMPLANTS

Inadequate glycemic control can hinder the success of dental implant procedures. Diabetes-related inhibition of collagen matrix formation and alterations in protein synthesis can affect bone production and repair. Insulin helps modulate normal skeletal growth by stimulating bone matrix synthesis. Through direct and indirect processes, insulin can alter bone turnover rates, decrease the number of osteoblasts and osteoclasts, and reduce osteocalcin. Changes in bone metabolism, the association of AGEs with extracellular matrix components, and level of glucose control may influence osseointegration and reduce the percentage of bone-to-implant contact (16).

PRACTICAL POINT

The timing of a patient's dental visit may affect the daily diabetes treatment program. Nurses may need to counsel patients about changes in food or medication schedules as determined by the procedure to be done and the length of recovery. Blood glucose checks should be done before the dental visit and after the procedure, and action should be taken to correct levels outside of the acceptable range for control.

The 1998 National Institutes of Health Consensus Development Conference Statement on Dental Implants underlines the importance of glucose control in patients seeking dental implants (17). Patients with inadequately controlled diabetes should not be considered candidates for these procedures. A careful preoperative assessment must determine that a patient has no contraindications, but at present there are no established guidelines for selecting candidates for dental implants in the diabetic population. A risk factor analysis for implant loss looks at a variety of issues: type of diabetes, duration of disease, diabetes treatment program, current and previous glycemic control, history of periodontitis and amount of tooth loss, smoking history, and poor wound-healing history.

In the initial evaluation, some dental centers perform a complete blood cell count, fasting glucose, A1C, prothrombin, and partial thromboplastin times. If metabolic control is clinically inadequate, the implant procedure is delayed until glucose levels are within the set parameters. To reduce the risk of infection, a 10-day regimen of a broad-spectrum antibiotic may be prescribed and initiated the day before the procedure (18).

Postoperatively, high circulating levels of glucose reduce wound healing and increase rates of infection, compromising the success of the implant procedure. Strict glucose control and meticulous oral hygiene are vital components of post-procedure care. During this time, patients are encouraged to stop smoking to reduce the risk of implant failure.

SUMMARY

Dental care needs to figure more prominently in the standards for periodic examinations and continuing care of people with diabetes. Just as nurses guide and encourage patients to have routine foot and eye examinations, they must also promote dental checkups as an important component of diabetes management. To help patients make this goal a reality, financial support for dental care must be more readily available to both the general population and individuals with chronic illness. As patient advocates, nurses must help payers to see the importance of dental health in preserving health and function in individuals with diabetes.

REFERENCES

1. Centers for Disease Control and Prevention: *The Prevention and Treatment of Complications of Diabetes, 1991.* Atlanta, GA, U.S. Department of Health and Human Services, Public Health Service, 1991
2. Tomar SL, Lester A: Dental and other health care visits among U.S. adults with diabetes. *Diabetes Care* 23:1505–1510, 2000
3. Pinson M, Hoffman WH, Garnick JJ, Litaker MS: Periodontal disease and type 1 diabetes mellitus in children and adolescents. *J Clin Periodontol* 22:118–123, 1995
4. Kao CH, Tsai SC, Sun SS: Scintigraphic evidence of poor salivary function in type 2 diabetes. *Diabetes Care* 24:952–953, 2001
5. Vernillo AT: Diabetes mellitus: relevance to dental treatment. *Oral Surg Oral Med Oral Pathol Oral Radiol Endod* 91:263–270, 2001
6. Hein C: "Getting it right" in long-term management of chronic periodontitis associated with diabetes, part 1. *Contemporary Oral Hygiene* 3:24–31, 2003
7. Haber J, Wattles J, Crowley M, Mandell R, Joshipura K, Kent RL: Evidence for cigarette smoking as a major risk factor for periodontal disease. *J Periodontol* 64:16–23, 1993

8. Ryan ME, Oana C, Kamer A: The influence of diabetes on the periodontal tissues. *J Am Dent Assoc* 143 (Suppl.):34s–40s, 2003

9. Mattson JS, Cerutis DR: Diabetes mellitus: a review of the literature and dental implications. *Compendium* 22:757–772, 2001

10. Tervonen T, Karjalainen K: Periodontal disease related to diabetics' status: a pilot study of the response to periodontal therapy in type 1 diabetes. *J Clin Periodontol* 24:505–510, 1997

11. Oringer RJ, Research, Science, and Therapy Committee of the American Academy of Periodontology: Modulation of the host response in periodontal therapy. *J Periodontol* 73:460–470, 2002

12. Iacopino AM: Periodontitis and diabetes interrelationships: role of inflammation. *Ann Periodontol* 6:125–137, 2001

13. Grossi SG: Treatment of periodontal disease and control of diabetes: an assessment of the evidence and need for future research. *Ann Periodontol* 6:138–145, 2001

14. Lalla RV, D'Ambrosio JA: Dental management considerations for the patient with diabetes mellitus. *J Am Dent Assoc* 132:1425–1432, 2001

15. Golden SH, Peart-Vigilance C, Kao WH, Brancati FL: Perioperative glycemic control and the risk of infectious complications in a cohort of adults with diabetes. *Diabetes Care* 22:1408–1414, 1999

16. Fiorellini JP, Nevins ML: Dental implant considerations in the diabetic patient. *Periodontol* 23:73–77, 2000

17. National Institutes of Health Consensus Development: Conference statement on dental implants June 13–15, 1998. *J Dent Educ* 52:824–827, 1998

18. Abdulwassie H, Dhanrajani PJ: Diabetes mellitus and dental implants: a clinical study. *Implant Dentistry* 11:83–85, 2002

*Ms. Spollett is an Adult Nurse Practitioner at Yale Diabetes Center, New Haven, CT.
Dr. Crape has a private practice in Milford, CT.*

13. Dermatological Changes Associated with Diabetes

GERALYN SPOLLETT, MSN, C-ANP, CDE

Just as diabetes interferes with the physiology of the microvasculature of the eye and kidney, the small vessels of the skin are similarly affected, which may lead to skin changes (1). Dyslipidemia and other metabolic changes associated with diabetes can also create dermatological changes. Autoimmune skin diseases such as vitiligo can occur in autoimmune, or type 1, diabetes. In rare cases, medications that are used in the treatment of diabetes can cause adverse skin reactions. In general, how the disruption of normal insulin and glucose metabolism affects the skin is not completely understood (1).

NECROBIOSIS LIPOIDICA DIABETICORUM

Necrobiosis lipoidica diabeticorum (NLD), one of the least common diabetic lesions, has no known etiology (Fig. 13.1). In general, this type of lesion is seen in individuals with diabetes of long duration, but its progression seems to have little to do with glucose control (1). NLD occurs in 0.3–1.6% of individuals with diabetes and is three times more common in women than in men (2). When the lesion occurs in people who do not have diabetes, many of these patients (~90%) go on to develop impaired glucose tolerance or have a family history of diabetes (3). Therefore, screening for diabetes in these individuals is highly recommended.

The NLD lesion progresses through a series of changes, beginning as a shiny, demarcated dusky pink plaque that is slightly elevated. Size varies from 1 to 3 cm to ~25 cm, and over time, it becomes redder and can take on a brownish tinge. As the weeks and months progress, it becomes atrophic, with a thin, shiny, slightly pigmented appearance. The center may have a yellowish tinge, indicating a loss of collagen or severe thinning of the skin, making the subcutaneous fat visible. The lesion may initially present as a series of closely grouped small plaques that coalesce into a larger plaque over time. Usually, the lesions are not painful but may be pruritic or tender (4). With thinning, the plaque becomes susceptible to ulceration, and the most minor trauma can cause a rupture. The resulting ulcers are painful and very difficult to heal. Approximately 20% of NLD lesions will resolve spontaneously after 6–12 years (5).

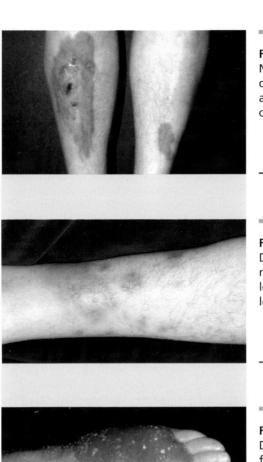

FIGURE 13.1
Necrobiosis lipoidica diabeticorum. Yellow tinge at the center of the lesion is caused by a lack of collagen.

FIGURE 13.2
Diabetic dermopathy. The most common dermatologic lesion usually seen on the lower extremities.

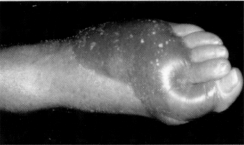

FIGURE 13.3
Diabetic bullae. Large fluid-filled sacs usually found on the hands are a marker for diabetes.

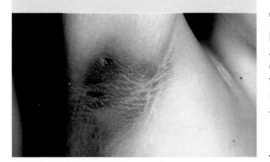

FIGURE 13.4
Acanthosis nigricans. The dark, velvety appearance of this condition is usually seen in the skin folds of the neck and axillae.

Classically, NLD occurs bilaterally on the pretibial or medial malleolar areas. Lesions can also present on the hands, forearms, abdomen, face, and scalp, but these locations are less associated with diabetes.

There are no standard guidelines for the treatment of NLD. Middle- to high-potency topical steroids with or without occlusion, intralesional injections of steroids at the active border, and, in some instances, systemic steroids have been used in the treatment of NLD (6). Other treatments such as cyclosporine, psoralen and ultraviolet A light (PUVA), high-dose nicotinamide, clofazimine, pentoxifylline, aspirin, and dipyridamole have been tried with varying rates of success (2). Laser treatment may help reduce bleeding and improve the appearance of the lesion (7). In severe cases, synthetic hydrocolloid dressings have given symptomatic relief. Specialized wound care clinics are best equipped to treat the ulcerated lesions and may use artificial skin substitutes in an attempt to resurface these areas.

GRANULOMA ANNULARE

Although granuloma annulare (GA) is not associated with diabetes, lesion presentation is so similar to NLD that a connection between GA and diabetes has been sought. The initial presentation is small, flesh-colored papule(s) that progress to one larger plaque. The dermal plaques have a ring border and a depressed center. The lesions may be pruritic but are not painful. Histological testing shows collagen degeneration, chronic inflammation, and fibrosis (6). Commonly, lesions appear over the extensor joint areas in children and young adults and may be more generally distributed in middle-aged to older adults. In its more generalized form, plaques are smaller, and hundreds of small lesions may be present. Controversy exists concerning the association of diabetes with this generalized form of GA. At this time, screening for diabetes is recommended for individuals with this form of GA.

Treatment for GA is similar to NLD: topical, intralesional, and general steroid use. Localized GA remits spontaneously without scarring, but the more generalized version has a longer course with rare spontaneous resolution (2). The duration is variable; 50% of patients are without lesions within 2 years, but 40% can experience reoccurrence at the same site (6).

DIABETIC DERMOPATHY

Diabetic dermopathy, also known as shin spots or pigmented pretibial papules, is by far the most common cutaneous manifestation of diabetes (Fig. 13.2). Although it can be present in individuals without diabetes, it is found in as many as 70% of people with diabetes. It occurs more frequently in men aged >50 years (2).

The pigmented shin spots, usually seen on the extensor surfaces of the lower legs, begin as round or oval red papules that progress to atrophic hyperpigmented macules. A fine scale over the surface of the macule is sometimes seen. The lesions are usually bilateral but have an asymmetric distribution. They may also appear on the forearms, thighs, and lateral malleoli (2). Histological findings indicate edema of the papillary dermis, thickened superficial blood vessels, extravasation of erythrocytes, and a mild lymphocytic infiltrate (8). Diabetic dermopathy differs from NLD in that the collagen change is much less marked and necrobiosis is absent (9). The lesions of diabetic dermopathy are asymptomatic.

Although some studies link diabetic dermopathy with the microvascular complications of diabetes, other studies have been unable to substantiate these findings.

Capillary changes may predispose to shin spots but are not the only cause of this condition (2). Blood glucose control is unrelated to the occurrence or progression of the problem, and there is no effective treatment for these lesions. New lesions appear while old lesions spontaneously heal and leave small scars in their place.

DIABETIC BULLAE

Diabetic bullae, also known as bullosis diabeticorum, are a clinically distinct marker for diabetes (Fig. 13.3) that are often reported in adults with diabetes of long duration and neuropathy. Usually confined to the hands and feet, the blisters occur spontaneously and can be a few millimeters to several centimeters in size.

There are three types of diabetic bullae: *1*) sterile and fluid filled, *2*) hemorrhagic, and *3*) multiple, nonscarring bullae on tanned skin. Of these, only the hemorrhagic type leaves scarring. The bullae resolve spontaneously without treatment in 2–3 weeks but may reoccur in the same or a different anatomical place.

Preventing infection is a major focus in caring for these lesions. Thorough cleaning, topical antibiotics, and clean dressings on a daily basis will reduce the occurrence of infection. The bullae fluid can be aspirated, but the blister roof should be preserved and used as a physiological cover for the wound.

ACANTHOSIS NIGRICANS

Acanthosis nigricans (AN) is characterized by velvety, light brown to black hyperpigmented plaques that appear in the folds of the skin (Fig. 13.4). The thickened skin is most commonly seen around the neck and axillae. Other affected areas include the groin, umbilicus, submammary regions, and hands. It initially presents with hyperpigmentation, which is then followed by a hypertrophy of the epidermis (8).

Although there are eight different forms of AN, the one most commonly seen in diabetes is associated with insulin resistance and obesity. The pathogenesis may be related to insulin-like growth factor receptors on the keratinocytes and dermal fibroblasts, stimulating growth (2). The dark color of these plaques is related to the thickness of the keratin-containing superficial epithelium. AN has been linked to impaired glucose tolerance in younger patients and, as a marker, can serve to alert providers to screen the patient for diabetes. Certain forms of AN are associated with carcinoma (stomach adenocarcinoma) and various endocrinopathies. The sudden appearance of AN after the age of 40 years is an ominous sign. When malignancy is present, the lesion develops suddenly and progresses rapidly. Despite a strong association with diabetes, all AN lesions warrant a workup to rule out underlying causes, the most common of which are pineal tumors, occult malignancies, stomach adenocarcinoma, and drug use (nicotinic acid, estrogen, corticosteroids) (6).

Lesions are usually asymptomatic. Although there is no specific treatment for AN related to diabetes, weight loss and improvement in glucose control, with a lowering of insulin resistance, can improve the condition. Retinoic and salicylic acid may help cosmetic appearance.

DIABETIC THICK SKIN

Diabetic thick skin has been reported in as many as 33% of individuals with diabetes (1) and has been divided into three categories: *1*) scleroderma-like changes of the hand associated with stiff joints and limited mobility, *2*) measurable skin thickness, and *3*) scleredema diabeticorum. The etiology of diabetic thick skin is not fully known. The skin has abnormal collagen accumulation that may be related to hyperglycemic accelerated nonenzymatic glycosylation. A second theory identifies insulin, acting as a growth factor, as causing an overproduction and buildup of collagen.

Tiny pebble-like papules that become confluent appear on the back of the hand, the knuckles, and along the fingernails. Patients may report difficulty completely extending fingers, and slight contractures of the palmar surface (Dupuytren's contracture) may be seen.

Diabetic scleredema (Fig. 13.5) is characterized by diffuse nonpitting induration of the skin with the loss of skin markings over the upper back, neck, and shoulders (2). It can extend to the face, arms, chest, and abdomen. The condition is usually asymptomatic, but the lack of skin flexibility may cause neck and back discomfort. Scleredema occurs in 2.5–14% of individuals with type 2 diabetes.

Improved glucose control and use of potent topical and intralesional steroids, penicillamine, intralesional insulin, bath PUVA, low-dose methotrexate, prostaglandin E1, and pentoxifylline have had limited therapeutic success in the treatment of scleredema (2).

XANTHOMA

Xanthomas usually appear as a consequence of hyperlipidemia, particularly hypertriglyceridemia associated with diabetes (Fig. 13.6). Triglyceride levels are often >800 mg/dl and may exceed 1,500 or 2,000 mg/dl (1). Cutaneous xanthomas are a result of an extracellular deposition of lipid in the form of cholesterol or triglycerides in the dermis or subcutaneous fat (4). Biopsy of the xanthomas will show lipid-laden macrophages in the mid-dermis. The eruptive lesions develop suddenly over the extensor surfaces of the arms, legs, and buttocks, originally as red papules but subsequently changing to yellow. The lesion may remain as scattered individual papules or may cluster and form a "rosette."

Diabetes and lipid control play key roles in the resolution of the lesions. If the patient is insulin depleted, as in diabetic ketoacidosis, a rapid correction of glucose levels will lead to a faster resolution of the lesions. However, if the problem is based on chronically elevated triglycerides, once correction of lipid chemistry is achieved, it may take several weeks before the lesions fully respond.

VITILIGO

Vitiligo, an absence of melanocytes that causes hypopigmentation of the skin, can be seen in patients with autoimmune diseases such as type 1 diabetes, Addison's disease, Hashimoto's thyroiditis, and pernicious anemia (Fig. 13.7). The lymphocytes attack the melanocytes, resulting in chalk-white lesions on the skin that are commonly found over extensor joints such as the elbow and knuckles and around orifices such as the mouth and eye. Although vitiligo can occur in children as well as adults and is found in 0.2–1.0% of the general population, it appears in ~5% of individuals with diabetes (1).

Most patients continue to see new patches of vitiligo throughout their lives. It is not symptomatic but can be disfiguring in darker-skinned people. There is no corrective treatment, but some benefit has been seen with potent topical steroid use.

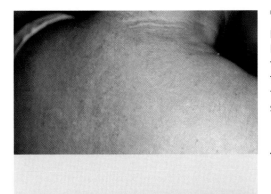

FIGURE 13.5
Diabetic scleredema. The thickened, nonpitting skin of this condition can affect the flexibility of the upper back, shoulders, and neck.

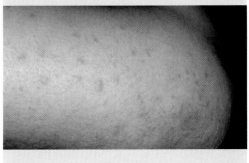

FIGURE 13.6
Xanthomas. This condition can result from elevated cholesterol, particularly hypertriglyceridemia. Note the pearly color of the lesions.

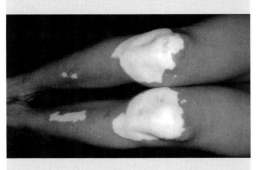

FIGURE 13.7
Vitiligo. Usually associated with autoimmune type 1 diabetes, loss of skin pigment accounts for the white color of this lesion.

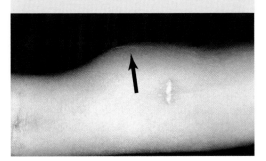

FIGURE 13.8
Lipohypertrophy. Usually appears in an area of repeated insulin injection.

SKIN INFECTION

Skin infections in patients with well-controlled diabetes occur at the same rate and severity as in the general population. However, those with suboptimal glycemic control have more frequent infections that are more severe and difficult to resolve. Approximately 20–50% of those with type 2 diabetes experience a skin infection (3). Elevated glucose levels cause numerous immunological dysfunctions that make the patient more vulnerable to infection and impede the healing process. With hyperglycemia, leukocytes are not able to move through the thickened capillary wall as effectively, phagocytic action is reduced, and chemotaxis is delayed, allowing an infection to worsen. Neuropathy and peripheral vascular disease can mask the symptoms of the infection, permitting it to advance unchecked. The presence of the infection further elevates glucose levels, contributing to the cycle of hyperglycemia and lengthening the recovery process.

Staphylococcal and fungal infections, particularly of the lower extremities, develop more often in patients with diabetes and are more resistant to therapy. For some patients, the skin infections become chronic problems, promoting skin breakdown and placing them at risk for more severe secondary infections.

Candida infections of the vagina, anogenital area, submammary regions, and axillae tend to be recurrent and occur most frequently in obese patients with type 2 diabetes. In men, the folds of the foreskin and coronal rim of the penis are sites for balanitis and phimosis. Difficult to keep clean and dry, these skinfold areas provide the ideal warm, moist environment for dermatophyte growth. The location of the infection makes applying topical antibacterial or antifungal creams an arduous task, and patients may not complete the full course of therapy, allowing some of the infective agent to persist.

If the patient suspects an infection, the health care provider should be notified immediately so that treatment can begin as soon as possible. In the individual with inadequately controlled diabetes, the course of therapy may be longer

---

PRACTICAL POINT

Prevention of skin infections begins with good personal hygiene, i.e., inspecting and washing areas at highest risk for bacterial or fungal growth. The patient may need assistance from a family member or may need to find creative solutions for accessing hard-to-reach areas, such as using a long-handled sponge to wash and a handheld hair dryer (set to low) to dry the area or a squirt bottle with warm water to help cleanse the anogenital area.

PRACTICAL POINT

Since many patients with neuropathy have impaired sensation, education regarding skin care must emphasize the need to assess the area for changes in color or temperature or the presence of swelling or discharge.

than in the general population, and the patient must understand that to eradicate the infection, the therapy must be used consistently and the course of medication or topical treatment completed.

> When caring for a patient with diabetes, it is important to remember that in areas of reduced blood flow such as the feet, systemic antibiotics used to treat skin infections have difficulty permeating the tissue and their effectiveness is reduced, necessitating a longer time frame for treatment.

Skin infections that involve the lower extremities can have severe consequences. Foot ulcers are a leading causative factor in amputations (8). The podiatric emergency and preventive foot care guidelines are discussed in CHAPTER 15. The importance of these guidelines in preventing foot infection or injuries that lead to infection cannot be overemphasized.

INSULIN ALLERGIES AND SKIN MANIFESTATIONS

Although rare, cutaneous reactions to insulin have been reported, usually as raised, warm, itchy nodules forming at the injection site that appear 15 min to 2 h postinjection. With the production of purified and recombinant insulins, the incidence of insulin allergy has been reduced. In some instances, the skin reaction is not to the insulin itself but to the latex of the vial stopper, the alcohol or cleanser used to prepare the injection site, or an intradermal rather than a subcutaneous injection.

True insulin allergy with systemic response such as urticaria or anaphylaxis is rare. Treatment involves a desensitization program that is generally carried out under medical observation.

Use of purified and recombinant insulin has reduced the occurrence of lipoatrophy, a hollowing of the skin at the injection site. More common is the problem of lipohypertrophy in areas of repeated insulin injections (Fig. 13.8). These large fatty-like deposits in the subcutaneous tissue can be disfiguring but are not physically painful. In fact, patients may continue to inject into the area because the sensation of administering the insulin is blunted. However, the continued use of a hypertrophied area may reduce insulin absorption and interfere with glucose control. Ceasing insulin injections at the hypertrophied site allows the skin to return to its normal state. Hypertrophy is avoided by rotating injection sites within anatomical areas and carefully observing the skin's reaction to injections.

Of the oral agents currently on the market, sulfonylureas are most likely to cause dermatological side effects. The sulfa component of the drug can produce an allergic reaction that usually presents as an uncomfortable "measles-like" maculopapular rash. The most common offenders are the first-generation sulfonylureas such as tolbutamide and chlorpropamide, medications that are rarely used. Occasionally, glyburide, a second-generation drug, has caused urticaria, photosensitivity, erythema, and pruritus; these symptoms disappear with drug discontinuation. Sensitivity to a sulfonylurea may indicate that the patient will react adversely to other sulfa medications. Caution should be used in prescribing any sulfa-containing medication.

SUMMARY

Preventive skin care education that centers on improved hygiene and early assessment and intervention for any suspected skin condition is a key component of nursing care. Many of the lesions associated with diabetes, such as NLD and diabetic bullae, have no prescribed protocol for treatment. The various trials of different forms of treatment, the consistent daily attention that the care of these lesions requires, and the long duration of the self-care process can be a heavy burden for the patient. Supportive nursing care and education enable the patient to understand the condition and be alert for any signs or symptoms of secondary infection.

In other skin conditions, such as xanthomas and injection site hypertrophy, addressing and treating the underlying cause is an essential component of care. For xanthomas, improved glucose control and lipid management must be achieved for resolution of the lesions to occur. In hypertrophy, patient education regarding insulin injection site rotation and its importance in both skin care and glucose control is central to the plan of care.

In AN, the nurse must realize that not all cases are related to diabetes and that sudden appearance and rapid progression of the lesion may indicate a life-threatening medical condition. Noting changes in size and texture of AN lesions and documenting them provides vital information for future assessment and analysis.

Patients with diabetes are just as susceptible to skin cancer as the general population. However, sunburns not only increase the risk of carcinoma, but they can also cause the breakdown of fragile skin, leading to infection, hyperglycemia, and a disruption of glucose control. The patient must be educated in sun protection guidelines to avoid these negative consequences.

REFERENCES

1. Reeves JRT: Skin changes associated with diabetes. In *Medical Management of Diabetes Mellitus.* Leahy JL, Clark NG, Cefalu WT, Eds. New York, Marcel Dekker, 2000, p. 539–558
2. Ferringer T, Miller OF: Cutaneous manifestations of diabetes mellitus. *Derm Clin North Am* 20:483–493, 2002
3. Paron NG, Lambert PW: Cutaneous manifestations of diabetes mellitus. *Prim Care* 27:371–383, 2000
4. Jelinek JE: Cutaneous markers of diabetes mellitus. In *The Skin in Diabetes.* Jelinek JE, Ed. Philadelphia, Lea and Febiger, 1986, p. 31–72
5. Sibbald RG, Landolt SJ, Toth D: Skin and diabetes. *Endocrinol Metab Clin North Am* 25:463–472, 1996
6. Habif TP, Campbell JL, Quitadamo MJ, Zug KA: Cutaneous manifestations of internal disease. In *Skin Diseases: Diagnosis and Treatment.* St. Louis, MO, Mosby, 2001, p. 458–471
7. Bello YM, Phillips TJ: Necrobiosis lipoidica. *Postgrad Med* 109:93–94, 2001
8. Chakrabarty A, Norman RA, Phillips TJ: Cutaneous manifestations of diabetes. *Wounds* 14:267–274, 2002
9. Sibbald RG, Schachter RK: The skin and diabetes mellitus. *Int J Dermatol* 23:567–584, 1984

Ms. Spollett is an Adult Nurse Practitioner at Yale Diabetes Center, New Haven, CT.

14. Peripheral and Autonomic Neuropathy

Wendy Kushion, RN, MSN, APRN-BC, CDE

Diabetic neuropathy is a chronic disorder that affects both the peripheral nervous system (sensory and motor) and the autonomic nervous system (ANS). It is the most common of all of the long-term complications and the least understood. Neuropathy usually has a slow progression and may appear with obvious symptoms, sometimes as the presenting symptom of previously undiagnosed diabetes, or it may be hidden and discovered only by careful testing. Symptoms of peripheral neuropathy (PN) often start with numbness and paresthesia in the toes and feet and later in the fingers and hands. Autonomic neuropathy affects innervation to all of the organs of the body and can cause dysfunction in any body part (1,2).

The precise pathogenesis of neuropathy in diabetes is unknown. Chronic hyperglycemia, insulin deficiency, nerve ischemia, microvascular disease, and nonenzymatic glycation have been suggested as the major causative factors in the development of neuropathy (2–4). Chronic hyperglycemia has historically been blamed and is reported to cause oxidative stress, which may cause nerve injury (5). Neuropathy may be present at the time of diagnosis or take years before symptoms arise. Most people with diabetes will develop symptoms of neuropathy over time, and these can cause minor to extreme physical symptoms.

PERIPHERAL NEUROPATHY

PN results from widely distributed lesions throughout the peripheral nerves. Distal symmetric polyneuropathy is the most widely recognized form of PN and the most easily recognized. The deficit is distributed over all sensorimotor nerves and starts in the most distal areas first, usually the toes and feet. PN usually begins with an early involvement of the long axons in the peripheral nerves, which is the characteristic lesion of neuropathy. Height plays a role because the longer the nerve fiber, the greater its vulnerability to injury (3,4).

Classes of PN are usually grouped into "diffuse" or "focal" types. Diffuse neuropathies include distal symmetric polyneuropathy and autonomic neuropathy. Focal neuropathies involve single or multiple peripheral nerves and are categorized as mononeuropathy, radiculopathy, or entrapment neuropathy.

Signs and Symptoms of Peripheral Neuropathy

- Pain and numbness
- "Glove and stocking" sensory loss
- Diminished deep tendon reflexes
- Diminished sense of position and light touch sensation
- Numbness, tingling, or feeling of cold feet
- Diminished or increased pain and temperature sensation
- Motor weakness
- Impaired balance
- Diminished proprioception and position sense
- Absent or reduced vibration sensation
- Ataxia
- Increased cutaneous hypersensitivity
- Extreme pain
- Distal muscle cramps
- Cranial nerve palsy
- Carpal tunnel and tarsal tunnel syndrome

Distal Symmetrical Polyneuropathy

This most common diffuse neuropathy begins in the toes and moves up the legs, causing a "stocking" pattern of sensory loss, with later upper-extremity "glove" sensory loss in the fingers and moving up the arms. Sensory deficits are more noticeable and common than motor deficits. Small-fiber sensory neurons are affected first, with loss of pain and temperature sensation. Large sensory fiber loss later occurs, with a loss of vibratory and light touch sensation, proprioception, and then gait and balance deficits. A diminished Achilles tendon reflex is also an early symptom (2,4,6). Motor weakness can occur in PN and appears as wasting of the small muscles of the hands and feet.

Testing. Testing includes a clinical assessment of sensitivity to light touch, position, Achilles tendon reflex, vibratory sensation (tuning fork), and sensation using a 10-g monofilament (see also CHAPTER 15). A thorough history of all symptoms and duration is essential to determine the extent of neuropathy. Nerve function tests may include quantitative sensory tests, nerve conduction studies, and electromyography. These tests evaluate the evidence of the specific sensory or motor nerve problem, its distribution and severity, and the underlying pathology (6).

Treatment. The initial and most effective treatment of PN is intensive glycemic control. The Diabetes Control and Complications Trial demonstrated that intensive insulin therapy decreases the development and progression of PN and may even reverse it (7). Alcohol use and cigarette smoking can also affect painful neuropathy, and patients should be advised to discontinue both. Pain management may include all forms of analgesics, including acetaminophen, nonsteroidal anti-inflammatory medications, and narcotics. Narcotics are typically avoided because of the risk of dependence. Tricyclic antidepressants may help with pain as well as insomnia, a frequent disturbance due to increased pain at night. Gabapentin has been demonstrated to be an effective treatment for painful PN but should be monitored closely because high doses can cause dizziness, lethargy, and supine hypertension. The dosage of gabapentin can vary widely (200–800 mg t.i.d.). The main treatment goal is the titration of medication to achieve efficacy with as few side effects as possible. Topical agents such as capsaicin, a derivative of hot peppers, have been shown to be effective by releasing substance P from local nerve endings (7). Recent new medications include duloxetine.

There is also evidence that α-lipoic acid and γ-linoleic acid can improve the sensory symptoms of diabetic polyneuropathy. α-Lipoic acid is a potent antioxidant and can be given both orally and intravenously. It has been used effectively in Germany for years and has been shown in international randomized controlled trials to effectively treat painful diabetic neuropathy (8,9). γ-Linoleic acid is a fatty acid found in evening primrose oil and has also been used to treat diabetic neuropathy. γ-Linoleic acid may improve problems with nerve membrane structure, impulse conduction, and nerve blood flow at doses of 360–480 mg/day (10). Although both of these acids have shown benefit in relieving the painful symptoms of diabetic neuropathy, further investigation is needed. For chronic unrelieved pain, referral to a pain management team may be appropriate.

Acute Painful Neuropathy

The main symptoms of this diffuse small-fiber neuropathy are pain and paresthesia. These symptoms are worse at night and are found in the feet more often than in the hands. The pain can be intense and is described as burning, stabbing, and a deep aching sensation. This form of neuropathy is more common in men and often subsides spontaneously but can also persist indefinitely and be debilitating, although the latter is rare (4).

Neuropathic Foot Ulcer

Trauma and damage to the foot can occur in distal symmetrical polyneuropathy because of the loss of sensitivity to pain, decreased proprioception, loss of muscle, and vascular changes. Because of the loss of feeling in the foot and repetitive trauma, ulceration can occur. The metatarsal heads are the most common sites, but ulcers can form in other areas of pressure. In the absence of pain, calluses form over the metatarsal areas and become thickened. The overlying skin breaks down, ulceration occurs, and the foot may become infected. Treatment should be prophylactic and include foot care education and identifying abnormal foot shape and weight bearing. However, once ulcers occur, treatment includes mechanical measures to reduce (or eliminate) improper weight bearing and fitting the patient with appropriate shoes. Debridement may be necessary to remove excess callus formation, and antibiotics will be needed if infection is present.

Charcot's Joints

Neuropathic arthropathy, or Charcot's joints, occurs with impaired pain recognition and proprioception but without motor loss. A picture is available on page 168 in CHAPTER 15. The foot appears swollen and red, with a flattened arch, and is usually painless and warm. The gait becomes abnormal, and repeated trauma occurs as a result. On X-ray examination, there may be multiple fractures, osteopenia, bone lysis, and osteomyelitis. The pulses often are strong and bounding, but these pulses are due to the shunting of blood and may lead to more problems such as excessive bone resorption and fractures. A podiatric or orthopedic referral is always necessary for the management of Charcot's joint and should be initiated as soon as possible to reduce foot disfiguration. Any symptoms of a red and hot foot in individuals with diabetes should be referred for an x-ray and assessment of Charcot joint.

Treatment. Treatment consists of reducing or eliminating weight bearing and preventing further structural damage. Antibiotics are needed if cellulitis or osteomyelitis is present. As in the treatment of neuropathic ulcers, proper shoes and mechanical devices will be necessary because the shape of the foot is usually grossly abnormal (3,4,6).

Proximal Motor Neuropathy

Proximal motor neuropathy, or diabetic amyotrophy, affects a single or multiple peripheral nerves. It is characterized by severe muscle atrophy in the limb girdle, weight loss, weakness and wasting of lower-extremity muscles, and pain in the thigh muscles, lumbar regions, or perineal regions. This syndrome is uncommon and usually occurs in older adults, the onset is usually acute, and complete or partial recovery occurs.

Cranial Neuropathies

Cranial neuropathies occur frequently, usually in older adults. The onset is abrupt, asymmetrical, and may be either painful or painless. The third cranial nerve is the most commonly affected, and symptoms include sudden headache, ptosis, and eye pain. Femoral and thoracic nerve ischemias can cause hip, thigh, chest, and abdominal pain. Bell's palsy (seventh nerve) can cause facial pain, drooping eyelid, and lacrimation. Recovery usually occurs in 6–8 weeks (4,6).

Radiculopathy

Radiculopathy is a sensory neuropathy (intercostal or truncal) with a dermatomal pain and loss of cutaneous sensation. A single sensory nerve root is affected and is almost always unilateral and asymmetrical with either hyperesthesia or paresthesia. This syndrome may be mistaken for acute abdominal crises, herniated disc, herpes zoster, or spinal cord compression. Spontaneous remission usually occurs within 3–6 months, and pain management will be necessary during that time (4,6).

Entrapment Neuropathies

Entrapment neuropathies (mononeuropathy/multiplex) are isolated peripheral nerve palsies that can cause focal nerve damage at common entrapment sites such as the wrist and palm, upper arm and elbow, or thigh. The risk of developing carpal tunnel syndrome is twice as common in individuals with diabetes. Diagnosis is made by electrodiagnostic studies. Treatment may be conservative, such as immobilization with a splint, or surgical, which is often minor in nature. However, untreated entrapment injuries can often lead to muscle atrophy of the hand and permanent disability.

AUTONOMIC NEUROPATHY

Autonomic neuropathy is a serious form of neuropathy that often goes unrecognized because of its slow onset and confusing symptoms. In patients with PN, 50% have asymptomatic autonomic neuropathy (4). Autonomic control for each organ system is usually divided between opposing sympathetic and parasympathetic systems. Usually, the parasympathetic nerve fibers are affected first, and within 5 years, sympathetic nervous system dysfunction appears. The ANS is a complex entity that consists of a reflex arc that is made up of a sensor, afferent nerve, central nervous system (CNS) component efferent nerve, nerve ending, and effector organ. Because autonomic control of each organ is divided between opposing parasympathetic and sympathetic innervation, a symptom such as tachycardia could be attributed to either a decrease in sympathetic function or an increase in parasympathetic function (6).

The development of autonomic neuropathy is often considered ominous because the mortality rate over a 3- to 5-year period is as high as 50–60% (4,6). Although the involvement of the ANS is often diffuse, symptoms may often be confined to a single organ system (6). The organ systems most often affected by autonomic neuropathy are the cardiovascular system, gastrointestinal tract, genitourinary system, sweat glands, adrenal medulla, and ocular pupil (1).

Abnormal Pupillary Function

Decreased parasympathetic tone produces a smaller-than-normal pupil. This can be diagnosed during a routine eye examination and/or with the aid of a measuring device called a pupillometer. No specific treatment is needed (6).

Gustatory Sweating

Abnormal profuse sweating occurs when eating certain foods, particularly cheese and foods that are spicy. Although this symptom is thought to be of no risk, it

Signs and Symptoms of Autonomic Neuropathy

- Tachycardia
- "Silent" myocardial infarction
- Decreased cardiac exercise performance
- Orthostatic hypotension
- Heat intolerance
- Esophageal dysfunction
- Gastroparesis
- Diarrhea and/or constipation
- Incontinence, urinary tract infections, and impaired bladder sensitivity
- Erectile dysfunction, retrograde ejaculation
- Dyspareunia
- Neurogenic bladder
- Gustatory sweating
- Symmetrical distal anhidrosis
- Hypoglycemia unawareness
- Decreased diameters of the pupils at rest

can be both bothersome and perplexing. Anticholinergic drugs may alleviate symptoms, although this may require a high dose, which can produce unwanted side effects (6).

Bladder Dysfunction

A sensory abnormality of the detrusor muscle is the earliest autonomic symptom to occur and results in impaired bladder sensation. This decreased sensation of bladder fullness and decreased urinary frequency can lead to urinary tract infections. It is the parasympathetic involvement that leads to decreased bladder contractions, causing individuals to have to strain to urinate. Urinary incontinence may also develop (6,7).

Asymptomatic urinary tract infections can occur. Periodic urinalysis is indicated to detect this. Also, symptoms of fever and rapid deterioration of blood glucose control may indicate urinary tract infections even in the absence of dysuria.

Tests of bladder function include postvoiding intravenous pyelogram, postvoiding catheterization, cystometry, sphincter electromyography, uroflometry, urethral pressure profile, and an electrophysiological test of bladder innervation (4,6). A postvoiding residual of >150 ml is diagnostic of abnormal bladder function. Suprapubic dullness to percussion over the bladder area can detect a full asymptomatic neurogenic bladder.

Treatment. Instructing individuals to urinate at least every 3–4 h, even though there may be no feeling of bladder fullness, will help to eliminate urinary tract infections. Medications such as bethanechol may help. Treatment should be aimed at reducing the number of urinary tract infections. If bladder emptying becomes difficult, self-catheterization may be necessary (7).

Erectile Dysfunction

Erectile dysfunction (ED), or impotence, is a frequent and disturbing symptom and may affect at least 50% of all men with diabetes. It is defined as the consistent inability to achieve or maintain an erection that permits intercourse. ED is also characterized by the absence of erections during sleep and early morning. It can be the earliest symptom of autonomic neuropathy (3,6,11). There is no difference in the incidence of ED between patients with type 1 diabetes and those with type 2 diabetes when matched for age (12). The sympathetic nerves mediate both orgasm and ejaculation. The parasympathetic nerves control erectile function. Impotence caused by autonomic neuropathy progresses gradually but may be permanent within 2 years. Changes in the vasculature of the penis may also play a role in sexual dysfunction and will need to be evaluated as well (3).

Diagnosis. Diagnosis is made by a detailed sexual history including rapidity of onset of symptoms and time of day of occurrences. It is important that possible adverse effects of drug therapy (e.g., some antihypertensives, antidepressants, tranquilizers), diseases (e.g., prostate, peripheral vascular), psychological problems, and other physical conditions (e.g., smoking, alcohol) be explored before diagnosing ED as caused by autonomic neuropathy.

Tests. Tests include nocturnal penile tumescence monitoring, which is used to differentiate between organic and psychogenic impotence. Other tests such as nerve conduction, vascular ultrasonography, pressure, and circumference measurements may also be used to obtain a diagnosis (6).

Treatment. Patients prefer to use oral medications for ED (see "Erectile Dysfunction Treatments," a patient handout in RESOURCES). Treatment may include the use of oral medications taken ~0.5–1 h before intercourse (vardenafil, sildenafil, and tadalafil). These medications work by inhibiting phosphodiesterase type 5 (PDE-5), which allows an increase in vasodilation and blood flow, resulting in penile rigidity. The cascade of chemical changes that lead to an erection is initiated during foreplay. Therefore, the PDE-5 inhibitors are only effective once sexual stimulation occurs. Most common side effects include flushing, headache, dyspepsia, and nasal congestion. High-fat-content meals eaten prior to the use of these drugs tend to slow the reaction time. Both vardenafil and sildenafil remain active in the system for ~4 h, and tadalafil can remain active for up to 36 h. Patients should not take the PDE-5 inhibitors more than once in a 24-h period. These drugs should not be prescribed for patients taking nitrate medications.

Papaverin and alprostadil are medicines that are injected into the corpus of the penis, which results in increased blood flow. Alprostadil as an injected medication is considered the "gold standard" by urologists. If an erection cannot be achieved through the injection of alprostadil, then there is little chance of restoring erectile function by any other medications. Alprostadil in pellet form can be placed intra-

---

> **PRACTICAL POINT**
>
> Discuss or initiate discussion of ED to determine whether the condition exists. Often, reluctance on the part of the patient to discuss ED will result in this condition going untreated. It is important to consider psychological factors as a cause. Questions about ability to experience nighttime or early morning erections may also help differentiate between organic and psychogenic ED. Vardenafil and sildenafil may not be used if a patient is using a nitrate, e.g., nitroglycerin.

urethrally and has the same effect.
The duration of the erection is from
0.5 to 2 h.

Mechanical vacuum devices and
surgically implanted penile prostheses
are also methods of treatment but
recently have been used less because
oral medications are more easily used
and are noninvasive (3,6). The vacuum device uses negative pressure to
draw blood into the penis. A ring is
then placed at the base of the penis to
retain the engorgement of the cavernosa. Patients using this device can achieve
satisfactory erections ~75% of the time (13). However, it is cumbersome and very
mechanical, and many men find it psychologically unappealing.

Penile implants have improved markedly over the past few years, and the
mechanical failures formerly associated with their use have been reduced. Infections resulting from the surgically implanted device are still of concern for men
with diabetes.

Female Sexual Dysfunction

The incidence of sexual dysfunction in women is as high as 30%, and the symptoms
are usually decreased vaginal lubrication, vaginal wall atrophy, and dyspareunia
(painful intercourse). The sympathetic nervous system mediates orgasm, whereas the
parasympathetic system affects vaginal lubrication (6).

It is more difficult to diagnose female sexual dysfunction because the symptoms
can be due to hormonal changes of menopause as well as psychogenic. Diagnosis
is made by careful history taking and report of painful intercourse and vaginal dryness. Treatment may include the use of vaginal lubricants and/or estrogen creams.

Cardiac Autonomic Neuropathy

The most frequent symptoms of cardiac autonomic neuropathy (CAN) are resting
tachycardia and postural hypotension. Other notable symptoms are exercise intolerance, painless myocardial infarction (due to cardiac denervation), and heat intolerance. Increased heart rate is due to vagal cardiac neuropathy and may cause
tachycardia to be at a fixed rate. Postural hypotension can be caused by a disturbance in the baroreceptors, which normally control blood pressure during a
change in position. Symptoms may be lightheadedness, syncope, and sudden
death. Cardiac arrest may occur in people with severe CAN, with the greatest
risk occurring during surgery. Parasympathetic cardiac dysfunction is seen first,
followed by sympathetic dysfunction (7,12). The increased frequency of sudden
death in patients with CAN might be attributed to cardiac arrhythmias, silent cardiac ischemia, sleep apnea, and abnormal response to hypoxia (3).

Tests to detect CAN are

- Resting heart rate: >100 bpm
- Beat-to-beat heart rate variation: measures variability of heart rate
- Valsalva maneuver: measures heart rate and peripheral vasoconstriction
  during strain

> **PRACTICAL POINT**
>
> Assess heart rate for tachycardia, blood pressure orthostatic measurements (lying, sitting, and standing), and history of symptoms of lightheadedness, weakness, fatigue, visual blurring, and neck pain. A thorough list of all antihypertensive medications taken and changes in therapy should be noted, especially if new symptoms develop.

- Heart rate response to standing: measures heart rate (tachycardia at beat 15 is normal and bradycardia at beat 30 is normal)
- Systolic blood pressure response to standing: abnormal when blood pressure falls >30 mmHg within the first 2 min of standing
- Diastolic blood pressure rise with sustained exercise: using a hand-gripped meter, the diastolic blood pressure should rise
- QT interval on electrocardiogram: measured according to a normal standard (4,12)

Treatment includes careful management of hypertension medications and steps to improve glycemic control. In treating postural hypotension, wearing elastic support stockings, increasing salt intake, and elevating the head of the bed during sleep have been helpful. Drug therapy may include fludrocortisone, sympathomimetics (e.g., clonidine), and pressor agents.

Gastropathy

Neuropathy of the gastrointestinal (GI) tract may involve any portion of the system from the esophagus to the rectum. It is estimated that as many as 75% of people with type 1 or 2 diabetes have neuropathy of the GI tract (12). Delayed gastric emptying, or gastroparesis, can lead to abnormal absorption of glucose and oral medications. The undigested food may remain in the stomach for hours after a meal (7). The result is suboptimal glucose control with hyperglycemia and/or hypoglycemia depending on the retention of food.

Treatment of this condition is aimed at controlling the potentially debilitating symptoms and improving glycemic control (14). Symptoms of gastropathy include heartburn or dysphagia, gastric esophageal reflux, early satiety, delayed gastric emptying and feelings of fullness, nausea and/or vomiting, constipation, diarrhea and/or incontinence of stool, and anorexia.

Treatment may include exercise, smoking cessation, small frequent meals, achieving excellent glucose control, liquid feedings (which are emptied more easily from the stomach), and avoidance of fatty foods and fiber. A nutritional assessment and counseling with a dietitian to include a calorie count and dietary adjustments may be necessary to ensure adequate intake (15). The following drugs have been shown to be useful as antiemetics and increase action on the smooth muscle to increase the rate of gastric emptying of both solids and liquids: metoclopramide, erythromycin, and domperidome (14,15).

Impaired Hypoglycemic Awareness and Hypoglycemia Unawareness

The response to hypoglycemia in people treated with insulin is mediated by the ANS. Impaired hypoglycemic awareness and hypoglycemia unawareness results in the inability of the person to recognize and treat hypoglycemia, with potential for injury or harm. The counterregulatory response consists of an increase in glucose

PRACTICAL POINT

People with diabetes may not realize that GI symptoms might be related to diabetes. Asking specific questions to reveal this information is important. Topics to discuss to obtain pertinent information include changes in appetite, feelings of fullness, unexplained nausea or vomiting, bloating, heartburn, abdominal cramping or pain, weight loss/gain, and diarrhea or constipation patterns. Because widely fluctuating blood glucose levels may also reveal gastropathy, a careful review of recent glucose control is essential, especially if it has deteriorated without apparent cause.

production from the liver, a decrease in peripheral glucose uptake, and the secretion of glucagon and epinephrine. In individuals with type 1 diabetes, the glucagon response to low blood glucose deteriorates 1–5 years after diagnosis. Epinephrine responses may also decrease with the duration of the disease. The combined absence of glucagon and epinephrine responses decreases counterregulation. The usual signs and symptoms of hypoglycemia (sweating and tachycardia) may be absent but may include confusion, lethargy, amnesia, mental irritability, and seizures (3,6).

Impaired hypoglycemic awareness and hypoglycemic unawareness can occur as a result of very tight blood glucose control and/or frequent episodes of hypoglycemia. It may be necessary to adjust targets for glycemia in order to improve hypoglycemia unawareness. Research suggests that preventing all hypoglycemia for ~3 weeks will allow the individual to regain their hypoglycemia awareness (16). There are now "hypoglycemia awareness" training programs (blood glucose awareness training is described in CHAPTER 17).

SUMMARY

Neuropathy is the most common chronic disorder in diabetes and is both complex and difficult to understand. Diabetes care, education, and management require a thorough assessment of the person's history, symptoms, and limitations. An understanding of the complexity of the various neuropathies is important in caring for and educating the person with these conditions. It is often the nurse who performs

PRACTICAL POINT

Individuals with hypoglycemia unawareness may have difficulty achieving glycemic control, and more frequent blood glucose monitoring is warranted. Situations that would put a person at high risk, such as driving, should not occur without a glucose check. Helping the patient recognize subtle symptoms that may indicate hypoglycemia, such as tingling around the mouth or a decreased ability to concentrate, that should then prompt a glucose check, is a critical component of patient education. Carrying SMBG equipment and portable hypoglycemia treatments at all times, such as glucose gel, juice boxes, or glucose tablets, is essential for safe management of this problem.

the initial assessment, and by knowing the questions to ask and seeking further information, quality care can be achieved for the patient.

REFERENCES

1. Vinik AI: Diagnosing diabetic autonomic neuropathy [Internet], 2004. Available from http://www.medscape.com/viewarticle/473205?src=search. Accessed 4 January 2005
2. Bailes BK: Diabetes mellitus and its chronic complications. *AORN J* 76: 266–276, 278–282 [quiz 283–286], 2002
3. Tarsy D, Freeman R: The nervous system and diabetes. In *Joslin's Diabetes Mellitus*. 13th ed. Kahn CR, Weir GC, Eds. Philadelphia, Lea & Febiger, 1994, p. 794–816
4. Vinik AI, Newlon P, Milicevic Z, McNitt P, Stansberry KB: Diabetic neuropathies: an overview of clinical aspects. In *Diabetes Mellitus: A Fundamental and Clinical Text*. LeRoith D, Taylor SI, Olefsky JM, Eds. Philadelphia, Lippincott-Raven, 1996, p. 737–739, p. 727–751
5. Schmeichel AM, Schmelzer JD, Low PA: Oxidative injury and apoptosis of dorsal root ganglion neurons in chronic experimental diabetic neuropathy. *Diabetes* 52:165–171, 2003
6. Greene DA, Feldman EL, Stevens MJ, Sima AAF, Albers JW, Pfeifer MA: Diabetic neuropathy. In *Ellenberg & Rifkin's Diabetes Mellitus*. 5th ed. Porte D, Sherwin RS, Eds. Stamford, CT, 1997, p. 1009–1074
7. Nathan DM, E Cagliero: Fuel metabolism. In *Endocrinology & Metabolism*. 4th ed. Felig P, Frohman LA, Eds. New York, McGraw-Hill, 2001, p. 827–927
8. Ziegler D, Reljanovic M, Mehnert H, Gries FA: Alpha lipoic acid in the treatment of diabetic polyneuropathy in Germany: current evidence from clinical trials. *Exp Clin Endocrinol Diabetes* 107:421–430, 1999
9. SYDNEY Trial Authors: The sensory symptoms of diabetic polyneuropathy are improved with α-lipoic acid: the SYDNEY trial. *Diabetes Care* 26:770–776, 2003
10. Shane-McWhorter L: Biological complementary therapies: a focus on botanical products in diabetes. *Diabetes Spectrum* 14:199–208, 2001
11. Goldstein I, DeTejeda IS: Erectile dysfunction in diabetes. In *Joslin's Diabetes Mellitus*. 13th ed. Kahn CR, Weir GC, Eds. Philadelphia, Lea & Febiger, 1994, p. 852–866
12. Unger RH, Foster DW: Diabetes mellitus. In *Williams Textbook of Endocrinology*. 9th ed. Wilson JD, Foster DW, Kronenberg HM, Larsen PR, Eds. Philadelphia, W. B. Saunders Company, 1998, p. 973–1060
13. Snow KJ, Guay A: Erectile dysfunction in diabetes mellitus. In *Medical Management of Diabetes Mellitus*. Leahy JL, Clark NG, Cefalu WT, Eds. New York, Marcel Dekker, 2000, p. 427–442
14. Bernstein G: The diabetic stomach: management strategies for clinicians and patients. *Diabetes Spectrum* 13:11–15, 2000
15. May RJ, Goyal RK: Effects of diabetes mellitus on the digestive system. In *Joslin's Diabetes Mellitus*. 13th ed. Kahn CR, Weir GC, Eds. Philadelphia, Lea & Febiger, 1994, p. 921–954
16. Cryer PE, Childs B: Negotiating the barrier to hypoglycemia in diabetes. *Diabetes Spectrum* 15:20–27, 2002

Ms. Kushion is the Manager and Clinical Nurse Specialist at Sparrow Regional Diabetes Center, Lansing, MI.

15. Evaluation and Management of the Diabetic Foot

George T. Liu, DPM, and John S. Steinberg, DPM

EPIDEMIOLOGY

The prevalence of diabetes in the U.S. has increased by 33% from 1990 to 1998 (1). Accordingly, the number of nontraumatic lower-extremity amputations has increased comparably. Reports have estimated that ~15% of patients with diabetes will develop a diabetic foot ulcer in their lifetimes (2,3). Consequently, 85% of nontraumatic lower-extremity amputations are preceded by the formation of a foot ulcer, making it the most common pivotal event (4,5). Foot complications account for 25% of diabetes-related admissions to hospitals (4–6), and an estimated 50% of those patients who undergo lower-extremity amputation will suffer a new amputation within 5 years (7,8).

Ulceration and amputation of the lower extremities pose a direct socioeconomic burden to both patients and society. Management for foot ulcers is estimated at $27,987 (U.S. dollars) per occurrence for the 2 years following diagnosis (9), and the average hospital cost incurred for diabetes-related lower-extremity amputation ranges from $20,000 to $27,930 (10–13). Studies have demonstrated a relationship between the presence of ulceration/amputation and a negative impact on function, self-perception, emotional health, and quality of life (14–18).

Recently, the initial presence of a foot ulcer was recognized as a marker of the diabetic disease state and not only as a local comorbid manifestation (19–21). In a recent study, 5-year mortality rates of diabetic patients with new-onset neuropathic, neuroischemic, and ischemic foot ulcers were 45%, 18%, and 55%, respectively (21). In a prospective study, diabetic patients with an ulcer were found to have a twofold increased risk of mortality compared with diabetic patients without a foot ulcer (19).

PATHOGENESIS OF DIABETIC FOOT PROBLEMS

Several pathological manifestations of diabetes contribute to ulceration and amputation of the diabetic foot. Sensory neuropathy is the most common reason for foot lesions encountered in the diabetic foot. This lack of protective sensation subjects the foot to increased risk of open injuries due to undetected trauma or repetitive low-grade stresses. Motor neuropathy causes muscle atrophy and subsequent imbalances of tendon pull across the foot joints. The resultant foot deformities, such as hammertoes, claw toes, and prominent plantar metatarsal heads, may serve as areas of irritation and pressure within tight shoes (Fig. 15.1). Additionally, abnormal plantar pressures develop as a result of these foot deformities and altered mechanics. Increased plantar pressure combined with sensory neuropathy may predispose the foot to ulceration (Fig. 15.2). Autonomic neuropathy in the foot may manifest as decreased sweating of the feet, predisposing the dorsal and plantar skin to dryness and fissures. A more serious manifestation of autonomic neuropathy in the foot is Charcot neuroarthropathy, in which destruction of the foot joints can cause severe foot deformities (Fig. 15.3). Another pathologic manifestation of long-term diabetes is nonenzymatic glycosylation. This process of glycosylation in diabetes stiffens soft tissues such as ligaments and tendons, causing limited joint mobility, which also leads to increased plantar pressures. In addition, peripheral arterial disease in patients with diabetes is more advanced and prevalent compared with that in individuals without diabetes. Poor tissue oxygenation together with impaired blood flow may slow the healing of foot wounds, delay the delivery of antibiotics, and, in severe cases, result in ischemic pain and gangrene.

FOOT ASSESSMENT AND EVALUATION

Assessment of high-risk conditions for ulceration and amputation in the diabetic foot is crucial in reducing the incidence of comorbid complications. A systems-based evaluation of the foot can identify early risk factors and identify appropriate interventions to prevent the progression toward the development of ulceration and amputation.

Vascular Assessment: Is There Adequate Blood Flow to the Foot?

Ischemia to the lower extremities impedes the immune response to infection, delivery of antibiotics, and healing of open wounds. Intermittent calf claudication, as identified by cramping of the calf muscles while walking, is an indication of relative ischemia, wherein the tissue demand for blood exceeds the available supply. Calf claudication is measured by city-block distances the patient is able to walk before intense cramping or tiredness of the leg ensues. Also measured is the amount of rest time required before walking can be comfortably initiated. Calf cramping during sleep (nocturnal leg cramping) is not intermittent calf claudication. Rest pain occurs in the advanced stages of ischemia and is characterized by intense pain and cramping primarily in the forefoot during sleep that is relieved only by placing the limb in a dependent position. Gangrene, ischemic tissue death, signifies end-stage peripheral vascular disease or absolute ischemia, in which the blood supply is completely inadequate for tissue survival.

Neurological Assessment: Is There Absence of Protective Sensation?

Indicators of clinical neuropathy may include the subjective presence of tingling, numbness, burning sensation, and/or formication (sensation of insects crawling on skin) that typically begins at the toes and fingertips. In advanced cases of sensory neuropathy, the symptomatic sensations progress proximally to a "stocking-and-glove" distribution.

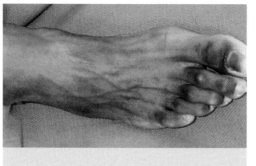

FIGURE 15.1
Retracted claw toes with prominent extensor tendons and depressed metatarsal head are a result of muscular imbalances from motor neuropathy.

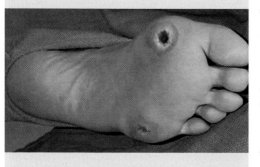

FIGURE 15.2
Depressed metatarsal heads create increased plantar pressures with walking. In the insensate foot, these focal pressures predispose skin to ulcerations.

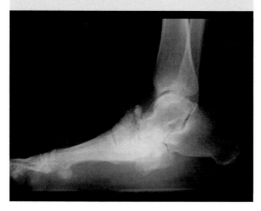

FIGURE 15.3
Clinically, Charcot foot presents with redness, swelling, heat, and severe deformity. Radiographic pictures demonstrate severe fracture dislocations accompanied with osteolysis and fragmentation in the foot joints.

Table 15.1 Examination of Vascular Status

Assessment	Potential Indication
Palpate femoral, popliteal, dorsalis pedis, and posterior tibial pulse	■ Absent pedal pulse may be an indication of poor inflow to the foot. ■ Palpating proximal arteries may help identify the level of lower arterial disease.
Feel for differences in skin temperature from proximal to distal; compare limbs	■ Coolness may indicate diminished circulatory perfusion. ■ Localized warmth may be an indication of infection or Charcot neuroarthropathy.
Inspect skin for atrophic, shiny, and taut appearances and digital hair growth	■ Loss of turgor and digital hair growth may be signs of poor cutaneous perfusion.
Evaluate digital capillary filling time	■ Normal refilling should be pink to color in 1–3 seconds. ■ Refilling that is ≥3–5 seconds may indicate arterial insufficiency. ■ Refilling that is immediate and bluish or purplish in color may indicate venous insufficiency.
Evaluate the following: ■ Elevational pallor by raising the leg above the level of the heart or 60° above horizontal for 1 min ■ Dependent rubor by lowering and hanging the lower extremity	■ In the elevated position, marked pallor to the sole and digits indicates arterial insufficiency. ■ When lowering the extremity, if it takes >10 seconds for the pink color to return or vein filling takes >15 seconds, arterial insufficiency should be suspected.
Inspect for areas of gangrene	■ Presence of gangrene is representative of end-stage vascular disease resulting in tissue death.

Evaluation for sensory neuropathy begins with assessment of protective sensation. The 5.07 Semmes-Weinstein monofilament wire (Fig. 15.4) has been the screening tool of choice for determining the loss of protective sensation with sensory neuropathy. This inexpensive and portable device can yield reproducible and predictive information regarding risk of ulcer formation (22). The 5.07 Semmes-Weinstein monofilament is calibrated to deliver 10 g of force to a designated testing site when sufficient force is applied, causing the wire to bend. The examination is performed with the subject's eyes closed. The patient is then asked to respond "yes" if any pressure from the monofilament wire is detected. Demonstrating the monofilament on the patient's proximal leg or palm may assist in identifying the type of sensation he or she is to detect. Ten sites are tested: plantar first, third, and fifth digits; plantar first, third, and fifth metatarsal heads; plantar medial and lateral midfoot; plantar heel; and dorsal midfoot. A clinical finding of four insensate sites was found to be 97% sensitive and 83% specific for detecting a loss of protective sensation (23,24).

Another testing modality used to assess loss of protective sensation is the biothesiometer. This instrument delivers different levels of vibration through an application tip tactor, which is usually applied to the distal pulp of the hallux. Voltage is

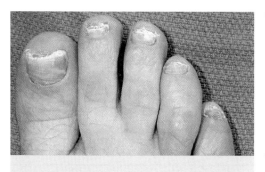

FIGURE 15.6
Fungally infected nails present with thickness, discoloration, and subungual debris. Thick nails may cause pressure to the nail bed within shoes, creating nail bed ulcerations.

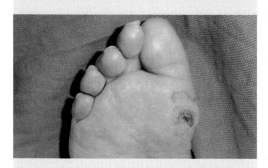

FIGURE 15.7
A hemorrhage beneath calluses may indicate the presence of a preulcerative lesion.

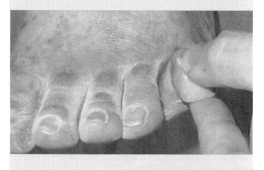

FIGURE 15.8
Web spaces of toes may retain moisture, which causes maceration. Chronic maceration may lead to skin breakdown.

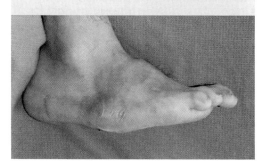

FIGURE 15.9
Collapse of the midfoot in Charcot foot will result in a "rocker bottom" deformity. The plantar bony prominence is subject to increased pressure and ulceration.

Dermatological Assessment: Is There Presence of Skin Pathology?

Among the many vital functions of the integumentary system, the skin serves as a barrier to protect the body from foreign pathogens. As previously discussed, open lesions to the foot serve as pathways of infection to the body. In the diabetic foot, absent protective sensation and foot deformity leave the skin susceptible to mechanical injury, resulting in skin breakdown. The presence of an open wound is the pivotal event for development of infection. Examination of the skin should identify areas of open injury, such as laceration or ulceration, and areas of low-grade mechanical irritation, such as that seen with a callus or corn.

Orthopedic and Biomechanical Assessment: Is There a Foot Deformity?

Structural and functional deformities of the foot may be sources of repetitive low-grade trauma during gait and within shoes. In the insensate foot, this continual trauma may lead to ulceration of the skin.

Table 15.3 Orthopedic Examination of Musculoskeletal Status

Assessment	Potential Indication
Observe for digital deformities (i.e., hammertoes, claw toes, and mallet toes)	■ Determine whether the deformity is flexible or rigid. Rigid deformities are more prone to irritation and skin breakdown within shoes. ■ Inspect for associated callus or corn formation along the bony prominences, an indication of low-grade irritation within shoe gear.
Identify bunion or Tailor's bunion (fifth metatarsophalangeal joint) deformity	■ Large bony protrusion of the metatarsal joint causing pressure in the area at risk of ulceration.
Inspect for prominent depressed metatarsal heads with an anteriorly displaced metatarsal fat pad	■ Prominent plantar metatarsal areas with loss of fat pad protection are subject to increased pressures. Diffuse callus formation may be present.
Identify midfoot deformities: low arch and high arch	■ Low arches may be seen with flatfoot deformities (pes planus). Inspect the plantar midfoot for any signs of callus formation or irritation. Collapse of the midfoot arch, with a "rocker bottom" deformity, may also be seen with Charcot neuroarthropathy (Fig. 15.9). This condition should be referred to a podiatrist or foot-and-ankle orthopedist for evaluation and treatment. ■ High arches may be seen with "intrinsic minus foot," in which atrophy of the intrinsic muscles of the foot and depression of the metatarsal heads gives a hollow appearance to the arch. This is accompanied with retracted digit and prominent extensor tendons. Observe the plantar metatarsal head area and heels for callus formation and irritation.
Identify rearfoot deformities: varus (inversion) or valgus (eversion)	■ Rigid varus or valgus rearfoot deformities at the heel may cause callus formation or irritation.

(continued)

Table 15.3 Orthopedic Examination of Musculoskeletal Status (*Continued*)

Assessment	Potential Indication
Identify prominences along joints or bones	■ Bony prominence may be the result of arthritic joint changes or bony injury. ■ Severe deformity may be seen in Charcot neuroarthropathy.
Identify previous foot amputations	■ Partial amputations of the foot alter the mechanics of gait and the normal distribution of plantar pressures, predisposing the foot to ulceration.
Assess the range of motion of joints for limited joint mobility	■ First metatarsophalangeal joint: 65° in dorsiflexion in the sagittal plane. ■ Subtalar joint: 10° eversion and 20° inversion in the frontal plane. ■ Ankle joint: 10° of dorsiflexion in the sagittal plane. ■ Limited joint range of motion of the lower-extremity joints reduces shock absorption capacity and translates increased plantar pressures to the foot. Limited joint mobility has been associated with increased risk of ulcer formation.

Shoe Assessment: Does the Patient Have Adequate Protective Footwear and Comply with Its Use?

Ideally, the role of footwear is to protect the feet from injury. By accommodating deformity and off-loading pressure, a proper set of footwear can prevent ulcer occurrence and recurrence, and patients must understand the importance of prevention and the role shoes and activity play. However, in the diabetic insensate foot, an ill-fitting shoe can be a source of repetitive injury. Also, examination of the shoe treads may reveal abnormal gait patterns and areas of increased pedal stress. Ideal footwear should be extra depth, with a wide toe box to accommodate digital deformities. Insoles should be custom molded and redistribute plantar pressures. Shoes should fit well, with little to no pistoning of the foot.

LABS AND TESTS

Few laboratory and advance testing modalities are used for routine assessment of the diabetic foot, and most ancillary tests are performed only when clinically indicated.

Radiographic evaluation for underlying osteomyelitis of the foot should be performed in the presence of chronic foot ulcerations that probe deep soft tissue or bone. Severe and acute foot deformities should be radiographically evaluated for fracture/dislocations and for Charcot neuroarthropathy. In the cases of severe clinical infection, foot radiographs may detect soft tissue gas and bony involvement.

Additionally, nuclear and advanced diagnostic imaging, such as bone scan, computed tomography, and magnetic resonance imaging, may be used to evaluate the presence of osteomyelitis. Noninvasive vascular evaluation of the lower-

Table 15.4 Footwear Evaluation

Assessment	Potential Indication
Inspect interior of shoe for foreign objects and exterior of the shoe for impaled sharp objects (Fig. 15.10)	▪ Sharp objects may injure the foot, predisposing to ulceration.
Inspect wear pattern of the shoe	▪ Wear patterns may be associated with abnormal gait and deformities of the foot.
Shoe fit	▪ Shoes should be well fitting. Tight shoes may create areas of pressure over the skin of bony prominences. Oversized or loose shoes will create pistoning within the shoe, which may produce areas of shear stress and irritation to the foot. ▪ Toe box of the shoe should be deep and wide enough to avoid digital pressure and irritation.
Inspect insoles for material fatigue and failure (bottoming out)	▪ If inner soles cannot be visually inspected, place a hand into the shoe to assess worn spots or areas where padding is weak and worn.

extremity arteries (arterial Dopplers, digital plethysmography, pulse volume recordings, and ankle-brachial and toe-brachial indexes) may be used to evaluate the quality of physiological blood flow. This examination is commonly performed in patients with diabetes who present with clinical signs and symptoms of ischemia in the lower extremity or an ischemic nonhealing wound. This examination is commonly performed before an arteriogram, which is an invasive test used to assess arterial runoff and target vessels for lower-extremity arterial bypass surgery.

TREATMENT

The goal of management of the diabetic foot is to address potential and presenting high-risk conditions associated with ulceration and amputation. Key treatment modalities include care of the nails, calluses, and skin; therapeutic footwear; and regular follow-up.

Nail care
▪ Mycotic and hypertrophic nails should be debrided to relieve potential pressure against the toe box in shoes. Reduction should be done by a health care professional with foot care training.
▪ Ingrowing and ingrown toenails should be treated with debridement of the offending margin or a partial nail avulsion by a health care professional with foot care training.

(continued)

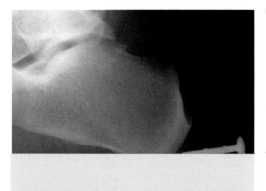

FIGURE 15.10
In the insensate foot, undetected impaled objects in the shoe are sources for repetitive injury.

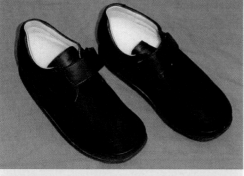

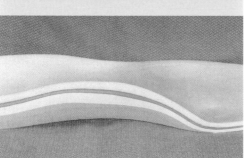

FIGURE 15.11
Extra-depth shoes with custom-molded inserts will accommodate minor foot deformities and attenuate focal plantar pressures.

- Ingrown nails with an infection (paronychia) often require debridement or avulsion of the offending nail margin and possible oral antibiotic therapy. This condition should be treated by a health care professional with foot care training.
- Elongated nails should be trimmed either transversely or along the contours of the distal toe pulp with care to maintain clearance of the nail border from the medial and lateral nail grooves. Patients may perform this nail reduction at home if the patient has normal nail type, good sensation, and adequate vision. If there is concern of self-injury, this care should be performed by a health care professional.

Callus care

- Thick calluses and corns should be reduced to prevent focal areas of pressure against the foot. Reduction is usually performed with a sharp blade by a health care professional with foot care training.
- Padding with soft cushioning devices, such as felt, moleskin, or viscoelastic material, may be applied to areas of callus reduction to reduce shear.
- Insole materials may be used to reduce plantar pressures at callus sites.
- Corns associated with rigid digital deformities may be accommodated with extra-depth or diabetic shoes with a soft toe box to reduce digital irritation.

Skin care

- Application of lotions and creams with mild keratolytics (e.g., 20 or 40% urea cream) may be used to penetrate and maintain moisture within thick dry skin.
- Clean between digital web spaces. Lamb's wool placed within the web spaces of toes may also be used to facilitate drying of macerated skin.
- Noninfected, clean ulcers should be gently scrubbed with a noncytotoxic, antiseptic solution and rinsed with normal saline. Debridement of the hyperkeratotic borders and necrotic tissue should be performed by a health care professional with training in foot care. Multiple dressing materials for wounds are available, but the dressing used should keep the wound site moist and protected from contamination.

Footwear

- The function of shoe gear in the diabetic foot is to reduce abnormal plantar pressures and to protect from external injury. Referral to a podiatrist or foot-and-ankle orthopedist is needed for prescription footwear. Consultation with a certified prosthetist/orthotist or shoe specialist will assist in selecting and developing

(continued)

the specific shoe design and fitting. Shoe selection should be based on level of risk.

– Sensate foot without deformity: commercial footwear.
– Sensory neuropathy: accommodative inserts and possibly a thera-peutic shoe if the patient's foot demonstrates areas of irritation with the present footwear.
– Sensory neuropathy and minor or flexible foot deformity: extra-depth shoe with custom-molded insert (Fig. 15.11).
– Severe rigid nonreducible foot deformity (e.g., quiescent Charcot foot): custom-molded shoe with custom-molded insert.
– Partial foot amputation: will often require a custom-molded filler/insert within either an extra-depth or a custom-molded shoe. Depending on the level of amputation, an ankle foot orthosis may be required to assist the patient in stability with walking.

Timing of follow-up care

■ Comprehensive foot examination for a diabetic patient should be performed annually to screen for high-risk conditions.
■ Patients with foot insensitivity should have their feet examined every 3–4 months.
■ Patients with foot insensitivity and deformity should have their feet examined every 2–3 months.
■ Patients with foot insensitivity, deformity, and history of ulceration or amputation should have their feet examined every 1–2 months.

PRACTICAL POINT

A culmination of individual factors contributes to the cumulative risk of developing foot ulcers (28).

■ Patients with sensory neuropathy were 1.7 times more likely to develop an ulcer.
■ Patients with neuropathy and deformity were 12.1 times more likely to develop an ulcer.
■ Patients with neuropathy, deformity, and history of amputation were 36.4 times more likely to develop an ulcer.
■ Presence of a callus in the diabetic foot is strongly associated with the site of ulcer formation (29).

EDUCATIONAL/BEHAVIORAL CONSIDERATIONS

Diabetes foot education has been shown to reduce foot complications associated with diabetes. Educating patients on daily monitoring and maintenance of the feet will aid in preventing complications and improve response time to potentially limb-threatening conditions.

Patient Daily Inspection

- Inspect feet, especially the soles, at least once per day for injury, callosities, and areas of redness. If the area of redness is associated with heat, swelling, pain, and pus accompanied with fever, chills, and night sweats, this condition should be reported immediately to a doctor or nurse. The use of a shatterproof mirror on the floor is recommended if the patient cannot bend his or her legs to visually inspect the feet.
- Inspect web spaces between toes for maceration and fissures.
- Inspect the interior and exterior of the shoe for foreign objects before wearing and note areas of wear and tear. Worn-out shoes may not be supportive and therefore unable to evenly distribute foot pressure across the sole.

Patient Daily Maintenance

- Do not walk barefoot (inside or outside the home). Always wear footwear recommended by a health care professional.
- Using lotions or creams recommended by a health care provider will help skin retain moisture and prevent cracking. Do not apply lotions to the web spaces between toes.
- Wash feet daily with mild soap and water. Test water temperature with elbow before submerging feet.
- Dry feet well, especially in the web spaces between toes, after washing to prevent maceration. Apply lamb's wool as instructed to the web spaces to facilitate drying of macerated skin.
- Wear cotton socks to absorb perspiration from the skin. Wearing clean, light-colored socks will help identify the presence of pus or blood from an undetected injury. Do not wear tight socks that constrict the circulation to the feet.
- Trim toenails either straight across or along the contours of the toe pulp to maintain nail clearance from adjacent skin and to reduce potential ingrown toenail formation.
- Small calluses may be reduced with a pumice stone, ideally after bathing when calluses are soft.
- Do not trim or cut nails or calluses if neuropathy is present, refer to a podiatrist.
- Do not use over-the-counter "medicated" corn and callus pads as they contain salicylic acid, which can injure the insensate foot. Nonmedicated corn and callus pads are acceptable as directed by a health care professional.
- Do not self-treat ingrown nails and associated infections and do not use sharp objects to reduce calluses. Seek the advice and help of a doctor or nurse.
- Open injuries of the foot should be cleansed with antiseptic solution and dressed. The condition should be reported immediately to the doctor or nurse for evaluation and treatment.
- Ulcer care should be performed as directed by a health care professional.

Addressing Barriers to Treatment and Lifestyle Changes

- Commonly reported reasons for poor patient adherence to treatment regimens are
  - inability to understand physicians' instructions (30)
  - difficulty remembering treatment regimen (31)
  - lack of social support for healthy lifestyle changes (32)
  - embarrassment when wearing protective therapeutic shoes because of appearance (33,34).
- Detailed explanations of the disease process and the rationale for treatment have been shown to improve compliance rates (30).
- Educate both patients and family members regarding diabetes and foot maintenance. Understanding the rationale for the patient's lifestyle changes will encourage cooperative behavior and improve the support of family members.
- Enrollment in a diabetes self-management education course (that also provides instruction for foot maintenance) (35,36), provision of simple instructions in a handout, and recruiting the assistance of a family member during the patient visit may improve compliance and overall outcomes.
- Evaluate the patient's ability to perform the daily self-examination, which may be limited by the following conditions:
  - inability to see his or her feet due to poor vision (37)
  - inability to reach with hands to examine feet (in this situation, recruiting the assistance of family members or home health nursing services may help provide this necessary daily inspection and care) (38).

ROLE OF NURSING

With the increased attention drawn to the multidisciplinary model of health care delivery to patients with diabetes, nurses of all specialties have played an integral role as an extension of vital primary care services and have provided ancillary patient support mechanisms.

Routine Foot Screenings

Routine foot screenings for diabetic patients in primary care settings are a fundamental and inexpensive means of prevention that are often neglected (39–43). Reports have shown that in primary care practices, diabetic foot examinations are performed only 10–23% of the time during a routine diabetes care visit (39,41,42). In a 78-chart review of six master's-level certified nurse practitioners in a primary ambulatory care center, a comprehensive foot examination based on American Diabetes Association foot care standards was documented for only 23.1% of diabetic patients (41). Additionally, a retrospective review of inpatient records revealed that a minimally acceptable evaluation of the acutely infected diabetic foot was performed for 14% of patients (44). Without routine screenings, high-risk conditions leading to diabetic foot complications cannot be identified. Altering practice patterns within the primary care setting, such as routinely removing the shoes and socks of patients during non–foot-related visits, has been shown to increase the likelihood of a foot examination more than threefold (45). Nurses play an important role in performing and facilitating foot screenings for high-risk conditions. Minimum requirements of the diabetic foot examination include evaluation of protective sensation, foot deformity and biomechanics, skin integrity, and vascular status (46).

Diabetic Foot Education

Studies have suggested that patient education improves foot care knowledge and behaviors that may reduce the incidence of complications in high-risk diabetic patients (35,36,47,48). In a randomized controlled study, patients attending a foot education session had a threefold decrease in ulceration and amputation rates after a 2-year follow-up period (35). Another randomized trial evaluating the outcome of diabetic patients who received group education compared with usual care by a general practitioner revealed a significant reduction in callus formation and minor skin injury at a 6-month follow-up (36). In preliminary evaluations, implementation of a support group that provides one-on-one and group interactive counseling and foot education to diabetic amputees and patients with chronic ulcerations has been shown to improve foot care behaviors, improve self-perceptions of health, and reduce the rate of reulceration and reamputation.

The Team Approach

A team approach to diabetic foot care is a coordinated method of addressing the multifaceted aspects of diabetic foot complications. Improved outcomes of diabetic foot care have been demonstrated with this organized approach. Patients who received intervention by a multidisciplinary diabetic foot team had 28% fewer reulcerations than a group who received standard foot care at a 2-year follow-up (49). Another study reported a 78% reduction in major amputations after implementation of a multidisciplinary program (50). Team members have included primary care physicians, podiatrists, nurse educators, nutritionists, diabetes nurses, shoe specialists, and vascular and orthopedic surgeons (4,49–52).

Interest in the development of nursing-based models of diabetes care has grown (53–55). In a university health system, nurse-provided screening, education, and treatment has been shown to be a potential cost- and resource-effective method of decreasing the rate of diabetic foot complications (55). One reported measure of behavior improvement from this study was a reduction in improper footwear use from 73 to 43% at the first follow-up visit.

SUMMARY

Amputations of the lower extremities are among the most dreaded complications of diabetes. An estimated 85% of foot amputations are preceded by a preventable ulceration. The diabetic foot is best managed by a team approach. Screening for high-risk conditions of the diabetic foot is a basic and fundamental tool to prevent foot ulceration and amputation. Patient education with diabetic foot care may also encourage behaviors and lifestyle changes that would reduce the foot complications of diabetes. Referral to a podiatrist or foot-and-ankle orthopedist should be made for specialized treatment and management of diabetic foot complications. Despite best efforts, however, foot ulcerations and amputations may occur. Whether for prevention or treatment, nursing personnel can provide an extension of much-needed services in screening and management of the diabetic foot. Nurses have played increasingly vital roles in the multidisciplinary team through screening, patient education, and treatment. With the exhaustion of medical resources for diabetes care, the development of nursing-based models of comprehensive diabetic foot care needs to be evaluated and validated with further clinical investigations.

REFERENCES

1. Mokdad A, Ford ES, Bowman BA, Nelson DE, Engelgau MM, Vinicor F, Marks JS: Diabetes Trends in the U.S.: 1990–1998. *Diabetes Care* 23: 1278–1283, 2000
2. Palumbo P, Melton L: Peripheral vascular disease and diabetes. In *Diabetes in America*. 1st ed. Harris M, Hamman R, Eds. Washington, DC, U.S. Govt. Printing Office, 1985, p. 1–21
3. Reiber G, Boyko E, Smith D: Lower extremity foot ulcers and amputations in diabetes. In *Diabetes in America*. 2nd ed. Harris M, Cowie C, Stern M, Boyko E, Reiber G, Bennett P, Eds. Washington, DC, U.S. Govt. Printing Office, 1995, p. 409–428
4. Apelqvist J, Ragnarson-Tennvall G, Persson U, Larsson J: Diabetic foot ulcers in a multidisciplinary setting: an economic analysis of primary healing and healing with amputation. *J Intern Med* 235:463–471, 1994
5. Pecoraro RE, Reiber GE, Burgess EM: Pathways to diabetic limb amputation: basis for prevention. *Diabetes Care* 13:513–521, 1990
6. Reiber GE, Pecoraro RE, Koepsell TD: Risk factors for amputation in patients with diabetes mellitus: a case-control study. *Ann Intern Med* 117:97–105, 1992
7. Goldner M: The fate of the second leg in the diabetic amputee. *Diabetes* 9: 100–103, 1960
8. Larsson J, Agardh CD, Apelqvist J, Stenstrom A: Long-term prognosis after healed amputation in patients with diabetes. *Clin Orthop* 350:149–158, 1998
9. Ramsey SD, Newton K, Blough D, McCulloch DK, Sandhu N, Reiber GE, Wagner EH: Incidence, outcomes, and cost of foot ulcers in patients with diabetes. *Diabetes Care* 22:382–387, 1999
10. Ashry HR, Lavery LA, Armstrong DG, Lavery DC, van Houtum WH: Cost of diabetes-related amputations in minorities. *J Foot Ankle Surg* 37:186–190, 1998
11. Bild DE, Selby JV, Sinnock P, Browner WS, Braveman P, Showstack JA: Lower-extremity amputation in people with diabetes: epidemiology and prevention. *Diabetes Care* 12:24–31, 1989
12. Fylling CP, Knighton DR: Amputation in the diabetic population: incidence, causes, cost, treatment, and prevention. *J Enterostomal Ther* 16:247–255, 1989
13. van Houtum WH, Lavery LA, Harkless LB: The costs of diabetes-related lower extremity amputations in the Netherlands. *Diabet Med* 12:777–781, 1995
14. Carrington AL, Mawdsley SK, Morley M, Kincey J, Boulton AJ: Psychological status of diabetic people with or without lower limb disability. *Diabetes Res Clin Pract* 32:19–25, 1996
15. Peters EJ, Childs MR, Wunderlich RP, Harkless LB, Armstrong DG, Lavery LA: Functional status of persons with diabetes-related lower-extremity amputations. *Diabetes Care* 24:1799–1804, 2001
16. Price P, Harding K: The impact of foot complications on health-related quality of life in patients with diabetes. *J Cutan Med Surg* 4:45–50, 2000
17. Ragnarson Tennvall G, Apelqvist J: Health-related quality of life in patients with diabetes mellitus and foot ulcers. *J Diabetes Complications* 14:235–241, 2000

18. Vileikyte L: Diabetic foot ulcers: a quality of life issue. *Diabetes Metab Res Rev* 17:246–249, 2001

19. Boyko EJ, Ahroni JH, Smith DG, Davignon D: Increased mortality associated with diabetic foot ulcer. *Diabet Med* 13:967–972, 1996

20. Chammas NK, Hill RL, Foster AV, Edmonds ME: Is neuropathic ulceration the key to understanding increased mortality due to ischaemic heart disease in diabetic foot ulcer patients? A population approach using a proportionate model. *J Int Med Res* 30:553–559, 2002

21. Moulik PK, Mtonga R, Gill GV: Amputation and mortality in new-onset diabetic foot ulcers stratified by etiology. *Diabetes Care* 26:491–494, 2003

22. Mayfield JA, Sugarman JR: The use of the Semmes-Weinstein monofilament and other threshold tests for preventing foot ulceration and amputation in persons with diabetes. *J Fam Pract* 49 (Suppl. 11):S17–S29, 2000

23. Armstrong DG, Lavery LA, Vela SA, Quebedeaux TL, Fleischli JG: Choosing a practical screening instrument to identify patients at risk for diabetic foot ulceration. *Arch Intern Med* 158:289–292, 1998

24. Mueller MJ: Identifying patients with diabetes mellitus who are at risk for lower-extremity complications: use of Semmes-Weinstein monofilaments. *Phys Ther* 76:68–71, 1996

25. Coppini DV, Bowtell PA, Weng C, Young PJ, Sonksen PH: Showing neuropathy is related to increased mortality in diabetic patients: a survival analysis using an accelerated failure time model. *J Clin Epidemiol* 53:519–523, 2000

26. Pham H, Armstrong DG, Harvey C, Harkless LB, Giurini JM, Veves A: Screening techniques to identify people at high risk for diabetic foot ulceration: a prospective multicenter trial. *Diabetes Care* 23:606–611, 2000

27. Young MJ, Breddy JL, Veves A, Boulton AJ: The prediction of diabetic neuropathic foot ulceration using vibration perception thresholds: a prospective study. *Diabetes Care* 17:557–560, 1994

28. Lavery LA, Armstrong DG, Vela SA, Quebedeaux TL, Fleischli JG: Practical criteria for screening patients at high risk for diabetic foot ulceration. *Arch Intern Med* 158:157–162, 1998

29. Murray HJ, Young MJ, Hollis S, Boulton AJ: The association between callus formation, high pressures and neuropathy in diabetic foot ulceration. *Diabet Med* 13:979–982, 1996

30. Davis M: Variations in patients' compliance with doctors' orders. *J Med Educ* 41:1037–1048, 1966

31. Fitzgerald JT, Anderson RM, Funnell MM, Arnold MS, Davis WK, Aman LC, Jacober SJ, Grunberger G: Differences in the impact of dietary restrictions on African Americans and Caucasians with NIDDM. *Diabetes Educ* 23:41–47, 1997

32. Tillotson LM, Smith MS: Locus of control, social support, and adherence to the diabetes regimen. *Diabetes Educ* 22:133–139, 1996

33. Breuer U: Diabetic patient's compliance with bespoke footwear after healing of neuropathic foot ulcers. *Diabete Metab* 20:415–419, 1994

34. Chantelau E, Kushner T, Spraul M: How effective is cushioned therapeutic footwear in protecting diabetic feet? A clinical study. *Diabet Med* 7:355–359, 1990

35. Malone JM, Snyder M, Anderson G, Bernhard VM, Holloway GA Jr, Bunt TJ: Prevention of amputation by diabetic education. *Am J Surg* 158:520–523, 1989

36. Pieber TR, Holler A, Siebenhofer A, Brunner GA, Semlitsch B, Schattenberg S, Zapotoczky H, Rainer W, Krejs GJ: Evaluation of a structured teaching

and treatment programme for type 2 diabetes in general practice in a rural area of Austria. *Diabet Med* 12:349–354, 1995

37. Crausaz FM, Clavel S, Liniger C, Albeanu A, Assal JP: Additional factors associated with plantar ulcers in diabetic neuropathy. *Diabet Med* 5:771–775, 1988

38. Thomson FJ, Masson EA: Can elderly diabetic patients co-operate with routine foot care? *Age Ageing* 21:333–337, 1992

39. Bailey TS, Yu HM, Rayfield EJ: Patterns of foot examination in a diabetes clinic. *Am J Med* 78:371–374, 1985

40. Chin MH, Cook S, Jin L, Drum ML, Harrison JF, Koppert J, Thiel F, Harrand AG, Schaefer CT, Takashima HT, Chiu SC: Barriers to providing diabetes care in community health centers. *Diabetes Care* 24:268–274, 2001

41. Fain JA, Melkus GD: Nurse practitioner practice patterns based on standards of medical care for patients with diabetes. *Diabetes Care* 17:879–881, 1994

42. Wylie-Rosett J, Walker EA, Shamoon H, Engel S, Basch C, Zybert P: Assessment of documented foot examinations for patients with diabetes in inner-city primary care clinics. *Arch Fam Med* 4:46–50, 1995

43. Zoorob RJ, Mainous AG 3rd: Practice patterns of rural family physicians based on the American Diabetes Association standards of care. *J Community Health* 21:175–182, 1996

44. Edelson GW, Armstrong DG, Lavery LA, Caicco G: The acutely infected diabetic foot is not adequately evaluated in an inpatient setting. *Arch Intern Med* 156:2373–2378, 1996

45. Cohen SJ: Potential barriers to diabetes care. *Diabetes Care* 6:499–500, 1983

46. American Diabetes Association: Preventive foot care in people with diabetes. *Foot Ankle Int* 21:76–77, 2000

47. Litzelman DK, Slemenda CW, Langefeld CD, Hays LM, Welch MA, Bild DE, Ford ES, Vinicor F: Reduction of lower extremity clinical abnormalities in patients with non-insulin-dependent diabetes mellitus: a randomized, controlled trial. *Ann Intern Med* 119:36–41, 1993

48. Ward A, Metz L, Oddone EZ, Edelman D: Foot education improves knowledge and satisfaction among patients at high risk for diabetic foot ulcer. *Diabetes Educ* 25:560–567, 1999

49. Dargis V, Pantelejeva O, Jonushaite A, Vileikyte L, Boulton AJ: Benefits of a multidisciplinary approach in the management of recurrent diabetic foot ulceration in Lithuania: a prospective study. *Diabetes Care* 22:1428–1431, 1999

50. Larsson J, Apelqvist J, Agardh CD, Stenstrom A: Decreasing incidence of major amputation in diabetic patients: a consequence of a multidisciplinary foot care team approach? *Diabet Med* 12:770–776, 1995

51. Edmonds ME, Blundell MP, Morris ME, Thomas EM, Cotton LT, Watkins PJ: Improved survival of the diabetic foot: the role of a specialized foot clinic. *Q J Med* 60:763–771, 1986

52. Frykberg RG: The team approach in diabetic foot management. *Adv Wound Care* 11:71–77, 1998

53. Davidson MB: Effect of nurse-directed diabetes care in a minority population. *Diabetes Care* 26:2281–2287, 2003

54. Jones PM: Quality improvement initiative to integrate teaching diabetes standards into home care visits. *Diabetes Educ* 28:1009–1020, 2002

55. Pinzur MS, Kernan-Schroeder D, Emanuele NV, Emanuel M: Development of a nurse-provided health system strategy for diabetic foot care. *Foot Ankle Int* 22:744–746, 2001

ADDITIONAL READING

Apelqvist J, Bakker K, van Houtum WH, Nabuurs-Franssen MH, Schaper NC: International consensus and practical guidelines on the management and the prevention of the diabetic foot: International Working Group on the Diabetic Foot. *Diabetes Metab Res Rev* 16 (Suppl. 1):S84–S92, 2000

Frykberg RG, Armstrong DG, Giurini J, Edwards A, Kravette M, Kravitz S, Ross C, Stavosky J, Stuck R, Vanore J: Diabetic foot disorders: a clinical practice guideline: American College of Foot and Ankle Surgeons. *J Foot Ankle Surg* 39 (Suppl. 5):S1–S60, 2000

Inlow S, Orsted H, Sibbald RG: Best practices for the prevention, diagnosis, and treatment of diabetic foot ulcers. *Ostomy Wound Manage* 46:55–68, 2000

Pinzur MS, Slovenkai MP, Trepman E: Guidelines for diabetic foot care: the Diabetes Committee of the American Orthopaedic Foot and Ankle Society. *Foot Ankle Int* 20:695–702, 1999

Schaper NC, Apelqvist J, Bakker K: The international consensus and practical guidelines on the management and prevention of the diabetic foot. *Curr Diabetes Rep* 3:475–479, 2003

Sykes MT, Godsey JB: Vascular evaluation of the problem diabetic foot. *Clin Podiatr Med Surg* 15:49–83, 1998

Dr. Liu is a Clinical Assistant Professor at the University of Texas Health Science Center at San Antonio, San Antonio, TX. Dr. Steinberg is an Assistant Professor at the University of Texas Health Science Center at San Antonio, San Antonio, TX, and Medical Director, Podiatry Clinic, at the Texas Diabetes Institute, San Antonio, TX.

DIABETES CARE
AND MANAGEMENT

16. Diabetes Education in the Management of Diabetes

MARTHA M. FUNNELL, MS, RN, CDE, AND
CAROLÉ R. MENSING, RN, MA, CDE

D iabetes self-management education (DSME) has long been considered a cornerstone of diabetes care. Because ~99% of the care is provided by the person with diabetes and his or her family members, effective care requires a partnership between an actively involved patient and the health care team (1). Education is critical for the patient to become involved and to make informed self-management decisions on a daily basis.

Most nurses think of diabetes education as a comprehensive program offered in an outpatient setting or by an inpatient diabetes nurse educator. In fact, each encounter with a person who has diabetes is an opportunity for education, and every nurse shares the responsibility for that education. Even when time is limited, nurses can create "teachable moments" to provide and reinforce needed information. For example, giving insulin to a hospitalized patient is an excellent time to assess and review insulin injection technique, treatment of hypoglycemia, insulin action times, and the need to wear or carry diabetes identification and glucose tablets. Doing a foot examination during an outpatient visit provides the opportunity to assess foot care self-management practices by asking, "What do you do to care for your feet at home?" and offering individualized foot care instruction.

EVIDENCE FOR DSME

Multiple meta-analyses and reviews have documented the effectiveness of DSME in improving knowledge, psychosocial outcomes, and health outcomes (2–8). The greatest predictive factor of the effectiveness of DSME is the amount of time spent with the educator, typically a nurse (4). Table 16.1 summarizes the key findings from these studies (5).

It is important to note that although no single educational program is more effective than others, interventions that incorporate effective and behavioral aspects produce better outcomes (10). Tailoring the interventions to the age and culture of the participants and including spouses and adult children may also increase DSME effectiveness, as has been shown for older African-American and Latino individuals with diabetes (7).

DSME is essential but not sufficient for the type of sustained behavior change required by a chronic illness such as diabetes (4,11). Without ongoing

---

Table 16.1 Effectiveness of DSME

Characteristics of effective interventions
- Regular reinforcement is more effective than one-time or short-term education.
- Patient participation and collaboration appear to produce more favorable results than didactic interventions.
- Group education is more effective than one-on-one education for lifestyle interventions and appears to be equally effective for improving knowledge and accuracy of self-monitoring of blood glucose (SMBG).
- Studies with short-term follow-up are more likely to demonstrate positive effects on glycemic control and behavioral outcomes than studies with long-term follow-up.

Effectiveness in clinical settings
- In the short term (<6 months), DSME improves knowledge levels, SMBG skills, and dietary habits (per self-report).
- In the short term (<6 months), glycemic control improves.
- Improved glycemic control does not appear to correspond to measured changes in knowledge or SMBG skills.
- Weight loss can be achieved with repetitive interventions or with short-term follow-up (<6 months).
- Physical activity levels are variably affected by interventions.
- Effects on lipids and blood pressure are variable but are more likely to be positive with interactive or individualized repetitive interventions.

Effectiveness in nonclinical settings
- Some evidence indicates that DSME is effective when given in community gathering places (e.g., churches and community centers) for adults with type 2 diabetes.
- The literature is insufficient to assess the effectiveness of DSME in the home for adults with diabetes (9).
- The literature is insufficient to assess the effectiveness of DSME in the workplace.

Reprinted with permission from Norris (5).

---

self-management support, most outcomes return to pre-education levels in ~6 months (4). Strategies that can be used to provide ongoing self-management support include self-directed goal setting, nurse care management, and use of lay or peer health workers and support groups.

Diabetes education has evolved in recent years from a didactic format to more theoretically based empowerment models that utilize approaches that recognize the principles of adult learning and acknowledge that the person with diabetes is the primary decision maker in his or her own care. Educational strategies have evolved as well to match this growing body of evidence and to meet quality standards to obtain reimbursement.

EDUCATIONAL PROCESS

Assessment

Individualization is a critical component of effective DSME. The first step in the process is assessment. Examples of questions to ask during the assessment process are listed in Table 16.2. The assessment is then used to develop the educational plan in collaboration with the participant. Areas of greatest concern

The educational process includes assessment, provision of content using appropriate strategies, documentation, and outcome evaluation. Each of these steps is necessary whether DSME is part of a comprehensive program or focused education is provided during hospitalization or routine outpatient visits.

and any questions identified by the patient need to be addressed at the beginning of the intervention. This helps tailor the educational program to that particular patient and increases both the efficiency and effectiveness of the DSME intervention. Beginning with "What questions do you have about . . ." or "What do you know about . . ." should be an effective way to start even a brief educational encounter.

Table 16.2 Examples of Educational Assessment Questions

- In what language do you prefer to speak? To read?
- What is your favorite way to learn (e.g., reading, discussion, videos, computers, group class, individual teaching)?
- Where do you get most of your information about health and diabetes?
- Do you have difficulty with your hearing or vision, such as reading regular-size print?
- How far did you go in school?
- Do you have any cultural or religious practices or beliefs that affect how you care for your health and diabetes?
- Do you ever have difficulty paying for your diabetes supplies or medicines?
- Do you have trouble remembering things?
- Have you ever known other people with diabetes? How did it affect them?
- Do you have health problems that you manage other than diabetes? What helps you to manage them?
- Have you ever lost weight or increased your physical activity? What helped you to make those changes? What got in your way?
- What areas of diabetes are you most interested in learning more about?
- What are you currently doing to manage your diabetes at home?
- On a scale of 1 to 10, with 10 being the most important, how important is managing diabetes in your life?
- How confident are you that you can manage your diabetes?
- How much stress are you experiencing in your life?
- Have you felt sad and blue most of the time for the past 2 weeks? Two months?
- What kind of support do you want and need from your family and friends to care for your diabetes?
- What kind of support do you receive from your family and friends to care for your diabetes?
- Who helps you the most to care for your diabetes?
- What is your greatest concern about your diabetes?
- What is the hardest thing for you in caring for your diabetes? What is the easiest?
- What were your thoughts/feelings when you first learned that you had diabetes? What are your thoughts/feelings now?
- How can I be most helpful to you?

A formal assessment needs to include a relevant medical history, cultural influences, health beliefs and attitudes, diabetes knowledge, self-management skills and behaviors, readiness to learn, language and literacy skills, cognitive ability, physical limitations, family support, and financial status (12).

Assessment is appropriate whether the patient is newly diagnosed or has lived with diabetes for some time. Even newly diagnosed adults have some level of knowledge or experience with diabetes. Assessing the level of information not only shows respect for the person and allows a true partnership to begin, but also provides the opportunity to clarify misconceptions and update old information.

Content

Table 16.3 outlines topic-specific content areas to be addressed in a comprehensive educational program (12). These content areas are written in behavioral terms to allow maximum creativity and flexibility in the teaching process. Specific areas to address with each patient are identified during the assessment. Ideally, all patients with diabetes are referred to an in-depth, comprehensive educational program, either at diagnosis or at some point during their life with diabetes. Even patients who have had diabetes for a number of years can benefit from a refresher course.

These content areas are applicable in all settings and can be provided at basic, intermediate, or advanced levels. Generally, the depth of the content needed determines the level rather than a particular topic. For example, basic or survival education for SMBG may only include the skills of testing and recording the results. Intermediate SMBG education may include interpretation of the results, and advanced SMBG education may include pattern management. Standardized curricula and goals for diabetes education are available to help nurses create programs that address all of the recommended content areas and to ensure consistency among instructors (see RESOURCES and "Additional Reading" at the end of this chapter). Many nurses find adapting these curricula to be more efficient than developing their own. These can also be useful for nurses who provide education on an ongoing basis to be sure that they are consistently addressing all of the critical content areas.

Table 16.3 DSME Content Areas

- Describing the diabetes disease process and treatment options
- Incorporating appropriate nutritional management
- Incorporating physical activity into lifestyle
- Using medications (if applicable) for therapeutic effectiveness
- Monitoring blood glucose and urine ketones (when appropriate) and using the results to improve control
- Preventing, detecting, and treating acute complications
- Preventing (through risk reduction behavior), detecting, and treating chronic complications
- Goal setting to promote health and problem solving for daily living
- Integrating psychosocial adjustment into daily life
- Promoting preconception care, management during pregnancy, and gestational diabetes management (if applicable)

Adapted from Mensing et al. (12).

The level of education is based on the assessment rather than length of time since diagnosis. In addition, patients may be at a basic level in one area and at an advanced level in others based on their self-management experience and past education. When there is only the opportunity to provide limited education, such as with hospitalized patients, asking what they know and want to know about diabetes, current practices and concerns about managing it at home, fears about diabetes, and what is hardest for them helps the nurse provide relevant targeted information in a short period of time. Referral to a comprehensive DSME program is an important part of discharge planning for these patients.

Educational Strategies

A variety of educational strategies have been tested and found to be effective. In general, strategies that are patient centered, engage and involve participants, and meet needs identified in the assessment are most effective. Framing information to meet patient-identified goals (e.g., have more energy, better quality of life) rather than focusing strictly on metabolic goals or risk reduction helps increase effectiveness. Incorporating behavioral and emotional aspects into all content areas is also important. For example, when teaching about SMBG, asking questions such as the following can help patients incorporate this behavior more easily.

- When will you check your blood glucose level?
- How will you check when you are away from home?
- How do others respond when you check your blood glucose in front of them?
- How would you like others to respond or show support?
- How do you feel/will you respond when a reading is higher or lower than you had hoped or anticipated?
- What can you do to help yourself check your blood glucose more faithfully?
- Would you like to set a goal for checking your blood glucose?

One strategy that has been used effectively is a question-based approach, with content presented in response to participant-identified issues (13–15). Content is monitored and recorded to be sure that all necessary areas are addressed. This approach helps ensure that participants remain engaged and actively involved in the discussion, take advantage of the experiences of other participants in the education program, and view it as "personal" (13).

Documentation

Documentation of education provided is needed to meet quality and accreditation standards. The documentation should include information about the content presented, the response of the patient, problems or barriers encountered, readiness to learn, and patient-selected goals. The documentation should provide enough information so that others can follow up and reinforce content as needed and assess goal attainment. Providing this information to the referring provider helps promote a team approach and allows additional reinforcement during patient visits. Developing a specific form that includes content areas, level of education provided, problems identified, and areas to reinforce helps promote consistent documentation and education by all health care providers.

Outcome Evaluation

Outcomes to be evaluated include individual patient outcomes and programmatic outcomes. Attainment of self-selected behavioral goals is the most important individual outcome to assess (16). It is more effective if this follow-up occurs in <6 months (3). Programmatic outcomes can include pre- and postmetabolic measures, screening for complications, self-care behaviors, quality of life or other validated psychosocial measures, and patient satisfaction. Knowledge tests can be useful for helping patients identify areas that need more attention, but are generally not adequate for program evaluation.

It is important to choose programmatic outcomes that are likely to be affected by the content and format of the DSME intervention. For example, if foot care is an area that is of particular relevance to the population and emphasized throughout the program, a pre- and postassessment of foot care behaviors would be an appropriate outcome measure. On the other hand, if the participants are primarily children, outcomes such as days missed from school due to diabetes are more appropriate than foot care.

Continuous quality improvement provides ongoing monitoring and allows adjustments and improvements on an ongoing basis (15). A DSME program advisory group or committee made up of key staff members, stakeholders, and patients is often a useful mechanism to ensure that this process occurs and that the program is modified accordingly.

INDIVIDUAL VERSUS GROUP EDUCATION

The provision of DSME is constantly changing and challenging for the nurse educator. Nurses are often most comfortable teaching patients individually at first, yet there are constraints with this approach. Time and money are two of the more compelling considerations in determining whether to provide a group or individual program. The time required for patients to attend such educational offerings and for nurse educators to set aside for the purpose of teaching is considerable, as are third-party reimbursement restrictions and self-payment abilities.

Group education is an important performance skill for nurses, and they are often encouraged by their patients, their own preferences, and their administrators to offer both individual and group opportunities. These approaches provide the educator and patient with a wider variety of experiences from which to learn skills and gain information. Group programs provide both the nurse and patients a wider variety of experiences to learn skills and gain information. The group sessions, like individual sessions, are based on the nurse's personal style and teaching preferences, the patients who are in attendance, as well as time available. Skills needed for effective group education include preparation (e.g., choice of teaching materials and resources), development of delivery options to enhance the content, assessment of the learners, and timely documentation tips (5,16). Nurses can provide counseling and problem solving in these settings without increasing the time spent (17). Nurses do not just teach information; they develop strategies and offer interesting alternatives and approaches to assist people to learn and to overcome obstacles.

Norris et al. (4) compared group and individual educational literature, concluding that the literature remains divided on the overall effectiveness of groups versus individual methods. They surmised that effects might be more positive for group delivery of lifestyle programs (for example, those that involve diet and physical activity). However, teaching self-care skills was effective in both group and individual sessions. For example, comparison of a group insulin-starter program when compared with individual education described a greater treatment satisfaction, yet similar glycemic control (18). The group setting is being recognized more and more as an effective method of education (7). Little information on cost-effectiveness exists, yet this aspect is often used as justification for group education. Although the group setting is being recognized more and more as an effective method of education (7), more study is needed to support one over the other.

Group education offers the nurse opportunities to learn a variety of new people skills, learn new perspectives on how to deliver the "same old information," share team creativity, and expand the team as a coordinated working unit. Whether educating in groups or individually, the most important factor is not the setting, but providing interesting interventions, an efficient learning process, and empowerment for both the teacher and the patient.

OTHER DELIVERY METHODS

Print materials, videotapes, CDs, DVDs, and computer learning programs can be a useful adjunct to the educational process. Materials are more effective when they are based on the needs of the target audience and on a formative evaluation, tailored to the age and cultural background of the target audience, written at a fifth- to sixth-grade reading level, and matched to a specific interest or need. Personalizing print materials by highlighting key areas or making handwritten notes helps increase their effectiveness. Print materials are available on the Internet from a variety of reputable sources, such as diabetes organizations (e.g., National Diabetes Information Clearinghouse [http://www.diabetes.niddk.nih.gov/intro/index.htm]). Downloading and providing these materials to patients has the advantage of offering more current information than keeping a number of booklets and brochures on hand.

Viewing a videotape or listening to a CD needs to be followed by asking patients if they have questions and evaluating their ability to apply the information to their own lives, situations, and treatment plans. Telephone follow-up for education, goal setting, and care management is also commonly used and effective (19–21).

Other technologies, such as the Internet and distance learning, show promise in preliminary studies but have not been used widely enough to be completely evaluated. Ask patients who have questions based on Internet information to bring the material to their appointment or education session. This will help you better understand their questions and evaluate the validity of the information.

RECOGNITION OF DSME

Standards for DSME were first developed in 1983 by key diabetes organizations, including the American Diabetes Association (ADA) and the American Association of Diabetes Educators. These standards were most recently revised and published in 2000 (12). The standards were based on current evidence and best practices. There are 10 standards that address the structure, process, and outcomes of DSME. Programs are required to include at least a registered nurse and registered dietitian as part of the program staff. Nutrition education and counseling may be provided as part of the program or through a separate referral to a registered dietitian or both.

The ADA created a process to recognize DSME programs that meet these national standards. Programs are required to apply and document that they meet the established review criteria. Referring patients to Recognized programs helps ensure that they receive comprehensive quality education that is likely to be reimbursed. A complete listing of Recognized programs can be found on the ADA web site (http://www.diabetes.org/for-health-professionals-and-scientists/recognition/edrecognition.jsp). In addition to the national ADA Recognition program, a few states offer certification for education programs through the Department of Community Health, and the Indian Health Service offers certification for programs provided by that agency.

CERTIFICATION FOR DIABETES EDUCATORS

All nurses who interact with patients are diabetes educators in some form. Registered nurses and other health care professionals can become certified diabetes educators and use the designation CDE. Certification is available from the National Certification Board for Diabetes Educators (NCBDE) (www.ncbde.org). Nurses who wish to become certified must meet the educational and experiential requirements of the NCBDE and pass a multidisciplinary examination. Recertification is required every 5 years through continuing education credits or retaking the examination. Certification provides documentation that the educator is qualified to provide education but does not directly affect reimbursement for services.

REIMBURSEMENT FOR DSME

Insurance coverage for DSME is available and mandated by most states in the U.S. This reimbursement is the direct result of significant advocacy efforts by the major diabetes organizations and the growing body of evidence supporting the effectiveness of DSME. Although requirements vary according to the state and the individual's health plan, most require ADA recognition or state certification to ensure quality. Although coverage is not yet universal, it is more available and accessible in recent years. Before referral, it is important for patients to check with their health insurance provider to determine the level of coverage available for them and the requirements for reimbursement. Most educational programs also have this information available.

Reimbursement for DSME was initiated by Medicare in 2001. Medicare requires a physician prescription and allows for 10 h of initial group training, unless the patient has special needs such as a hearing impairment, which creates an additional allowance for individual education. One hour of this time is set aside for the assessment. Two hours of follow-up per year may be provided individually or in groups. Patients are qualified if they are newly diagnosed, did not receive education at the time of diagnosis, or are at significant risk for complications of diabetes. Patients must also have had an elevated glycated hemoglobin A_{1c} (>8.5%) on two consecutive measurements taken ≥3 months apart. Other eligibility criteria include taking diabetes medication for the first time or switching from oral medications to insulin or being at high risk for complications based on hospitalization, emergency visits, or signs of complications (22).

SUMMARY

DSME is a critical element of quality diabetes care (23). Patients must have information to actively participate in their own care and to form a partnership with the health care team. DSME is effective when provided by nurses using strategies and interventions that incorporate the current evidence for effective teaching. Providing ongoing self-management support using behavioral strategies such as goal setting helps patients maintain needed health behaviors. The national standards and recognition or certification help ensure quality and support reimbursement.

The future health and outcomes of people with diabetes depends on their ability to effectively manage diabetes on a daily basis. Nurses play a key role in ensuring that patients recognize the importance of their role in managing their diabetes, the need for education, and have the requisite skills to effectively control it on a daily basis. Nurses need to take advantage of every encounter with patients to provide and reinforce education and the importance of self-management for their outcomes and future health. Providing information regarding third-party reimbursement and referring patients to programs that meet the national standards for DSME helps ensure that patients have access to this vital service.

REFERENCES

1. VonKorff M, Gruman J, Schaefer J, Curry SJ, Wagner EH: Collaborative management of chronic illness. *Ann Intern Med* 127:1097–1102, 1997
2. Brown S: Interventions to promote diabetes self-management: state of the science. *Diabetes Educ* 25 (Suppl.):52–61, 1999
3. Norris SL, Engelgau MM, Narayan KM: Effectiveness of self-management training in type 2 diabetes. *Diabetes Care* 24:561–587, 2001
4. Norris SL, Lau J, Smith SJ, Schmid CH, Engelgau MM: Self-management education for adults with type 2 diabetes: a meta-analysis of the effect on glycemic control. *Diabetes Care* 25:1159–1171, 2002
5. Norris SL: Self-management education in type 2 diabetes: what works? *Pract Diabetol* 22:7–13, 2003
6. Barlow J, Wright C, Sheasby J, Turner A, Hainsworth J: Self-management approaches for people with chronic conditions: a review. *Patient Educ Couns* 48:177–187, 2002
7. Sarkisian CA, Brown AAF, Norris CK, Wintz R, Mangione CM: A systematic review of diabetes self-care interventions for older, African American or Latino adults. *Diabetes Educ* 28:467–479, 2003
8. Clement S: Diabetes self-management education. *Diabetes Care* 18:1204–1214, 1995
9. Norris SL, Nichols PJ, Caspersen CJ, Glasgow RE, Engelgau MM, Jack L, Snyder SR, Carande-Kulis VG, Isham G, Garfield S, Briss P, McCulloch D: Increasing diabetes self-management education in community settings: a systematic review. *Am J Prev Med* 22 (Suppl. 4):39–66, 2002
10. Roter DL, Hall JA, Merisca R, Nordstrom B, Cretin D, Svarstad B: Effectiveness of interventions to improve patient compliance: a meta-analysis. *Med Care* 36:1138–1161, 1998
11. Piette JD, Glasgow RE: Education and self-monitoring of blood glucose. In *Evidence-Based Diabetes Care*. Gerstein HC, Haynes RB, Eds. Ontario, Canada, Decker, 2001, p. 207–251
12. Mensing C, Boucher J, Cypress M, Weigner K, Barta P, Hosey G, Koper W, Lasichak A, Lamb B, Mangan M, Norman J, Tanja J, Yauk L, Wisdom K, Adams C: National standards for diabetes self-management education. *Diabetes Care* 23:682–689, 2000
13. Anderson RM, Funnell MM, Nwankwo R, Gillard ML, Fitzgerald JT: Evaluation of a problem-based culturally specific, patient education program for African Americans with diabetes (Abstract). *Diabetes* 50 (Suppl. 2):A195, 2000

14. Deakin TA, Cade JE, Williams DRR, Greenwood DC: Empowered patients: better diabetes control, greater freedom to eat, no weight gain (Abstract). International Diabetes Federation 16th Annual Meeting, A90, 2003

15. Skinner TC, Cradock S, Arundel F, Graham WL: Lifestyle and behavior: four theories and a philosophy: self-management education for individuals newly diagnosed with type 2 diabetes. *Diabetes Spectrum* 16:75–80, 2003

16. Mensing CR, Norris SL: Group education in diabetes: effectiveness and implementation. *Diabetes Spectrum* 16:96–103, 2003

17. King EB, Schlundt DG, Pichert JW, Kinzer CK, Backer BA: Improving the skills of health professionals in engaging patients in diabetes-related problem solving. *J Contin Educ Health Prof* 22:94–102, 2002

18. Erskine P, Daly H, Idris I, Scott A: Patient preference and metabolic outcomes after starting insulin in groups compared with one-to-one specialist nurse teaching (Abstract). *Diabetes* 51 (Suppl. 2):A77, 2002

19. Piette JD, McPhee SJ, Weinberger M, Mah CA, Kraemer FB: Use of automated telephone disease management calls in an ethnically diverse sample of low-income patients with diabetes. *Diabetes Care* 22:1302–1309, 1999

20. Renders CM, Valk GD, Griffin SJ, Wagner EH, Eijk JThM van, Assendelft WJJ: Interventions to improve the management of diabetes mellitus in primary care, outpatient, and community settings (Cochrane Review). In *The Cochrane Library, Issue 4*. Chichester, UK, John Wiley & Sons, 2004

21. Norris SL, Nichols PJ, Caspersen CJ, Glasgow RE, Engelgau MM, Jack L, Snyder SR, Carande-Kulis VG, Isham G, Garfield S, Briss P, McCulloch D, Task Force on Community Preventive Services: The effectiveness of disease and case management for people with diabetes: a systematic review. *Am J Prev Med* 22 (Suppl. 4):15–38, 2002

22. Funnell MM: Reimbursement for diabetes self-management education. *Pract Diabetol* 20:45–46, 2001

23. American Diabetes Association: Standards of medical care in diabetes (Position Statement). *Diabetes Care* 28 (Suppl. 1):S4–S36, 2005

ADDITIONAL READING

American Diabetes Association: *Diabetes Education and Recognition Resource* (CD-ROM). 2nd ed. Alexandria, VA, American Diabetes Association, 2002

Franz MJ, Reader D, Monk A: Implementing Group and Individual Medical Nutrition Therapy for Diabetes. Alexandria, VA, American Diabetes Association, 2003

Funnell MM, Haas LB: Standards for diabetes self-management education programs: a technical review. *Diabetes Care* 18:100–116, 1995

Funnell MM, Lasichak AJ, Burkhart NT, Gillard ML, Nwankwo R: *101 Tips for Diabetes Self-Management Education*. Alexandria, VA, American Diabetes Association, 2002

Funnell MM, Lasichak AJ, Arnold MS, Barr PB: *Life with Diabetes: A Series of Teaching Outlines*. 3rd ed. Alexandria, VA, American Diabetes Association, 2004

Funnell MM, Arnold MS, Lasichak AJ, Barr PB (Eds.): *Type 2 Diabetes: A Series of Teaching Outlines*. Alexandria, VA, American Diabetes Association, 2002

Johnson PD, Anderson BA, Burkhart NT, White NS, Barr PA, Funnell MM: *Teenagers with Type 1 Diabetes: A Curriculum for Adolescents, Families, and Health Professionals*. Alexandria, VA, American Diabetes Association, 2000

Kanzer-Lewis G: *Patient Education: You Can Do It!* Alexandria, VA, American Diabetes Association, 2003

Siminerio L, McLaughlin S, Polonsky W: *Diabetes Education Goals*. 3rd ed. Alexandria, VA, American Diabetes Association, 2003

Ms. Funnell is a Clinical Nurse Specialist at the Michigan Diabetes Research and Training Center, University of Michigan, Ann Arbor, MI. Ms. Mensing is the Diabetes Clinical Nurse Specialist, Coordinator, at the Diabetes Self-Management Program, University of Connecticut, Farmington Campus, Farmington, CT.

Work on this article was supported in part by grant numbers NIH5P60 DK20572 and 1R18OK062323 from the National Institute of Diabetes and Digestive and Kidney Diseases of the National Institutes of Health.

17. Behavioral Strategies for Improving Self-Management

KATIE WEINGER, EdD, RN, AND SHEILA J. MCMURRICH, BA

Many health care professionals now recognize that health education involves more than just providing information. Diabetes education is a perfect example. The goal of diabetes education is to help individuals with diabetes live well. This goal is met by assisting those with diabetes integrate diabetes care into their lifestyles and, when necessary, adapt their lifestyle to healthy living guidelines and treatment requirements.

Accordingly, diabetes care and education are all about behavior, i.e., helping reinforce some behaviors and change others. Because change can be slow and frustrating, nurses caring for individuals with diabetes face the important challenge of effectively supporting patients in their efforts to live well with diabetes. This chapter discusses several aspects of behavioral approaches in the treatment of diabetes: general principles that apply to most interventions and strategies, useful tools and strategies for diabetes and education, four phases of psychological responses to diabetes, and examples of validated behavioral programs.

GENERAL PRINCIPLES IMPORTANT TO BEHAVIORAL STRATEGIES FOR DIABETES

Understand That Diabetes Is a Chronic Illness

Diabetes treatment and education do not fit neatly into the acute care model (1). Although acute episodes may arise and need immediate attention, diabetes is primarily a chronic illness that requires lifestyle adjustments and long-term prevention strategies to ensure maintenance of health. While much of the education and training for nurses occurs in hospital environments and is centered on an acute care model, several general principles may help these health care professionals make the transition to a chronic care model.

Use Empowerment in Diabetes

Empowerment in diabetes is a more philosophical approach to the care and support of individual diabetes patients than the more community-oriented public health model of empowerment. Empowerment is an approach to clinical practice that emphasizes "helping people discover and use their innate abilities to gain mastery over their diabetes" (2). Empowerment means that individuals with diabetes have the tools, such as knowledge, control, resources, and experience, to implement and evaluate their self-management practices (2). Most therapeutic communication skills and principles of adult learning described here are consistent with this philosophy of empowerment.

People with Diabetes Are in Charge of Their Own Care

One of the most important underlying principles of diabetes treatment is that individuals with diabetes, not their health care teams, provide the majority of care for their diabetes. Once this fact is accepted, behavioral approaches become logical methods to support patients in their diabetes self-management. Some health care professionals, particularly those schooled in an acute care approach, may struggle with this concept. Nurses need to conceptualize their role as one who helps the patient learn to solve problems rather than one who solves problems for the patient.

Health Education, Like Adult Education, Must Be Directly Relevant to the Learner

Nurses must remember that patients are learning about diabetes because they have it. Patients are more likely to remember information that they see as relevant to them and that affects how they live, work, play, and relate to others. The key is their perception; information must be presented in such a way that individuals with diabetes can immediately understand how information and recommended self-care tasks apply to them.

STRATEGIES AND TOOLS

Orienting Patients to the Health Care System

Although health care professionals spend years training for their profession, patients receive no formal instruction in how to be a patient. Yet, being a patient is a distinct and important role that will affect their lives. Over time, patients will develop an idea of their roles based on information from their own prior experience, the media, and intended and unintended cues from their health care providers and support staff. For example, if someone with diabetes has had a negative experience when dealing with a physician or nurse, they may "learn" that the health care team should only be contacted for dire emergencies. Without any guidelines as to when it is appropriate to contact the health care team, they may become reluctant to contact the health care team for help or advice. Therefore, orienting patients to diabetes treatment and providing guidelines on how best to use a health care team are important.

Building a Respectful Collaborative Relationship

The philosophy of empowerment and many of the tools described below contribute to the establishment of a mutually respectful relationship with patients (2). The health care provider and the patient should mutually agree on the agenda for an education appointment. As an educator, you may want to cover specific topics, but the patient will not be able to devote full attention to the issues you want to cover if he or she is concerned about other issues. Listening to a patient's concerns and validating your understanding through reflection and summarization are extremely important tools to use in developing a collaborative relationship. Table 17.1 lists several useful communication techniques.

Remember that the patient's task is to learn self-management, not simply to receive advice. People with diabetes must learn how to manage diabetes and problem solve and will not benefit from having problems solved for them. Although advice is often important, before giving advice, consider whether first clarifying the problem through discussion and then trying to problem solve would better serve the patient. Giving advice too quickly may stifle the relationship by emphasizing the nurse as the knowledgeable one and the patient as the passive recipient of knowledge. In this case, the health care professional, not the person with diabetes, is in control; passive knowledge rarely translates to behavior change.

Table 17.1 Useful Communication Techniques

Setting a mutually acceptable agenda	Begin an appointment by finding out what the patient wants to talk about. An agenda should include items important to the patient as well as items that you think are important. Be sure the number and depth of the agenda items fit within the time frame of the meeting.
Open-ended questions	Allow the patient to verbalize feelings and provide information in their own words by asking open-ended questions. Some examples are ■ "Tell me about. . . ." ■ "How are you doing with taking your medications?" ■ "What about your meal plan is working?" ■ "What problems are you having taking care of your diabetes?"
Listening	Actively listen while consciously focusing on what the person means. This is not as easy as it sounds. Many people tend to think about what they will say next instead of focusing on what the patient is actually saying. Two useful tools for listening are reflection and summarizing. **Reflection (3)** Repeat or paraphrase the statement back to the person but in the tone of a question. ■ "You are having trouble with your exercise plan?" ■ "You are frustrated with your treatment recommendations?" **Summarizing (3)** Summarizing the general idea of the patient's conversation shows that you have been listening and that you understand. It also provides an opportunity to correct any misunderstandings. If the patient has outlined a plan or made other positive steps, summarizing can help reinforce their progress.

Assessment

The goal of behavioral assessment is to understand patients' points of view and their specific questions and perceptions about diabetes, its treatment, and their health status. The behavioral assessment begins with open-ended questions that elicit knowledge of treatment recommendations and self-care tasks as well as attitudes, barriers, and support for diabetes self-management (Table 17.2). Reflection as a follow-up to open-ended questions often helps the patient verbalize issues and identify barriers to successful self-care (3).

Goal Setting

When asked what their goals for diabetes care are, most people think in broad, sweeping terms. Commonly stated goals are to "lose weight," "improve glycemic control," or "check glucose more often." However, sweeping goals often do not

Table 17.2 Important Behavioral Assessment Areas

Area	Comments
Knowledge of self-care recommendations	The rationale for and frequency of doing self-care behaviors is central, rather than knowledge of pathophysiology.
Attitudes toward diabetes and self-care tasks	Does the patient perceive self-care tasks as important? On a scale of 1 to 10, how important is it for the patient to take care of his or her diabetes? Is the person feeling overwhelmed? The Problem Areas in Diabetes survey (4,5) can be used to start conversation.
Depression	Depression is common in diabetes but underrecognized and undertreated. If a person is tearful, sad, or extremely angry, a referral to a mental health professional may be necessary.
Cognitive status	Over time, diabetes may affect memory, and aging certainly affects memory. Be aware of signs of lack of understanding. Have the person summarize important points before leaving, providing key points in writing.
Readiness, ability, and intention to make necessary changes	Does the patient feel that changing behavior is necessary or important? Until a person is ready, behavior is difficult to change, and maintenance of a behavior change is even more difficult.
Family and other support	Does the person feel alone with their diabetes or overwhelmed by family nagging ("diabetes police")? Does the person with diabetes receive the amount of emotional support and the amount of help that he or she wants (6)?
Literacy	Assess whether and in what language(s) the person can read. Remember that most people read at least one to two grade levels below their highest grade achieved. Reading ability is not necessarily equated with level of intelligence.

affect behavior because they are long term and difficult to put into operation. Such broad goals should be acknowledged and used to set short-term goals that are realistic, achievable, and measurable (7,8). Identifying the steps to be taken to achieve the goal is important. Effective evaluation recognizes the amount or percentage of the goal achieved rather than simply determining whether the goal was met. For example, a patient who walked for 30 min 3 days a week instead of the desired 5 days achieved 60% of his or her goal. Evaluation, more than just a check to see whether goals are met, should also be an opportunity for patients to assess their plan. Did they meet their goals because of their plan or in spite of it? If the latter is true, then they need to think about revising their plan. Once goals are met, patients need to develop a maintenance plan or set new goals.

Use of Structured Activities

Several tools, such as glucose monitors and pedometers, help engage people in their diabetes self-care. If used correctly, these tools can improve self-management because they help people learn about the body's response to diabetes and its treatment. Two important rules apply to this type of equipment. First, all information is valuable. Thus, when a glucose reading is high, patients must learn to acknowledge the importance of knowing that information so they can take action. Similarly, knowing that a treatment is not working is important. If a patient's eating habits are not healthy, then that is also important to know. Only with knowledge can changes be made. Inadvertent verbal and nonverbal negative messages about high glucose readings may foster avoidance of glucose monitoring. The second rule is that patients must understand what to do with the information; if they do not, they will not use it. Pedometers are very popular among people with diabetes as well as the general population, mainly because they provide information that is relatively easy to understand and are easy to use. On the other hand, glucose monitoring is not as intuitive, particularly for individuals with type 2 diabetes. However, if they use a glucose meter to learn how medications, food, or exercise affects their blood glucose, monitoring can be more relevant and less frustrating.

FOUR PHASES OF PSYCHOLOGICAL RESPONSE TO DIABETES

The emotional or psychological response of a person with diabetes can influence the success of behavioral approaches. Psychological responses follow a general progression of four phases from the time of diagnosis until complications are so dominant that they may overshadow diabetes care (9,10).

Diagnosis

A person with newly diagnosed diabetes struggles to learn about this chronic illness, to figure out how life will change, and to incorporate the diagnosis into his or her persona. Meanwhile, the individual also strives to maintain life as it is already known.

A person recently diagnosed with type 1 diabetes can be so overwhelmed trying to process the fact of the diagnosis that he or she may not be able to internalize any additional information provided. Repetition of all information is important. A contact telephone number and a clearly written handout that repeats all key points are extremely useful for the person to have at home. Schedule follow-up sessions within 1 month to assess how the person is doing and to reinforce important self-care behaviors.

For individuals with newly diagnosed type 1 diabetes, survival skills are important. Patients must learn how to handle equipment and give themselves injections with either a syringe or a pen. Repetitive practice is very helpful. Although one demonstration by the educator may be adequate, many practice sessions under the watchful guidance of an educator are typically more useful. Patients should feel comfortable handling the equipment and drawing up the correct dose before leaving the office.

The ability to learn new information and skills may also be compromised in individuals newly diagnosed with type 2 diabetes if the diagnosis is accompanied by severe comorbidity. Depending on the patient's age, support systems, and cognitive status, several educational sessions may be necessary to help the patient understand the care and implications of diabetes.

Individuals with type 2 diabetes without comorbidities may consider the diagnosis of diabetes to be a normal part of aging, simply "taking another pill." Such individuals may lack the motivation to make important lifestyle changes.

Prevention Period

During this phase, the person with diabetes is expected to implement lifestyle changes to stay healthy and prevent complications. However, the patient experiences no immediate distressful symptoms. This lack of symptoms may diminish motivation for lifestyle adjustments, particularly for individuals whose coping styles include procrastination and denial. Several validated behavioral interventions may be useful during this phase. Training in coping skills helps healthy adolescents who are receiving intensive treatment improve their diabetes self-management skills. Motivational interviewing may be used to help patients recognize the importance of self-management tasks and thus move toward improving their self-care behaviors (11) (Table 17.3).

Worry About Complications/Early Complications

Individuals who have not maintained glycemic control within targets may begin to worry about complications, particularly if they have signs of early complications. This phase often triggers patients to take action to regain control of their diabetes; this response, if unfulfilled or unstructured, may result in burnout (6). Feelings of being overwhelmed by diabetes self-care, of being controlled by diabetes, and of constantly worrying about taking care of diabetes and perhaps becoming unmotivated or unwilling to continue with diabetes self-care practices are evidence of diabetes burnout. Cognitive behavioral techniques and motivational interviewing are useful interventions to help address negative attitudes and perceptions that interfere with self-care (Table 17.3).

Complications Dominate

When individuals with diabetes develop one or more serious complications, they may seek treatment from subspecialists who treat the complication but not the underlying diabetes. Thus, the patient is faced with several different illnesses with which to cope instead of focusing on one integrated diabetes treatment program.

Table 17.3 Examples of Successful Behavioral Intervention Programs

Program Name	Description
Blood Glucose Awareness Training (12)	Eight-week group education with homework assignments designed to help participants with type 1 diabetes prevent glucose fluctuations by early recognition or anticipation and treatment of hypoglycemia and hyperglycemia. Blood glucose awareness training is helpful for individuals with hypoglycemia unawareness.
Coping Skills Training (13)	Small-group program designed to help adolescents develop more positive coping strategies to help them manage the stresses of diabetes and its treatment. Coping skills training uses role-playing and scenarios to engage teens in learning how to cope with typical life situations.
Motivational Interviewing (3,11,14)	Developed in the treatment of addictions, motivational interviewing is currently being investigated for use in the treatment of diabetes. In the treatment of diabetes, this approach uses interviewing techniques and therapeutic approaches to help patients become more ready to change their self-management behaviors. Motivational interviewing is mainly used in one-on-one interactions.
Cognitive Behavioral Therapy (15,16)	In the treatment of diabetes, this type of therapy is used in group education sessions to help people with diabetes change their negative attitudes and thought habits to more positive approaches to diabetes self-management.

PRACTICAL POINT

People with diabetes may exhibit a variety of symptoms and may flow in and out of these phases of psychological response at different times. Simply labeling an individual as "noncompliant" when they are having difficulty coping with their disease and self-management regimen does a disservice to patients and does little to assist in improving their health. An assessment of behavior and emotions can help identify problem areas for intervention or referral.

SUMMARY

Reinforcing some behaviors and changing others is a key component of diabetes care and education. Endorsing the philosophy that the patient is in charge of his or her diabetes and providing the person with the tools and knowledge necessary to manage his or her own care provide the foundation for the nurse's role in the treatment of diabetes. Supporting others in the management of their diabetes requires the nurse to develop skillful communication techniques and use other behavioral interventions.

REFERENCES

1. Anderson RM, Funnell MM: Using the empowerment approach to help patients change behavior. In *Practical Psychology for Diabetes Clinicians*. 2nd ed.

Anderson BJ, Rubin RR, Eds. Alexandria, VA, American Diabetes Association, 2002, p. 3–12

2. Anderson B, Funnell M: *The Art of Empowerment: Stories and Strategies for Diabetes Educators.* 2nd ed. Alexandria, VA, American Diabetes Association, 2005

3. Rollnick S, Mason P, Butler C: *Health Behavior Change: A Guide For Practitioners.* Edinburgh, UK, Churchill Livingstone, 1999

4. Polonsky WH, Anderson BJ, Lohrer PA, Welch G, Jacobson AM, Aponte JE, Schwartz CE: Assessment of diabetes-related distress. *Diabetes Care* 18: 754–760, 1995

5. Welch GW, Jacobson AM, Polonsky WH: The Problem Areas in Diabetes (PAID) scale: an examination of its clinical utility. *Diabetes Care* 20:760–766, 1997

6. Polonsky WH: *Diabetes Burnout: What To Do When You Can't Take It Anymore.* Alexandria, VA, American Diabetes Association, 1999

7. Davis M, Eshelman ER, McKay M: *The Relaxation & Stress Reduction Workbook.* Oakland, CA, New Harbinger Publications, 1988

8. Strecher VJ, Seijts GH, Kok GJ, Latham GP, Glasgow R, DeVellis B, Meertens RM, Bulger DW: Goal setting as a strategy for health behavior change. *Health Educ Q* 22:190–201, 1995

9. Hamburg BA, Inoff GE: Coping with predictable crises of diabetes. *Diabetes Care* 6:409–416, 1983

10. Jacobson AM, Weinger K: Psychosocial complications in diabetes. In *Medical Management of Diabetes Mellitus.* Leahy JL, Clark NG, Cefalu WT, Eds. New York, Marcel Dekker, 2000, p. 559–572

11. Miller WR, Rollnick S: *Motivational Interviewing: Preparing People for Change.* Miller WR, Rollnick S, Eds. New York, Guilford Press, 2002, p. 3–198

12. Cox D, Gonder-Frederick L, Polonsky W, Schlundt D, Julian D, Clarke W: A multicenter evaluation of blood glucose awareness training II. *Diabetes Care* 18:523–528, 1995

13. Grey M, Boland EA, Davidson M, Li J, Tamborlane WV: Coping skills training for youth with diabetes mellitus has long-lasting effects on metabolic control and quality of life. *J Pediatr* 137:107–113, 2000

14. Zweben A, Zuckoff A: Motivational interviewing and treatment adherence. In *Motivational Interviewing: Preparing People for Change.* Miller WR, Rollnick S, Eds. New York, Guilford Press, 2002, p. 299–319

15. Van der Ven N, Weinger K, Snoek F: Cognitive behavior therapy in diabetes: an opportunity to help people with diabetes improve their self-management. *Diabetes Voice* 47:10–13, 2002

16. Snoek FJ, van der Ven NC, Lubach CH, Chatrou M, Ader HJ, Heine RJ, Jacobson AM: Effects of cognitive behavioral group training (CBGT) in adult patients with poorly controlled insulin-dependent (type 1) diabetes: a pilot study. *Patient Educ Couns* 45:143–148, 2001

Dr. Weinger is an Assistant Professor, Department of Psychology, at Harvard Medical School, Boston, MA, and an Investigator at the Section on Behavioral and Mental Health Research, Joslin Diabetes Center, Boston, MA. She also directs the Center for Innovation in Diabetes Education and the Office of Research Fellow Affairs at Joslin Diabetes Center, Boston, MA. Ms. McMurrich is a Research Assistant at the Section on Behavioral and Mental Health Research, Joslin Diabetes Center, Boston, MA.

18. Cultural Context of Diabetes Education and Care

GAIL D'ERAMO MELKUS, EDD, C-ANP, CDE, FAAN, AND
KELLEY NEWLIN, MSN, ANP

Diabetes affects individuals across the lifespan from infancy to old age, independent of sex, socioeconomic status, and ethnicity. This diversity is represented in the increasing number of individuals living with diabetes in the U.S. and worldwide. Although diabetes does not discriminate in terms of whom it affects, type 2 diabetes and its related complications are disproportionately present among American ethnic minorities (1). In fact, recent studies on health disparities provide evidence that ethnic minority and vulnerable populations often do not receive adequate care, including diabetes care (2). Disparate care may result from a mismatch in illness experiences between patients and providers that are based on a range of cultural factors such as religion, ethnic background, and personal history.

Diabetes self-management and related metabolic outcomes are associated with the development of diabetes-related complications (3,4). Thus, optimal glycemic control is the goal of diabetes care and patient education interventions. The complexity of disease management necessitates the active involvement of the patient (and often the family as well) in daily decisions regarding dietary intake, physical activity, and medications in an effort to achieve optimal glycemic control and prevent complications. Individual and family response to these daily demands of living with diabetes is central to self-management and its related outcomes. Participation that results in successful adherence to the therapeutic regimen depends on a number of important factors, such as patient satisfaction with the provider and setting and perceived benefit of adherence on health status (5). An individual's personal response and participation in self-management are often based on a complex set of health beliefs, perceptions, and practices that are culturally embedded (6). Because of increasing cultural diversity among Americans, rising incidence and prevalence of diabetes, and complexity of self-management, cultural considerations must be addressed in the context of delivering quality diabetes care and education.

The American Diabetes Association (ADA), the American Association of Diabetes Educators (AADE), and the Centers for Disease Control and Prevention (CDC) strongly recommend that diabetes education and care address cultural factors. The ADA and CDC clinical care guidelines and the AADE standards for diabetes education underscore the significant influence that cultural factors may have in adherence to prescribed regimens of self-care and, in turn, physiological outcomes (7,8).

CONCEPTUAL PERSPECTIVES

Culture is a concept that is derived from anthropological and sociological concepts. Leininger, a nursing anthropologist, defines culture as the "learned and shared beliefs, values, and lifeways of a designated or particular group that are generally transmitted intergenerationally and influence one's thinking and action modes" (9). Mechanic, a medical sociologist, proposes that great variation exists in behaviors among people within a particular cultural group; therefore, observed cultural patterns may be considered only rough approximations of how people act in specific contexts (10). Thus, among any ethnic or cultural group there is a great degree of within-group variation in terms of socioeconomic status, traditions, concepts of health and illness, and personal identity. Based on both anthropological and sociological concepts, the Office of Minority Health, U.S. Department of Health and Human Services, defines culture as "integrated patterns of human behavior that include language, thoughts, communications, actions, customs, beliefs, values, and institutions of racial, ethnic, religious, or social groups" (11). It is important to note, however, that membership within a given cultural group may or may not delineate a person's ethnic affiliation.

ETHNICITY

Ethnicity more specifically defines a person's race, religion, national or geographic origin, or symbolic identification. It is important to note that although there is no scientific or biological basis of race, the terms *race* and *racism* have meaning as social constructs and therefore have social connotations that differ from ethnicity (12). Although cultural competency is necessary for providing diabetes care and education to any given group, cultural assessment of each patient is necessary to prevent cultural stereotyping.

Often, the term *cultural competence* is used interchangeably with *cultural sensitivity, cultural awareness, cultural congruence, cultural relevance,* and other related terms, suggesting that these terms are synonymous. They are in fact conceptually distinct. Cultural sensitivity or awareness refers to the examination of a person's own assumptions regarding other cultural groups and becoming aware of how these notions might affect perceptions and prejudices of culturally different groups (13). Cultural congruence refers to a match between the delivery of care and the cultural values, beliefs, and patterned behavior of the care recipients (14). Cultural relevance involves the perception of the care recipient in terms of the cultural appropriateness of the delivery of health services. Cultural competence, as suggested by the Office of Minority Health (11), involves the actual integration of consistent behaviors, attitudes, and policies in the delivery of health care in cross-cultural situations. This involves blending congruent behaviors, attitudes, and policies in systems, in agencies, among professionals, and in therapeutic interventions to effectively work within cross-cultural contexts involving the beliefs, behaviors, communication patterns, and needs of health care consumers and their communities (15). A recent review of the literature on culturally competent health care interventions found a compelling number of studies that demonstrated significantly improved outcomes for patients with diabetes and other health problems after receiving culturally competent or relevant interventions compared with others who did not receive such care (16).

Cultural Health Beliefs and Practices

Beliefs of health and illness are derived from heritage and cultural phenomena that vary among cultural, religious, and ethnic groups. As already stated, there is great within- and between-group diversity among any given group, lending to a multicultural identity for many individuals. Thus, the domains of culture may vary based on the extent to which an individual has become acculturated to the dominant culture and the degree to which individuals have maintained their traditional heritage (17). Studies have shown that the more acculturated an individual is, the more likely he or she is to exhibit autonomy in the patient role and with patient-provider interactions (18,19), consistent with the American model of health care delivery. However, even when patient autonomy is present, individuals from different ethnic groups often rely on family involvement in the context of illness regardless of their personal cultural identity. This is particularly true of Native Americans, whose family-centeredness is constant regardless of acculturation level, tribal affiliation, and family lifestyle (traditional or bicultural) (20).

Spiritual and Religious Beliefs and Practices

Spirituality and religion are prominent cultural factors across American ethnic groups, demonstrating constancy independent of other culturally related factors. In fact, most Americans (97%) consider themselves spiritual, religious, or both (21). Furthermore, many Americans indicate that spirituality and/or religion are important components of health, reporting the use of prayer in a medical context (67%) and desire for physicians to be "spiritually attuned to them" (70%) (22).

Spirituality and religion, although often used interchangeably, are conceptually different but related terms. *Spirituality*, as a broader term, is often defined by such attributes as transcendence, hope, strength, identification of meaning and purpose in life, and interconnectedness with others, God, or a higher power (23–26). Spirituality is further referred to as a source of peace, coping, and guidance (25). *Religion* may be conceived of as an organized system of beliefs and practices that provides intellectual, behavioral, and social forms to spiritual expression and thereby nurtures a relationship with God or a higher power (23,24,26).

Spirituality and/or religion often shape health care beliefs and practices (Table 18.1). Yet, across and within ethnicities, such health beliefs and practices are interfused with ethnically based values and traditions to varying degrees, which further influence a person's orientation or approach to health and illness. Across ethnicities, distinct spiritual and/or religious health beliefs and practices are apparent.

To illustrate, Native Americans, although belonging to >300 individual tribal traditions, tend to view health or wellness as harmony with natural, social, and supernatural environments (27). Illness or disharmony may be treated by traditional religious practices, involving, for example, cleansing sweats, prayer, and the intervention of a medicine man or woman (28,29). However, certain illnesses, such

Table 18.1 Religious Health Beliefs, Practices/Restrictions, and Dietary Habits Relevant to Diabetes Care

Religious Groups	Religious Health Beliefs	Religious Health Care Practices/Restrictions Relevant to Diabetes Care	Religious Dietary Habits Relevant to Diabetes Care
Adventist, Seventh Day	■ Body is the temple of God ■ Healthy living is essential (48) ■ Healing may be achieved through both divine and medical interventions (27,49)	■ Prayer ■ Anointing of the Sick, involving prayer and anointing with oil by the clergy ■ Holy Communion (48) ■ No restrictions on medications ■ Some sects may prohibit narcotics and/or stimulants (27) ■ No restrictions on surgical procedures, including amputations ■ Emphasis on physical medicine, rehabilitation, and therapeutic diets (27,49)	■ Vegetarian diet is common ■ Nonvegetarian members may refrain from pork, shellfish, and some birds (27,49) ■ Alcohol, coffee, and tea are proscribed (27) ■ Fasting may be practiced by individual churches to varying degrees ■ Fasting is not recommended if it is likely to have an adverse effect on health (49)
American Indian religions	■ Wellness reflects harmony (29) ■ Illness reflects disharmony with nature, social, and supernatural environments (27) ■ Creator reveals guidance to achieve restoration of harmony ■ Individual responsible for following Creator's guidance and thereby personal health (27,29)	■ Varies according to tribe ■ Some tribes participate in sweat ceremonies, involving singing, sharing, prayer, and contemplation. Participation in sweat ceremonies promotes spiritual and physical cleansing, physical transcendence, and receptivity to ancestral wisdom ■ Peyote used as a sacrament within the Native American Church. Peyote promotes spiritual guidance and may stimulate inner cleansing/release (27) ■ Prayers for harmony with nature and for health (29) ■ Use of a Medicine Man or Woman to heal through prayers, ceremonies, and/or spiritual powers of ancestors,	■ Blessed food is believed to be free of harmful substances (28) ■ Following spiritual rituals, berries, corn, and dried meats may be consumed (27)

Table 18.1 Religious Health Beliefs, Practices/Restrictions, and Dietary Habits Relevant to Diabetes Care (*Continued*)

Religious Groups	Religious Health Beliefs	Religious Health Care Practices/Restrictions Relevant to Diabetes Care	Religious Dietary Habits Relevant to Diabetes Care
		often complementing traditional western medicine (27,50)	
Buddhism	■ Illness due to karma or the result of actions in this or a previous life (27) ■ Healing not achieved through faith ■ Healing and recovery promoted by peace and liberation from anxiety experienced through awakening to Buddha's wisdom (27,49)	■ Specific practices and restrictions not dictated ■ Practices determined on an individual basis (27,49) ■ Practices that contribute to Enlightenment are encouraged ■ Medical procedures that may prolong life and attainment of Enlightenment are encouraged (49)	■ Moderate diet is encouraged (49)
Catholicism	■ Body is the temple of the Holy Spirit ■ Health is a gift from God ■ Illness may result from sin (27) ■ Christ has the power to forgive sins and heal illness ■ Christ's healing presence is active through the sacraments and prayer ■ Care for personal health and the health of others is encouraged	■ Sacrament of the Sick (anointing, communion, and blessing by a priest) (49) ■ Sacrament of Holy Communion (receiving the Eucharist—a consecrated wafer—for health and healing) ■ Prayer and/or laying on of hands (48,49) ■ Medications encouraged if benefits exceed risks (49) ■ Amputations are acceptable if they are for the good of the whole person (49)	■ Foods and beverages to be used in moderation and in a manner not detrimental to health ■ Healthy adults are encouraged to abstain from meat and meat products on Ash Wednesday, Good Friday, and all Fridays during Lent (48)
Islam	■ Life is a gift from God, or Allah ■ Illness reflects God's will ■ Illness may serve as a means for expiating sin and strengthening character	■ Daily prayer and reading or listening to the Qur'an in combination with medical treatment (51) ■ Faith healing is acceptable in the context of deteriorating physiological and mental	■ Pork, alcohol, and some shellfish are proscribed (27,48) ■ Permissible meat must be blessed and properly slaughtered (48) *(continued)*

Table 18.1 Religious Health Beliefs, Practices/Restrictions, and Dietary Habits Relevant to Diabetes Care (*Continued*)

Religious Groups	Religious Health Beliefs	Religious Health Care Practices/Restrictions Relevant to Diabetes Care	Religious Dietary Habits Relevant to Diabetes Care
	■ God shows mercy and compassion by providing cures (27,51)	health as a supplement to medical treatment (27,49) ■ Prescribed medications are not restricted, including pork derivatives ■ Amputations are not restricted (49) ■ Feminine modesty and feminine preference for female clinicians (48) ■ During the *month* of Ramadan, a patient may not take medication between dawn and sunset (52)	■ Dietary moderation is expected (27) ■ Fasting from dawn to sunset during the entire *month* of Ramadan. Children, elderly, infirm, and pregnant or nursing women are exempt (48)
Judaism	■ Illness may result from sin ■ God's given wisdom responsible for medical discoveries that modify/eliminate disease or suffering ■ Jewish law requires Jews to seek medical services to promote health and healing (27,53)	■ Praying independently or in community to God ■ Commandment of visiting the sick (27,53) ■ No medication restrictions (27) ■ On the weekly Sabbath (sunset Friday to sunset Saturday), ultra-Orthodox Jews may refrain from taking medications if viewed as not life threatening (53) ■ Consultation with a Rabbi in health care decisions is encouraged (27) ■ Beliefs related to amputations vary widely (49)	■ Wine is appropriate and acceptable in moderation (53) ■ Orthodox and some Conservative and Reform Jews follow kosher laws, including no consumption of predatory fowl, pork products, shellfish, fish without fins or scales, and animal products not ritually slaughtered (48) ■ Rosh Hashanah may be initiated by eating apples and honey (53) ■ On Yom Kippur, Jews fast for 24 h unless prevented by medical reasons ■ During Passover, leavened products are not eaten (48)

Table 18.1 Religious Health Beliefs, Practices/Restrictions, and Dietary Habits Relevant to Diabetes Care (*Continued*)

Religious Groups	Religious Health Beliefs	Religious Health Care Practices/Restrictions Relevant to Diabetes Care	Religious Dietary Habits Relevant to Diabetes Care
Protestantism	■ Varied beliefs about health and illness ■ Individuals are encouraged to formulate beliefs according to conscious and not formal religious authority (27)	■ Scripture reading and personal prayer common among many Protestants ■ Holy Communion ■ Anointing of the Sick (e.g., Church of Brethren and Lutheran traditions) ■ Prayer and/or laying on of hands for divine healing often in conjunction with medical treatment (e.g., Assemblies of God and Church of Nazarene traditions) (48,49)	■ Abstinence from alcohol is encouraged by some Protestant faiths (e.g., Baptist, Church of Nazarene, and Mennonite traditions) ■ Fasting is not required among the Protestant faiths ■ Episcopalians may abstain from meat on Fridays (48)

as diabetes, may be considered "non-Indian" diseases. In such cases, traditional western medicine may be preferred and may be incorporated with traditional practices (28).

In contrast, spiritual and/or religious African Americans may view illness in relation to God or Jesus. God or Jesus may be conceived as the divine physician or supreme healer (30). Predominantly Protestant, a number of African Americans believe God's health prescriptions and healing powers are revealed in the Bible (31). Also, God's healing powers may be realized through faith and related religious and/or spiritual practices such as prayer, scripture reading, and laying on of hands (25,30). Traditional folk remedies dating back to slavery may be integrated with faith practices (30,32).

Within any given ethnic group, spiritual and/or religious health beliefs and practices are similarly diverse. America's Hispanic population, for example, consists of individuals of Mexican, Cuban, Puerto Rican, Central American, and South American descent, among others. Within this broadly defined ethnic population, spiritual and/or religious health beliefs and practices may be heterogeneous, despite the predominance of Catholicism. A number of Cuban Americans blend Catholicism with Yoruba tribal beliefs and practices into a religion called Santeria (also known as Regla de Ocha). Believers of Santeria may seek healing assistance from a santero, or priest, which commonly involves spells, magic, and animal sacrifice (33,34). Likewise, some Puerto-Rican Americans integrate elements of Catholicism with African and Indian beliefs, practicing Espiritismo. In the context of illness, espiritistas, or spiritual healers, may be called on to use healing practices such as topical herbs, aromatic ointments or liquids, and prayers (35,36).

   The diversity of cultural health beliefs and practices, including those related to religion and spirituality, necessitates that a comprehensive cultural assessment be conducted as part of the diabetes education and care process.

CULTURAL ASSESSMENT

A cultural assessment addresses patient beliefs and practices in the context of the larger reference group, the family, and the individual. Culturally competent education and care requires skills of individualized cross-cultural communication, assessment, interpretation, and intervention (37). These skills are the basis of the cultural and linguistically competent care recommended by the Office of Minority Health in newly published guidelines aimed at decreasing health disparities (38) (Table 18.2).

Self-Assessment

The first step in cross-cultural communication and counseling is self-assessment. Health care providers will have to identify cultural assumptions by reviewing their own social, religious, and personal beliefs and practices, particularly those related to health and illness. Diabetes education and care are focused on self-management of dietary intake, physical activity, medications, and screening and care practices for prevention of complications, e.g., eye examinations, foot care, dental care. Therefore, nurses and other health care providers who are involved in diabetes education and care must self-evaluate their own attitudes, beliefs, values, and norms that are related to having a chronic illness such as diabetes.

Dietary Practices

Diet and nutrition therapy is a core component of education and care for people with diabetes, and for the majority of individuals with type 2 diabetes, such care

---

Table 18.2 Standards for Culturally and Linguistically Appropriate Services Summarized by Themes

Standards 1–3: Culturally Competent Care
- Ensure diverse staff
- Ongoing training of staff

Standards 4–7: Language Access Services
- Bilingual staff
- Interpreter services
- Printed patient materials

Standards 8–14: Operational Support for Cultural Competence
- Community collaborations
- Demographic database
- Organizational assessment

From U.S. Office of Minority Health, Department of Health and Human Services (38).

PRACTICAL POINT

Four steps to cross-cultural counseling

1. Self-evaluation of own culture
   - Review past and present social, religious, and personal beliefs and attitudes about health, illness, food, and food use
2. Learn patient culture
   - Research written materials
   - Talk with friends or colleagues of the same ethnic group as the patient
   - Eat in a restaurant or visit a food store of the patient's ethnic background
3. Interview patient
   - Offer opportunities for family and/or significant other(s) to participate as appropriate
4. Analyze information and plan intervention
   - Identify cultural beliefs, practices, traditions, food preferences, meals, and patterns of eating
   - Incorporate findings into management strategy
   - Involve the patient in setting goals

---

is focused on dietary modification for the purpose of weight loss and maintenance. Attitudes and beliefs about eating, body shape, and weight will influence the process and outcomes of nutrition therapy as well as physical activity recommendations. In conducting an assessment of personal attitudes toward patterns of food use, shape, and weight, health care providers should acknowledge their own cultural assumptions and preferences, which may differ from those of other ethnic groups. In terms of weight and shape, white women often experience the greatest social pressure for thinness, whereas black women may not perceive weight as a problem when compared with a reference group of other black women (39,40). In some cultures, eating and overweight are equated with good health and thinness with illness. Based on such assumptions, suggestions to change dietary patterns and food preferences may be met with resistance.

Attitudes and practices related to types of food also differ among groups, and taking time to learn about a patient's culture is another important aspect of cross-cultural counseling. For example, in certain European countries, corn is animal feed unfit for human consumption, whereas corn is a core food with spiritual connotations for some Native-American groups (lending to the belief by Americans in general that corn is used as both livestock feed and human food). Core foods and conventional methods of preparation are important factors for consideration in planning cross-cultural dietary interventions. Japanese, Chinese, Korean, and other Asian groups, like many Hispanic groups, use rice as a core food, whereas Italians use pasta and Native Americans use cornmeal. Many African Americans, including those of Caribbean descent, enjoy fried foods, whereas West Africans use stews. It is important to note, however, that many African Americans, like various other groups living in or from the southern U.S. region, may be accustomed to fried foods because it is conventional for southern-style cooking. The cultural context of regional cooking needs to be considered as well as ethnic and religious practices to avoid making generalized assumptions of food practices.

In many ethnic cultural groups, dietary practices and religious and/or spiritual beliefs are related. Chinese people with chronic illness use dietary manipulation based on the concepts of Yin-Yang to restore balance and health (41). Yin conditions (negative, dark, and cold) of Yin organs such as the heart, lung, liver, spleen, and kidney are treated with Yang, or hot, foods such as ginger or beef. Yang conditions (positive, light, and warm) of the Yang organs such as the stomach, gallbladder, intestines, and bladder are treated with Yin, or cold, foods such as coconut or pork. This association of hot and cold foods with health and illness is also found among Mexican and Filipino people. For instance, chest pain is considered a cold disease brought on by cold air or cold foods, such as tropical fruits, fresh vegetables, or dairy products, and is treated with hot foods, such as herbal teas, soups, and temperate-zone fruit. Some African Americans rely on folk medicine remedies such as blueberry tea, peach tree leaves tea, lemon juice, vinegar, and aloe vera to lower blood glucose or prevent diabetes-related complications (42,43).

COMMUNICATION AND INTERACTION

Interactions between patients and health care providers are heavily influenced by the personal beliefs and communication strategies of both parties. This communication consists of both verbal and nonverbal expression. Cultural differences in eye contact, touching behaviors, and personal space vary among cultures. For example, some Native Americans believe that avoidance of eye contact is a sign of respect and that a handshake is a sign of courtesy (20). The goals of communication between the patient and health care provider are to *1*) create a good interpersonal relationship; *2*) exchange information, which consists of giving and receiving information; and *3*) make treatment decisions. These goals of communication are difficult to achieve when language and cultural barriers exist, underscoring the need for cultural literacy and linguistic competency (44). A recent study to identify barriers in the provision of diabetes care in 42 Midwestern community health centers found that providers frequently identified language or cultural barriers as elements that hinder the quality of patient education (45). Health care providers can evaluate their cultural and linguistic competencies by using the *Inventory for Assessing the Process of Cultural Competence Among Health Care Professionals* (46) (see also the "Additional Reading" provided at the end of this chapter).

SUMMARY

The goal of diabetes patient education and care is to assist the patient and family with self-management that results in optimal glycemic control and improved quality of life. In recognizing the increasing diversity of individuals affected by diabetes, culturally competent care must be incorporated into clinical practice and education programs. It has been written that "although the knowledge of differences between cultures may be useful, the knowledge of the *what* of health and illness in different cultures does not reveal the *how* of being in the care experience as it is actually lived" (47). Cross-cultural counseling is an opening step in the long process of understanding and facilitating cultural diversity and specificity in the context of culturally competent diabetes education and care. The Healthy People 2010 (www.healthypeople.gov) goal of equitable health care for all people can only be met through a combination of approaches that minimizes the barriers for individuals from different cultural, ethnic, racial, and socioeconomic backgrounds and results in the delivery of culturally competent care.

REFERENCES

1. National Center for Health Statistics, Division of Health, Promotion Statistics: Data 2010: The Healthy People 2010 Database [Internet]. Available from http://wonder.cdc.gov/data2010. Accessed 24 March 2005
2. Flaskerud JH, Lesser J, Dixon E, Anderson N, Conde F, Kim S, Koniak-Griffin D, Strehlow A, Tullmann D, Verzemnieks I: Health disparities among vulnerable populations: evolution of knowledge over five decades in Nursing Research publications. *Nurs Res* 5192:74–84, 2002
3. Diabetes Control and Complications Trial Research Group: The effect of intensive diabetes treatment on the development and progression of long-term complications in insulin-dependent diabetes mellitus. *N Engl J Med* 329:977–986, 1993
4. UK Prospective Diabetes Study Group: Tight blood pressure control and risk of macrovascular and microvascular complications in type 2 diabetes (UKPDS 38). *BMJ* 317:703–723, 1998
5. Haynes RB, McKibbon KA, Kanani R: Systematic review of randomized trials of interventions to assist patients to follow prescriptions for medications. *Lancet* 348:383–386, 1996
6. Steffenson MS, Colker L: Intercultural misunderstandings about health care: recall of descriptions of illness and treatment. *Soc Sci Med* 16:1949–1954, 1982
7. American Diabetes Association: Standards of medical care in diabetes (Position Statement). *Diabetes Care* 28 (Suppl. 1):S4–S36, 2005
8. Centers for Disease Control and Prevention: The prevention and treatment of complications of diabetes mellitus: a guide for primary care practitioners, [Internet] 2003. Available from http://www.cdc.gov/diabetes/pubs/complications/psyc.htm. Accessed September 2003
9. Leininger M: What is transcultural nursing and culturally competent care? *J Transcult Nurs* 10:9, 1999
10. Mechanic D: *Medical Sociology: A Selective View.* New York, The Free Press, 1968
11. Goode T: Promoting cultural diversity and cultural competency. *Closing the Gap: Newsletter of the Office of Minority Health.* 6–7 January 2000
12. Tripp-Reimer T: Cultural interventions for ethnic groups of color. In *Handbook of Clinical Nursing Research.* Hinshaw AS, Feetham SL, Shaver JL, Eds. Thousand Oaks, CA, Sage, 1999
13. Brach C, Fraser I: Can cultural competency reduce racial and ethnic health disparities? A review and conceptual model. *Med Care Res Rev* 57 (Suppl. 1): 181–217, 2000
14. Cross TL, Bazron BJ, Dennis KW, Isaacs MR: *Towards a Culturally Competent System of Care: A Monograph on Effective Services for Minority Children Who Are Emotionally Disturbed.* Washington, DC, Child and Assistance Center, Georgetown University Child Development Center, 1989
15. Meleis A: Culturally competent care (Letter). *J Transcult Nurs* 10:12, 1999
16. Kehoe KA, Melkus GD, Newlin K: Culture within the context of care: an integrative review. *Ethn Dis* 13:344–353, 2003
17. Spector RE: *Cultural Diversity in Health and Illness.* 4th ed. Stamford, CT, Appleton and Lange, 1996

18. Blacknall L, Murphy S, Frank G, Michel V, Azen S: Ethnicity and attitudes toward patient autonomy. *JAMA* 274:820–825, 1995
19. Degazon C: Ethnic identification, social support and coping strategies among three groups of ethnic African elders. *J Cult Divers* 1:79–86, 1994
20. Seideman R, Jacobson S, Primeaux M, Burns P, Weatherby F: Assessing American Indian families. *MCN Am J Matern Child Nurs* 21:274–279, 1996
21. Gallup News Service: *Religion and Values: New Index Tracks Spiritual State of the Union.* 28 January 2003
22. Gallup News Service: *Religion and Values: Religion May Do a Body Good.* 28 May 2002
23. Burkhardt M: Spirituality: an analysis of the concept. *Holist Nurs Pract* 3:69–77, 1989
24. Meraviglia M: Critical analysis of spirituality and its empirical indicators. *J Holist Nurs* 17:18–33, 1999
25. Newlin K, Knafl K, Melkus GD: African-American spirituality: a concept analysis. *Adv Nurs Sci* 25:57–70, 2002
26. Emblen J: Religion and spirituality defined according to current use in nursing literature. *J Prof Nurs* 18:41–47, 1992
27. Minarik PA: Diversity among spiritual and religious beliefs. In *Culture & Nursing Care: A Pocket Guide.* Lipson JG, Dibble SL, Minarik PA, Eds. San Francisco, CA, UCSF Nursing Press, 1996, p. B1–B21
28. Kramer J: American Indians. In *Culture & Nursing Care: A Pocket Guide.* Lipson JG, Dibble SL, Minarik PA, Eds. San Francisco, CA, UCSF Nursing Press, 1996, p. 11–22
29. Still O, Hodgins D: Navajo Indians. In *Transcultural Health Care.* 2nd ed. Purnell LD, Paulanka BJ, Eds. Philadelphia, FA Davis, 2003, p. 284–306
30. Glanville CL: People of African American heritage. In *Transcultural Health Care.* 2nd ed. Purnell LD, Paulanka BJ, Eds. Philadelphia, FA Davis, 2003, p. 40–53
31. Morgan MG: African Americans and culture care. In *Transcultural Nursing: Concepts, Theories, Research and Practice.* 3rd ed. Leininger M, McFarland MR, Eds. New York, McGraw-Hill, 2002, p. 313–324
32. Locks S, Boateng L: Black/African Americans. In *Culture & Nursing Care: A Pocket Guide.* Lipson JG, Dibble SL, Minarik PA, Eds. San Francisco, CA, UCSF Nursing Press, 1996, p. 37–43
33. Varela L: Cubans. In *Culture & Nursing Care: A Pocket Guide.* Lipson JG, Dibble SL, Minarik PA, Eds. San Francisco, CA, UCSF Nursing Press, 1996, p. 91–100
34. Purnell LD: People of Cuban heritage. In *Transcultural Health Care.* 2nd ed. Purnell, LD, Paulanka BJ, Eds. Philadelphia, FA Davis, 2003, p. 122–137
35. Juarbe T: Puerto Ricans. In *Culture & Nursing Care: A Pocket Guide.* Lipson JG, Dibble SL, Minarik PA, Eds. San Francisco, CA, UCSF Nursing Press, 1996, p. 222–228
36. Juarbe TC: People of Puerto Rican heritage. In *Transcultural Health Care.* 2nd ed. Purnell, LD, Paulanka BJ, Eds. Philadelphia, FA Davis, 2003, p. 307–326
37. Lipson JG: Culturally competent nursing care. In *Culture & Nursing Care: A Pocket Guide.* Lipson JG, Dibble SL, Minarik PA, Eds. San Francisco, CA, UCSF Nursing Press, 1996, p. 1–6
38. Department of Health and Human Services, U.S. Office of Minority Health: Standards for culturally and linguistically appropriate services (CLAS). *Closing The Gap: Newsletter of the Office of Minority Health.* February/March 2001, p. 3

39. Cassell J: Social anthropology and nutrition: a different look at obesity in America. *J Am Diet Assoc* 95:424–427, 1995
40. Kumanyika SK, Wilson JF, Guilford-Davenport M: Weight-related attitudes and behaviors of black women. *J Am Diet Assoc* 93:416–422, 1993
41. Hwu Y, Coates V, Boore J: The health behaviours of Chinese people with chronic illness. *Int J Nurs Stud* 28:629–641, 2000
42. Anderson-Loftin W, Moneyham L: Long-term disease management needs of Southern African Americans with diabetes. *Diabetes Educ* 26:821–832, 2000
43. Anderson-Loftin W, Barnett S, Sullivan P, Summers Bunn P, Tavakoll A: Culturally competent dietary education for southern rural African Americans with diabetes. *Diabetes Educ* 28:245–257, 2002
44. Vandervort EB, Melkus GD: Linguistic services in ambulatory clinics. *J Transcult Nurs* 14:358–366, 2003
45. Chin M, Auerbach SB, Cook S, Harrison J, Koppert J, Jin J, Thiel F, Karrison T, Harrand A, Schaefer C, Takashima H, Eghert N, Chiu S, McNabb W: Quality of diabetes care in community health centers. *Am J Public Health* 90:431–434, 2000
46. Campinha-Bacote J: *Inventory for Assessing the Process of Cultural Competence Among Health Care Professionals.* Cincinnati, OH, Transcultural C.A.R.E. Association, 1998
47. Smith C: The lived experience of care within the context of cultural diversity. *J Holist Nurs* 12:282–290, 1994
48. Gerardi R: Western spirituality and health care. In *Spiritual Dimensions of Nursing Practice.* Carson V, Ed. Philadelphia, W. B. Saunders, 1989, p. 76–112
49. Andrews MM, Hanson PA: Religion, culture, and nursing. In *Transcultural Concepts in Nursing Care.* 4th ed. Andrews MM, Boyle JS, Eds. Philadelphia, Lippincott Williams & Wilkins, 2003, p. 432–502
50. Tom-Orme L: Transcultural nursing and health care among Native American peoples. In *Transcultural Nursing: Concepts, Theories, Research and Practice.* 3rd ed. Leininger M, McFarland MR, Eds. New York, McGraw-Hill, 2002, p. 429–440
51. Kulwicki AD: People of Arab heritage. In *Transcultural Health Care.* 2nd ed. Purnell LD, Paulanka BJ, Eds. Philadelphia, FA Davis, 2003, p. 90–105
52. Henley A, Schott J: *Culture, Religion, and Patient Care in a Multi-Ethnic Society.* London, Age Concern England, 1999
53. Selekman J: People of Jewish heritage. In *Transcultural Health Care.* 2nd ed. Purnell LD, Paulanka BJ, Eds. Philadelphia, FA Davis, 2003, p. 234–248

ADDITIONAL READING

Mason JL: *Cultural Competence Self-Assessment Questionnaire: A Manual for Users.* Portland, OR, Portland State University, 1995

Dr. D'Eramo Melkus is the Independence Foundation Professor of Nursing at Yale University School of Nursing, New Haven, CT. Ms. Newlin is a Doctoral Student at Yale University School of Nursing, New Haven, CT.

19. Economic Costs of Diabetes

Geralyn Spollett, MSN, C-ANP, CDE

Diabetes is a costly disease. The expenditure of health care dollars, the reduction in productivity, and other indirect expenses are estimated to be five times greater among people with diabetes than health-related expenses among the general population. According to a 2003 American Diabetes Association (ADA) statement (1), direct and indirect expenditures attributable to diabetes were estimated at $132 billion in 2002. This is a conservative estimate that does not reflect many of the associated costs of diabetes care. Data regarding the cost of diabetes care can also be found on the ADA web site (www.diabetes.org).

Diabetes is the sixth leading cause of death by disease in the U.S. At present, it is estimated that there are >13 million people diagnosed with this disease. This figure does not include individuals who do not know they have the disease or who did not report their diagnosis to the U.S. Census Bureau. It also does not include women with gestational diabetes. Lost productivity among this group based on lost workdays, restricted activity days, prevalence of permanent disability, and mortality attributable to diabetes cost the U.S. economy an estimated $40 billion in 2002. However, this may be an underestimated figure. Men and women with diabetes are less likely to be in the labor force than those without diabetes because a higher proportion of individuals with diabetes have disabilities, such as vision loss, kidney failure, and amputations, that prohibit full-time or part-time employment.

Currently, the age-group with the largest incidence of diabetes comprises individuals ≥55 years old. The prevalence of diabetes continues to increase with age. Certain ethnic and racial minority groups are also disproportionately affected by diabetes, and the growth rates of disease within these groups in addition to the aging of the population indicate that the number of people with diabetes could increase to 17.4 million by 2020, with an estimated annual cost of $192 billion. This cost does not take into consideration adjustments in the cost of living or the effect that increasing rates of obesity may have on the total number of individuals diagnosed with type 2 diabetes.

The economic burden of diabetes will become greater over time. By 2020, the size of the population with diabetes is projected to increase by 44%. The overall prevalence rate for diagnosed cases of diabetes is expected to grow from 4.2% in 2002 to 5.2% in 2020. The rates of racial and ethnic minorities affected by diabetes will double, and the incidence of diabetes among individuals aged 45–64 years is projected to increase by 46%.

USE OF HEALTH CARE RESOURCES

Use of health care resources is higher among individuals with diabetes than in the general population. People with diabetes are at greater risk for a host of medical complications that are directly or indirectly related to diabetes. Various neurological, cardiovascular, peripheral, vascular, renal, endocrine, and ophthalmic diseases can be associated with diabetes, and underlying diabetes may worsen their presentation and/or progression. The number of inpatient stays, nursing home occupancies, and home health care visits are all higher in the diabetic population. It is also estimated that inpatient days and outpatient visits for treatment of diabetes and its comorbidities tend to be more expensive than other disease states. The complexities of caring for individuals with multiple illnesses, complications, and medications that require frequent and periodic monitoring, observation, and follow-up make caring for diabetes a very costly disease. These comorbidities not only increase care costs, but they limit the earning potential of the person with diabetes, resulting in higher health care bills and reduced income with which to pay them.

The Social Security Disability Insurance (SSDI) program assists disabled workers by providing benefits to them, their spouse, and/or their children. In 2002, the calculated number of individuals aged 18–64 years who received SSDI attributed to diabetes-related disability topped 230,000 people; of those, 122,000 listed diabetes as the primary basis of disability. The U.S. government estimates that each case of permanent disability results in an average of $42,462 in lost earnings per year.

In a study of economic costs in diabetes conducted by the ADA (1), three trends were identified:

- Most of the health care use attributable to diabetes is for the treatment of general medical conditions in which the primary diagnosis is neither diabetes nor a related chronic complication.
- Of the chronic complications associated with diabetes, cardiovascular disease accounts for the largest proportion of health care use attributable to diabetes.
- Diabetes accounts for a sizable increase in the use of health care services.

In 2002, $23.2 billion was spent for health care events with a primary diagnosis of uncomplicated diabetes. This figure also included dollars spent for diabetes-related supplies. More than $1 of every $10 spent on health care in the U.S. is attributable to diabetes. The total cost of insulin, insulin-related supplies, and oral agents is approximately $12 billion. The estimated cost to provide health care to people with diabetes exceeded $160 billion in 2002. However, this figure does not

---

HOW MUCH DOES IT COST TO HAVE DIABETES?

On average, in the year 2002, the per capita expenditure for diabetes care was $13,243. In comparison, health care expenditures for a person without diabetes were approximately $2,560. Because the people with diabetes were older than individuals in the general population, this figure may be overstated. The ADA adjusted this figure for age and found that a ratio of ~2.4 to 1 seemed more accurate for health care expenditures among people with and without diabetes.

include certain services such as podiatry, dentistry, optometry, and nutrition coun-seling, which are necessary components of diabetes care.

Of the 186,000 people with diabetes who died in 2002, 58% had cardiovascular disease listed as the primary cause. Renal disease accounted for ~2,000 deaths. Other causes listed were cerebrovascular disease or diabetes. Dialysis, coronary bypass surgeries, stroke, and cardiac rehabilitation are expensive tertiary care interven-tions aimed at extending life. As evidenced by the rate of mortality in these areas, people with diabetes, many of whom have cardiovascular, renal, or cerebrovascular complications, use a high proportion of health care dollars and resources. These costs do not factor in pain and suffering or family sacrifice and support.

ADDRESSING THE PROBLEM

Improving diabetes care outcomes, thereby decreasing the incidence of chronic complications, can reduce the devastatingly high socioeconomic burden of dia-betes. Research such as that from the Diabetes Control and Complications Trial and the U.K. Prospective Diabetes Study has demonstrated the importance of glycemic control in reducing the rates of many chronic complications such as renal and eye disease. Each 10% increase in glycated hemoglobin A_{1c} is associated with a 20% increase in the rate of microalbuminuria and a 56% increase in the rate of retinopathy (2).

Because cardiovascular disease accounts for ~50% of deaths attributable to diabetes, control of cardiovascular risk factors will reduce health care costs and increase productivity among individuals with diabetes. Improved blood pressure control has a significant impact on preventing vascular and renal disease and may be equal to glycemic control in preventing chronic complications. Lipid screening and treatment of dyslipidemias can prevent myocardial and cerebrovascular mor-tality. Smoking cessation is critical to preserving cardiovascular health. More time and energy need to be dedicated to informing people with diabetes of the high health risks associated with smoking.

Countries that have adopted diabetes care programs that include prevention strategies taught by a health care team at the national, provincial, or county lev-els were able to improve the quality of care and optimize human and economic resources (3). For the U.S. to adequately meet the economic challenge of pre-venting and treating diabetes in the next decade, the current health care delivery system will need to shift care practices toward more fully encompassing the lifestyle issues and cardiovascular risk factors that contribute so heavily to the inci-dence of diabetes (see also "Keeping Medicine Costs Under Control," a patient handout in RESOURCES).

REFERENCES

1. American Diabetes Association: Economic costs of diabetes in the U.S. in 2002 (Position Statement). *Diabetes Care* 26:917–932, 2003
2. Vijan S, Hofer TP, Hayward RA: Estimated benefits of glycemic control in micro-vascular complications in type 2 diabetes. *Ann Intern Med* 127:788–795, 1997
3. Gagliardino JJ, Williams R, Clark CM: Using hospitalization rates to track the economic costs and benefits of improved diabetes care in the Americas: a proposal for health policy makers. *Diabetes Care* 23:1844–1846, 2000

Ms. Spollett is an Adult Nurse Practitioner at Yale Diabetes Center, New Haven, CT.

20. Alternative and Complementary Medicine

Diana W. Guthrie, PhD, FAAN, ARNP, BC-ADM, CDE

Complementary and alternative medicine (CAM) has existed throughout time. People have tried numerous remedies or treatments for various ailments, some with success and some to the detriment of the recipient. CAM therapy, as it is commonly known, has increased in popularity because of recognition that it can be useful and perhaps even cost-effective. Senator Thomas Harkins of Iowa became a supporter of CAM after he had health problems related to allergies (1). After a series of treatments in the 1980s provided no relief, he was goaded into trying a CAM therapist. According to Senator Harkins, the results were positive and his "allergies [were] cured." He co-submitted a bill to Congress that created the Office of Alternative Medicine (OAM). The first call for grants by OAM resulted in the submission of 455 proposals, 30 of which were subsequently funded. Gradually, CAM centers took their place not only as centers for research training, but also as grantees for specific research proposals. At the end of the 1990s, OAM became the National Center for Complementary and Alternative Medicine (NCCAM).

Two significant papers showed that the public had an interest in using alternative therapies. The benchmark article by Eisenberg et al. (2) titled "Unconventional Medicine in the United States" was followed 5 years later by another publication from the same group that focused on changes in the use and opinions of CAM over time (3). CAM use was working its way into the minds, if not the hearts, of more health care professionals (4).

Complementary therapies are those used along with standard practices. Therapies (modalities) such as any of the energy therapies, massage, acupuncture, and the use of various herbs, vitamins, and/or minerals alongside standard practice are considered complementary therapy. These might include the more familiar medical nutrition therapies, exercise, and relaxation techniques. Using these modalities in place of standard practice, particularly medication, is considered alternative therapy. Meal planning and exercise can be considered an alternative form of medicine, one that was found to be more effective than medication in the prevention of type 2 diabetes in the Diabetes Prevention Program (5). In that study, appropriate food choices and exercise were successfully used in place of medication in the earliest forms of type 2 diabetes.

The use of CAM therapies in diabetes dates back centuries. The early Greek treatise, which described diabetes as a "melting down" into the urine, stated that diabetes was treated with fasting, specific food choices, water restriction, or the use of herbs. Any treatment that reduced the flow of urine was included in the early treatments.

CAM EFFECT ON BLOOD GLUCOSE

Today, there are >400 herbs known to lower blood glucose levels and some that actually raise blood glucose levels (Table 20.1; 6). Much of the concern regarding the use of CAM therapies is centered on the self-administration of herbs without adequate knowledge of their efficacy and safety. In addition, the purity and concentration of packaged herbs is not regulated and may be inconsistent.

Herbs and plants lower blood glucose levels through a variety of physiological responses. Some, such as guar gum, decrease the absorption of food and increase the feeling of fullness (6). Others, such as ginseng, increase metabolism but may also add weight from increased muscle growth (7). Increasing fiber in the meal plan, as can be done using fenugreek seeds, might aid in lowering blood glucose levels and can be especially beneficial for someone who has type 2 diabetes (8,9).

CAM EFFECT ON COMPLICATIONS

CAM therapy may be of some use when the associated complications of diabetes are present. If polyneuropathy is present, then a trial of α-lipoic acid might be helpful, especially if normalization of blood glucose levels has not fully relieved the burning or tingling sensation in the extremities. Milk thistle, which is known

Table 20.1 Effects of Plants and Herbs on Blood Glucose

Plants That May Lower Blood Glucose	Plants That May Raise Blood Glucose
Aloe: dried exudates	Cocoa: seeds
Banana: flowers and roots	Coffee: seeds
Barley: sprouts	Cola: seeds
Bilberry: leaves	Mahuang: plant
Bitter melon: fruit	Rosemary: leaves
Carob: bean gum	Tea: leaves
Cashew: leaves	
Cucumber: fruit	
Cumin: seed	
Dandelion: plant	
Eucalyptus: leaves	
Fenugreek: seeds	
Garlic: cloves	
Ginseng: roots	
Guar gum: seeds and pods	
Juniper: berries	
Kidney beans: immature pods	
Mulberry: leaves	
Onion: bulbs	
Prickly pear: cactus plant	
Reijshi mushroom: body	
Spinach: leaves	
Wheat: leaves	

to have hepatoprotective effects, might be very useful if the person has developed some mild liver enzyme changes because of statin medication.

SAFETY ISSUES

The patient should discuss all herb use with the health care team. Overuse or increased amounts of certain herbs can cause unfavorable reactions. Examples are impaction from the use of guar gum, diarrhea from the use of dandelion, or toxic responses. Table 20.2 lists unsafe herbs (10), Table 20.3 lists moderately unsafe herbs (7), and Table 20.4 lists modalities that have been shown to be useful for people with diabetes (11).

Caution should be exercised when recommending use of herbs or dietary supplements because some are not standardized regarding purity or strength. Safe dosages should be considered when advising the use of these products. (A useful web site is www.prescribersletter.com, which has a natural medicine database on the usage of herbs and supplements and safety issues.) Additionally, these supplements may be regulated by state practice acts; check your local guidelines before prescribing.

Pain is known to raise blood glucose, and fever may further raise blood glucose levels. Anything that reduces pain, such as standard medication, massage, or acupuncture, could also lower blood glucose levels. Anxious infants have responded with lower blood glucose levels when massage was used (12). The use of biofeedback to speed up the learning process when teaching relaxation techniques was also found to lower blood glucose and to aid in increased circulation (13). Anxiety and its corresponding stressors are known to result in increased glucose levels. However, if a person becomes very agitated, there is a possibility that glucose levels will decrease.

ASSESSMENT

The NCCAM has divided CAM therapies into five categories (Table 20.5). These therapies cover the use of nutrition, i.e., herbs, vitamins, minerals, and various modalities, from Chinese medicine to magnetic therapy.

Each of these therapeutic areas may directly or indirectly have an effect on diabetes. Some may counteract a medication or foster higher blood glucose levels rather than having the desired lowering effect. Factors such as renal and hepatic clearance need to be considered when prescribing these therapies for a person with diabetes. Certain herbal therapies may not be excreted properly from the body and over time build up to toxic levels. It is unknown how some of these herbs might affect the diabetes medications currently being used. This requires further study.

Table 20.2 Unsafe Herbs

Chaparral: liver damage
Ephedra (Mahuang): raises blood glucose, raises blood pressure, toxic
Hydrangea: leaves contain cyanide
Poke root: vomiting
Sassafras: carcinogenic, liver damage
Yohimbine: raises blood pressure, increases anxiety

Table 20.3 Moderately Unsafe Herbs

Bearberry: not to be used in pregnancy or for prostate disorders
Black/blue cohosh: not to be used during pregnancy or chronic illnesses (might affect blood glucose levels)
Boneset: toxicity possible in large doses
Comfrey: liver damage
Juniper: kidney disease, not for use in pregnancy
Licorice: not for use in pregnancy, diabetes, heart disease, or hypertension
Lobelia: not to be used in pregnancy
Wormwood: not to be used in pregnancy

Table 20.4 Useful Modalities for People with Diabetes

Nutrients: ω-3 and -6 fatty acids (γ-linolenic acid), bulk laxatives (such as bran, psyllium, and methylcellulose)
Vitamins: B, C, D, E (dosage not >400 IU)
Minerals: chromium, magnesium, vanadium, zinc
Herbs (topical or oral): basil, bilberry, bitter melon, capsaicin, fenugreek, ginko biloba, panax ginseng, gymnema sylvestre, milk thistle, nopal
Body-based methods: massage, chiropractic, reflexology
Energy therapies: acupressure (acupuncture), healing touch, Reiki, therapeutic touch

Table 20.5 NCCAM Therapy Categories

1. Alternative medical systems: Chinese medicine, Ayurveda
2. Mind-body interventions: prayer, meditation, music, support groups
3. Biologically based therapies: dietary supplements, herbal products
4. Manipulative and body-based methods: chiropractic, massage
5. Energy therapies: yoga, healing touch
    a. Biofield therapies: qigong, Reiki, therapeutic touch
    b. Bioelectromagnetic-based therapies: electromagnetic fields, alternating or direct current fields

---

PRACTICAL POINT

Factors to consider when choosing a CAM therapy for someone with diabetes:
- Is the kidney and hepatic function normal?
- Will there be an effect on blood pressure?
- How will the therapy affect blood glucose levels?

ENERGY-BASED AND BODY-BASED METHODS

Last, relaxation therapies or energy therapies might aid in lowering glucose levels. Massage- or biofeedback-enhanced relaxation training may result in less labile blood glucose levels or overall lowered blood glucose levels, especially in type 1 diabetes.

Table 20.6 describes some common types of CAM and will help the nurse decide which therapeutic modality will be most effective in the plan of care. No single CAM modality will be appropriate for every patient. Choosing one or two specific modalities depends on the need(s) as determined by the assessment of the person. If the person is in pain, one of the energy or massage therapies might be in order and could be accompanied by an herb for use in aromatherapy. Less pain and lowered blood glucose levels may occur.

Determining the effectiveness of a CAM therapy requires a trial period. For instance, if a person begins taking α-lipoic acid for polyneuropathy, then a trial period of 2–3 months is needed using therapeutic levels. If no response is seen in that time, there is no value in continuing the therapy, and another therapy may be tried. No single CAM modality is appropriate or effective for all people. In a 2001 survey of health care professionals who recommend CAM therapy, the providers indicated that they prescribed the same therapy for a specific condition 34% of the time. This survey would indicate that health care professionals are individualizing CAM prescriptions (15).

EDUCATIONAL AND BEHAVIORAL CONSIDERATIONS

Education should accompany any chosen modality and include an explanation of what it is, its intended therapeutic effect, and the time needed to achieve the expected outcome (see "A Step-by-Step Approach to Complementary Therapies" and "Guidelines for Using Vitamin, Mineral, and Herbal Supplements," patient handouts in RESOURCES). Side effects and possible adverse reactions must also be discussed and the person alerted to signs or symptoms that require immediate action. In people with diabetes, the effect of the CAM modality on both acute and chronic complications will need to be reviewed.

Assessing a Person for CAM

When assessing a person for CAM, the nurse should do the following:
- Take a thorough history of daily intake of food and fluids.
- Include current or past use of herbs, supplements, or other types of CAM.
- Determine whether there are problems with various body systems.
- List stressors that might be found at home, school, or work.
- Identify and explore religious and social beliefs.
- Aid the person in identifying present coping mechanisms that are already in use.
- Determine what might be of use or acceptable for the individual, e.g., daily meditation to lower blood pressure, lower pulse rate, and lead to the more effective use of oxygen (14).

Once this assessment is complete, the nurse can determine which modalities are best suited for the patient.

Table 20.6 Common Types of CAM

CAM Type	Description
Acupuncture	Insertion of very fine needles into or along various pathways called meridians to enhance the flow of energy.
Aromatherapy	The use of various oils to aid in, depending on the oil, antibacterial action, antiviral action, harmonizing moods, relaxation, joint and muscle improvement, and diuretic action, among others.
Biofeedback	Any type of information that enhances the learning process and supports healing, e.g., body temperature, an indicator of relaxation and improved blood circulation.
Healing touch	A variety of techniques that increase the body's energy output or modulate this energy into more useful patterns.
Hypnotherapy	A technique for self-learning to assist in peace of mind and of body through the use of suggestion.
Magnetic therapy	Altering the body's responses through the use of magnetic energy.
Massage	Manipulation of the muscles, joints, and, indirectly, the nerves to promote healing, e.g., various forms of massage using body meridians (shiatsu), a particular pattern of massage (Swedish), or a greater focus on the joints and muscles attached to such joints (Thai).
Reflexology	Massage and manipulation of the reflexes of the feet (or hands) to correspond to the needs in various parts of the body for the purpose of rebalancing the body.
Reiki	Supporting the flow of energy throughout the body for the purpose of healing.
Therapeutic touch	A set use of physical and nonphysical contacts for the purpose of relieving pain, reducing inflammation, and enhancing relaxation, i.e., centering, assessing, modulating, and smoothing.
Yoga	Another energy therapy with the purpose of uniting the flow of physical, mental, and spiritual energy for improving health and well-being.

Some of these modalities have not been adequately studied or not studied in relation to diabetes. The American Diabetes Association (ADA) has established guidelines regarding the use of unproven therapies (16). Therapies are classified as clearly effective, somewhat effective, unknown or unproven but possibly promising, or clearly ineffective. Operationally, the ADA considers the therapeutic modality to be safe and effective if it has been approved by the U.S. Food and Drug Administration, is supported by at least two independent well-controlled studies that have been published in a peer-reviewed scientific publication, endorsed or recommended by the ADA Professional Practice Committee, or endorsed by a relevant or appropriate medical specialty organization.

The physical, mental, and emotional state of the person should be weighed against the chosen therapy. Treatment should include a team effort between the health care professional, the person with diabetes, and, if needed, a certified professional in the field of CAM therapy (such professionals can be found through the American Holistic Nurses Association [www.ahna.org] and the Healing Touch Association International). Education should be updated as new treatments become available or as new information regarding current CAM is discovered. The therapeutic plan may need to be adjusted.

SUMMARY

The Internet has become a source of information and education, but not necessarily in a way that is safe for someone with a chronic condition. The reading level of most CAM information on the Internet is at an eleventh grade level (17). Greater misunderstanding can occur when the language is not thoroughly understood by the patient. Reviewing these materials with the patient is necessary to ensure adequate understanding. Although CAM therapy for people with diabetes is comparable with that for individuals without diabetes, only 20% of individuals with diabetes reported that they were using CAM therapy to treat their diabetes (18).

Reimbursement has become another area of concern. Even though third-party payment is increasing for such modalities as chiropractic, acupuncture, and therapeutic massage (19), there are still many more modalities that are not supported by insurance carriers. According to a 2002 article (20), Medicaid reimbursement for the use of CAM therapies is increasing. This increase allows individuals who are unable to pay out of pocket to also experience complementary or alternate treatments for their diabetes management.

CAM has had a significant impact on today's medicine and nursing care (21). Patients seek information regarding CAM and its use in their health care regimen and expect that their provider will be able to respond appropriately. Physicians and nurses will need to foster communication with their patients about CAM therapy and provide sufficient information for adequate and safe decision making (22). For safe use of such modalities, health care professionals should have a working knowledge of the prescribed CAM or be able to consult or refer to a certified professional in that field.

Eisenberg (23) recognized that there is a role for CAM in psychiatry. Health care professionals in this field, as in other medical fields, face problems if they do not provide sufficient information to patients for adequate and safe decisions to be made.

Ethical considerations must also be taken into account when using CAM. The patient has the right to be informed of the various therapeutic modalities available for the treatment of his or her disease. The health care provider must be open to discussion of CAM modalities and allow the patient to pursue alternative methods, if appropriate. The provider also has the responsibility to inform the patient of unintended consequences or deleterious effects caused by the initiation of CAM or the discontinuation of proven medical therapies (24). As public interest increases, more patients and health care professionals will turn to the use of CAM, and these ethical considerations must be met (25).

Sociology of the use of CAM therapies has emerged (26). This development leads to the need for relevant research to clearly determine the use, problems, and promises of this field. Resources such as useful books and Internet sites as well as monographs and literature databases may be found (27). Not only is rigorous research needed from the standpoint of the effective use of these therapies, but it is especially salient for the field of diabetes, wherein potential problems might occur due to the diabetes disease state (28). NCCAM is supportive of such research and welcomes proposals, especially those that document the specific needs found in diabetes care.

REFERENCES

1. NCCAM web site. Available from http://nccam.nih.gov. Accessed 1 January 2005
2. Eisenberg DM, Kessler RC, Foster C, Norlock RE, Calkins DR, DelBance TL: Unconventional medicine in the United States: prevalence, cost and patterns of use. *N Engl J Med* 328:246–252, 1993
3. Eisenberg DM, Davis RB, Ettner SL, Appel S, Wilkey S, Van-Rompay MI, Kessler RC: Trends in alternative medicine use in the United States. *JAMA* 280:1569–1575, 1998
4. Eisenberg DM, Kessler RC, Van-Rompay MI, Kaptchuk TJ, Wilkey SA, Appel S, David RB: Perceptions about complementary therapies relative to conventional therapies among adults who use both: results from a national survey. *Ann Intern Med* 135:344–351, 2001
5. Pastors JG, Warshaw H, Daly A, Franz M, Kulkarni K: The evidence for the effectiveness of medical nutrition therapy in diabetes management. *Diabetes Care* 25:608–613, 2002
6. Shane-McWhorter L: Biological complementary therapies: a focus on botanical products in diabetes. In *Annual Review of Diabetes 2002.* Alexandria, VA, American Diabetes Association, 2002, p. 136–145
7. Vuksan V, Sievenpiper JL, Koo VY, Francis T, Beljan-Zdravkovic U, Xu Z, Vidgen E: American ginseng (*Panax quinquefolius L*) reduces postprandial glycemia in nondiabetic subjects and subjects with type 2 diabetes mellitus. *Arch Intern Med* 160:1009–1013, 2000
8. Pavithran K: Fenugreek in diabetes mellitus (Letter). *J Assoc Physicians India* 42:33–35, 1994
9. Puri D: Fenugreek in diabetes mellitus (Letter). *J Assoc Physicians India* 47:255–256, 1999
10. Tyler VE: *The Honest Herbal.* New York, Pharmaceutical Products, 1993
11. Guthrie D, Huebscher R, Shuler P, Rauckhorst L, Miller H: Endocrine concerns. In *Natural, Alternative, and Complementary Health Care Practices.* Huebscher R, Shuler P, Eds. St. Louis, MO, Mosby, 2004, p. 658–713
12. Field TM, Hernandez-Reif M, LaGreca A, Shaw K, Schanberg S, Kuhn C: Massage therapy lowers blood glucose levels in children with diabetes. *Diabetes Spectrum* 10:237–239, 1997
13. Rice BI, Schindler JV: Effect of thermal biofeedback assisted relaxation training for blood circulation in lower extremities of a population with diabetes. *Diabetes Care* 15:853–858, 1992
14. Benson H, Steward EM: *The Wellness Book: The Comprehensive Guide to Maintaining Health and Treating Stress Related Illness.* New York, Simon & Shuster, 1993
15. Long L, Huntley A, Ernst E: Which complementary and alternative therapies benefit which conditions? A survey of the opinions of 223 professional organizations. *Complement Ther Med* 9:178–185, 2001
16. American Diabetes Association: Unproven therapies (Position Statement). *Diabetes Care* 27 (Suppl. 1):S135, 2004
17. Sagaram S, Walji M, Bernstam E: Evaluating the prevalence, content and readability of complementary and alternative medicine (CAM) web pages on the Internet. *Proc AMIA Symp* 672–676, 2002
18. Yeh GY, Eisenberg DM, Davis RB, Phillips RS: Use of complementary and alternative medicine among persons with diabetes mellitus: results of a national survey. *Am J Public Health* 92:1648–1652, 2002

19. Cleary-Guida MB, Okvat HA, Oz MC, Ting W: A regional survey of health insurance coverage for complementary and alternative medicine: current status and future ramifications. *J Altern Complement Med* 7:269–173, 2001
20. Steyer TE, Freed GL, Lantz PM: Medicaid reimbursement for alternative therapies. *Altern Ther Health Med* 8:84–88, 2002
21. Egan CD: Addressing use of herbal medicine in the primary care setting. *J Am Acad Nurse Pract* 14:166–171, 2002
22. Corbin-Winslow L, Shapiro H: Physicians want education about complementary and alternative medicine to enhance communication with their patients. *Arch Intern Med* 162:1176–1181, 2002
23. Eisenberg L: Complementary and alternative medicine: what is its role? *Harv Rev Psychiatry* 10:221–230, 2002
24. Kaler MM, Ravella PC: Staying on the ethical high ground with complementary and alternative medicine. *Nurse Pract* 27:38–42, 2002
25. Jonas WB: Advising patients on the use of complementary and alternative medicine. *Appl Psychophysiol Biofeedback* 26:205–214, 2001
26. Tovey P, Adams J: Nostalgic and nostophobic referencing and the authentication of nurses' use of complementary therapies. *Soc Sci Med* 56:1469–1480, 2003
27. Kiefer D, Shah S, Gardiner P, Wechkin H: Finding information on herbal therapy: a guide to useful sources for clinicians. *Altern Ther Health Med* 7:74–78, 2001
28. Kinsel JF, Straus SE: Complementary and alternative therapeutics: rigorous research is needed to support claims. *Ann Rev Pharmacol Toxicol* 43:463–484, 2003

ADDITIONAL READING

Dossey BM, Keegan L, Guzzetta CE: *Holistic Nursing: A Handbook for Practice.* 3rd ed. Gaithersburg, MD, Aspen, 2000
Guthrie DW: *Alternative and Complementary Diabetes Care.* New York, Wiley, 2002
Huebscher R, Shuler P: *Natural, Alternative, and Complementary Health Care Practices.* St. Louis, MO, Mosby, 2004
Kuhn MA: *Complementary Therapies for Health Care Providers.* Baltimore, MD, Lippincott Williams & Wilkins, 1999
Physicians' Desk Reference for Herbal Medicines. 2nd ed. Montvale, NJ, Medical Economics, 2000
Physicians' Desk Reference for Nutritional Supplements. Montvale, NJ, Medical Economics, 2001
Snyder M, Lindquist R (Eds.): *Complementary/Alternative Therapies in Nursing.* 4th ed. New York, Springer, 2002
Yeh GY, Eisenberg DM, Kaptchuk TJ, Phillips RS: Systematic review of herbs and dietary supplements for glycemic control in diabetes. *Diabetes Care* 26:1277–1294, 2003

Dr. Guthrie is a Diabetes Nurse Specialist/Practitioner at Mid-America Diabetes Associates, Wichita, KS.

21. Living with Diabetes

DIANA RHILEY, LCMFT, CDE

L iving with diabetes is a daily challenge. The nature of the regimen—frequent blood glucose monitoring, meal planning, exercising, and scheduling medication—creates the need for constant vigilance on the part of the person with diabetes. There are tremendous payoffs for these efforts, including fewer and less frequent complications of diabetes, but such efforts are not without cost. Patients often express a sense of loss of freedom, spontaneity, or food choices and the feeling that diabetes management is taking over their lives. Diabetes may affect relationships, limit social interactions, and present the fear that even with hard work, bad things can happen.

The health care professional becomes part of the individual's health care team and support system. This may be a short-term relationship for nurses in a short-stay hospital or a long-term relationship for the nurse in the clinic or home health care setting. The role of the nurse may be pivotal in assisting the patient in self-care management skills and in the psychosocial adaptation to a life-changing illness. Many courageous people successfully live with diabetes because of the skills, relationships, and strategies they have developed to cope with the day-to-day challenges of diabetes.

The individual with diabetes sometimes feels more comfortable confiding in a nurse or nonphysician health care professional. Therefore, the role of the nurse is important in assessing an individual's ability to adjust, cope, and manage his or her diabetes effectively. Assessment involves careful observation, probing questions, and attention to the types of responses.

PRACTICAL POINT

Diabetes doesn't take a day off. Diabetes is a disease of many details. It is not surprising that it is difficult to maintain vigilance to the regimen day in and day out. The nurse plays an important role as coach and advocate.

EVALUATING LEVEL OF ADAPTATION

Table 21.1 identifies several key questions that the nurse can use to assess the individual's level of knowledge about diabetes, perceived stress level, family dynamics, attitudes about life, and potential for depression, diabetes burnout, or denial.

REDUCING DIABETES BURNOUT

The term *diabetes burnout* is accepted as the description for the individual with diabetes who has developed a feeling of failure and chronic frustration. One study

Table 21.1 Key Questions and Observations Regarding Adaptation

Assessment Areas	Specific Questions and Observations
Knowledge and attitude toward diabetes	What can the patient tell you about his or her regimen? Is he or she able to describe the diabetes regimen accurately? What is the patient's attitude when talking about diabetes and the diabetes regimen? What is this discussion's effect on the patient? Does he or she get tearful or angry? Is he or she proud of their ability to self-manage? Are there past personal or family experiences that are meaningful to the patient and influence his or her attitudes toward diabetes and self-care issues?
Current stress level	What are the current stressors in the patient's life in addition to diabetes? Work? Finances? Relationships?
Family dynamics and support systems	What are the family dynamics? Are interactions pleasant and loving or are they cold and distant? Do other family members show knowledge of the regimen and take part in it? Are family members overly protective and indulgent? Do family members tend to nag, creating a situation in which the patient may resist doing the things that are in his or her best interest? If the patient lives alone, where does the support come from? Is there a close extended family, helpful neighbors, supportive friends, and a supportive health care team or health care professionals?
Attitude about life	What is the patient's overall attitude toward life? Does he or she make reference to his or her faith or spiritual life? How has the person coped with personal challenges in the past?
Depression	Do you see any signs of depression or anxiety? Is the patient sleeping through the night? Has the patient's eating pattern changed beyond just what the diabetes recommendations include? Has the patient lost interest in the things he or she would have been excited about previously? Has the patient restricted social activities or withdrawn from friends, significant others, etc.? Does the patient talk of worrying about things?
Denial or burnout	Does the patient show any signs of denial or burnout or express feelings of being overwhelmed? Is the patient unable to incorporate changes in his or her treatment program? Does he or she tend to minimize diabetes? Or does the patient justify or rationalize away the poor choices he or she has made?

reported that ~60% of patients sampled reported at least one serious diabetes-related concern (1,2).

RECOGNIZING DIABETES BURNOUT

Burnout may create feelings of being alone or overwhelmed and of failure. Poor self-care and poor follow-up with the health care professional are other common symptoms. The patient may feel that diabetes controls his or her life. Strategies identified to alleviate diabetes burnout are included in Table 21.2.

Table 21.2 Strategies to Assist in Reducing Diabetes Burnout

Skills	Suggested Strategies
Establish a strong collaborative relationship	It may be very helpful to the patient for the health care professional to acknowledge the patient's struggles, applaud successes, and strive for frequent visits to help the patient through the time of burnout.
Negotiate goals	The health care professional can help the patient reestablish goals that are measurable and achievable. Start with what the patient is already doing and add to it in small steps. Make sure to help the individual develop simple goals that are realistic.
Pay attention to strong negative feelings	Listen intently and acknowledge or validate. Acknowledging the patient's feelings is a very powerful tool. This means that the health care professional must listen intently to identify and label those feelings and then normalize those feelings when possible. If this continues to be a roadblock after repeated attempts by the health care professional, consider a referral to a mental health professional.
Optimize social support	Loving, supportive relationships with others who take an interest in diabetes management can be a great antidote to diabetes burnout. Other parts of this chapter also address the role of the support system.
Engage the patient in active problem solving	1) Implement only one change at a time. 2) Focus on a behavior that can become a habit. 3) When possible, use the environment as a reminder to do a behavior, e.g., putting vitamins next to the coffeemaker (2).

PRACTICAL POINT

Adapting to Newly Diagnosed Diabetes

The patient who is newly diagnosed has special needs and considerations. Table 21.3 provides suggested questions and observations to assist in supporting the patient who has recently been diagnosed with diabetes. This is a critical time for supporting and empowering the patient in preparation for self-care management. The messages that the patient with newly diagnosed diabetes receives at this moment will be remembered for a lifetime. It is important to provide accurate, positive information to the patient and family.

ADAPTING TO COMPLICATIONS

The patient with complications from diabetes has special considerations. It will be important to assess the level of pain and his or her ability to cope with the complications. Table 21.4 lists assessment areas and questions and observations for individuals with complications.

Individuals who develop diabetes-related complications face many challenges, particularly accommodating limitations and loss, such as alterations in vision or mobility. The process of adjusting to a complication may be similar to the individual's adjustment to the diagnosis of diabetes. Many of the assessment items used at the time of diagnosis may be useful when assessing a patient with a new complication, such as the onset of renal failure or the significant visual changes associated with retinopathy. The psychological implications of a diabetes-related complication might be devastating and result in self-blame, rage, and feelings of failure or depression. The RESOURCES section of this book has a list of organizations that can provide materials and support for the patient dealing with visual changes or amputations.

DEPRESSION

At some point during the process of dealing with diabetes, many patients will experience depression (see CHAPTER 22). It may not be recognized, particularly because some of the symptoms of depression, e.g., fatigue, feelings of hopelessness, and lack of appetite, resemble poorly controlled diabetes or hyperglycemia. There is a tendency to underdiagnose or undertreat depression in patients with chronic illness. Because depression has been shown to contribute independently to the complications of diabetes, in addition to its contribution to hyperglycemia, health care professionals must be aware of its presence (3). Using a simple and quick screening tool for depression such as the Beck Depression Scale or Zung Depression Scale gives the provider an opportunity to recognize, refer, or provide treatment (see RESOURCES for an online screening tool).

The health care provider must be supportive and help the patient recognize that depression is a medical problem and must be treated as such. For some patients, being diagnosed with depression carries a stigma, and they may resist counseling and medication therapy. In these cases, it is critical that the health care provider help the patient understand that the stress of living with a chronic

Table 21.3 Specific Assessment Questions for the Newly Diagnosed Patient

Assessment Areas	Questions and Observations
Education	Who will provide the patient's education? Does the patient have access to certified diabetes educators? If hospitalized, will there be more intensive education after discharge? If a Certified Diabetes Educator (CDE) is providing inpatient education, ask the patient about what he or she is learning. Is the patient retaining the information? Are family members involved in the education?
Patient structure	Does the patient appear to have a way of organizing himself or herself? Does the patient prefer structure? Or does structure and schedule feel confining and something he or she will come to resent? Does the patient have a schedule and routine in his or her daily life? Is this a chaotic time in the patient's life, when structure is changing, e.g., new job, moving, breakup of a relationship?
Ability to change	Is the patient beginning to process change? Is he or she talking about what will be different and how such changes will be implemented? Can the patient discuss implementing the recommendations into his or her current lifestyle?
Support system	Who makes up the patient's support system? Can the patient easily access them? What is their proximity to the patient? Are they willing to be involved? Will they be present for education?
Ability to ask for help	Is the patient good at asking for help when needed? Or does something prevent him or her from asking for support or information from others? If the patient is unclear about something, will he or she ask for clarification? If the patient is having a hypoglycemic event, will he or she seek assistance?

Table 21.4 Specific Questions and Observations for a Patient With Diabetes Complications

Assessment Areas	Questions and Observations
Severity	What is the complication? How severe is the complication? Does it interfere with the patient's lifestyle? If so, how has the patient adapted?
Pain level	Is the patient experiencing physical discomfort in relation to the complication? If so, how much? It may be necessary to use a pain severity scale.
Support system and coping skills	It is crucial to assess the patient's coping skills and support system. These will be key indicators as to how the client will handle the complication and assimilate it into his or her future.

illness can result in depression and that this is not unusual and neither is it a reflection of his or her character (see RESOURCES for information on these tools and the patient handout, "How Can We Help You?").

SUPPORT SYSTEMS

It is difficult to face a chronic disease and make and maintain numerous lifestyle changes without a support system. Affirmation and validation by others can assist the individual with diabetes in continuing effective health care behaviors.

At the same time, diabetes can cause a strain on relationships. A support person may begin to resent an individual who does not follow all of the recommendations and is not the "perfect patient." Some individuals may feel that it is their responsibility to make sure the person with diabetes takes better care of himself or herself. They may begin to nag and constantly watch the person with diabetes. Keeping in mind the degree of dependency present, the support person and the person with diabetes need to talk about their mutual expectations in the management of diabetes. Without open, honest communication, the relationship can evolve into a game and a tool with which to hurt each other. The support person needs to be aware of his or her feelings about diabetes, such as fear, resentment, anger, etc. It is often these kinds of feelings that drive one toward overprotective or smothering behavior. If a codependent or other unhealthy relationship is suspected, referral to a mental health professional is recommended.

COPING SKILLS

Coping skills are a necessary tool for a person to acknowledge and accept the difficulties of managing diabetes. Table 21.5 outlines specific skills that may be beneficial to the individual with diabetes and his or her family.

Table 21.5 Behaviors to Enhance Coping Skills

Skill	Specific Behaviors
Self-talk as a foundation for attitude	Listen to the patient's exact language, it is a direct link to his or her attitude: • *Encourage motivating and successful speech:* Does the patient use words that include hope and are encouraging? A patient's self-efficacy is crucial to his or her success, so it is important to know if he or she feels able to do the things asked of him or her and to do them over the long term. • *Words lead to attitude:* The patient's words are a good clue as to how he or she sees this process playing out. Encourage patients to change their words to match a successful attitude.
Assertiveness	Assertiveness is an extremely important skill for people with diabetes. Assertiveness includes the following behaviors: • *Expressing feelings rather than holding them in and taking ownership of these feelings:* Encourage discussion about feelings of frustrations or resentment.

(continued)

Table 21.5 Behaviors to Enhance Coping Skills (*Continued*)

Skill	Specific Behaviors
	■ *Saying "no" when he or she really means it:* They need to set and maintain protective limits around their time and energy in order to preserve good health.
	■ *Asking questions:* The patient needs to be able to ask for clarification. Not asking may be a sign of being overwhelmed or depressed.
	■ *Asking for assistance when needed:* The ability to ask for assistance demonstrates that the patient has balanced the dependence/independence behavior dichotomy and knows how and when to seek help.
Problem solving	Problem solving is a skill that helps the patient maintain a sense of empowerment. Problem solving includes the following steps, which are done together with the patient:
	■ *Develop a clear definition of the problem:* What is the issue? What does the patient want to happen?
	■ *Brainstorm possible solutions:* Identify realistic goals, and guide the patient toward selecting his or her own resolution.
	■ *Utilize reasonable solutions:* Identify what is possible within the patient's power and implement that plan.
	■ *Engage in active problem solving:* Include the three steps used for active problem solving in Table 21.2.
Goal setting and time management	Diabetes requires a significant amount of time for self-care activities, and therefore the priority given it by a patient is tantamount to the success of the treatment regimen:
	■ *Assess the priority of diabetes self-care:* Where on the patient's priority list is diabetes care? Is it high enough to make a commitment to it? It will be difficult for the patient to make a time commitment to these tasks unless these goals are given significant priority.
	■ *Determine an approach for reluctant individuals:* The use of motivational interviewing and skills, such as agenda setting, rapport building, negotiating, building readiness to change, and assessment of importance and confidence, may be helpful when working with a reluctant patient (4,5).
Support system	Help the patient identify the person or people who can play the following roles in his or her life:
	■ Someone who can help with the day-to-day "mechanics" of diabetes, e.g., cooking and meal planning, keeping prescriptions filled, being an exercise partner?
	■ Someone with whom the patient can share frustrations and achievements?
	■ Someone who can run interference in situations that wear the patient down or that the patient continually finds frustrating?
Manage stress	Help individuals identify different methods for coping or managing stress (see also "Stress Management Tools," a patient handout in RESOURCES). For example, ask them what they like to do to relax or what they do when they feel very stressed. Some people like to listen to music, read a book, or talk with a friend.

Table 21.5 Behaviors to Enhance Coping Skills (*Continued*)

Skill	Specific Behaviors
	Other types of stress management skills are: ■ *Exercise:* Exercise creates many benefits for everyone. Not only is it a large part of a successful diabetes management regimen, but it also pays huge rewards as part of a stress management program. The more consistent the exercise, the greater the benefit. ■ *Relaxation:* Begin with progressive relaxation. This is the alternate tensing and relaxing of muscle groups to really be able to know the difference between tense and relaxed muscles. Work with large motor muscles and progress to fine motor muscles. Autogenic relaxation focuses on producing physical sensations that are associated with relaxation. Imagining body parts as feeling heavy and warm can reduce the tension in the body. Imagery is the creation of a relaxing scene in the mind in which the person feels free and relaxed and totally removed from pressure and worry. Using relaxation successfully requires practice sessions of ~20 min twice daily for 6 weeks. Before that, it may be difficult to implement the benefits of relaxation in the middle of a stressful moment. ■ *Biofeedback:* Biofeedback is the monitoring of a bodily function such as heart rate, brain waves, or hand temperature. In the learning process, it is coupled with relaxation so that a patient can learn to create the conditions that help calm the body.

SUMMARY

A nurse can play a key role in assisting the individual to live successfully with diabetes. To help individuals with diabetes, it is essential that nurses provide current and accurate diabetes information or be able to refer the patient to someone with appropriate expertise. The American Diabetes Association, the American Association of Diabetes Educators, and a local CDE are good resources.

Interactions with the patient may only be for a limited time. Unless the patient has requested that information be kept confidential, the health care team should be apprised of any changes or concerns regarding individual patients. It is important that the patient receives the same messages from each of his or her health care professionals. Any information obtained from the assessments that causes concern should be directed to the patient's primary health care provider and certified diabetes educators. Interactions with the patient may broaden the primary health care provider's understanding of the patient and help him or her better meet the patient's needs. It may be appropriate to encourage a social services or mental health consultation.

Frequent interactions with patients, however brief, may also be vital in encouraging the patient to maintain a continued commitment to diabetes care. Because of the investment of time and interest on the part of the health care provider, the patient may find that living with diabetes can be easier.

REFERENCES

1. Anderson B, Rubin R (Eds.): *Practical Psychology for Diabetes Clinicians*. 2nd ed. Alexandria, VA, American Diabetes Association, 2002
2. Polonsky WH: Understanding and treating patients with diabetes burnout. In *Practical Psychology for Diabetes Clinicians*. 2nd ed. Anderson B, Rubin R, Eds. Alexandria, VA, American Diabetes Association, 2002, p. 219–228
3. Lustman PJ, Singh PK, Clouse RE: Recognizing and managing depression in patients with diabetes. In *Practical Psychology for Diabetes Clinicians*. 2nd ed. Anderson B, Rubin R, Eds. Alexandria, VA, American Diabetes Association, 2002, p. 229–238
4. Rollnick S, Mason P, Butler C: *Health Behavior Change: A Guide for Practitioners*. London, Churchill Livingstone, 1999
5. Miller WR, Rollnick S: *Motivational Interviewing: Preparing People for Change*. 2nd ed. New York, Guilford Press, 2002

ADDITIONAL READING

American Diabetes Association: *Caring for the Diabetic Soul*. Alexandria, VA, American Diabetes Association, 1997
Anderson B, Funnell M: *The Art of Empowerment: Stories and Strategies for Diabetes Educators*. 2nd ed. Alexandria, VA, American Diabetes Association, 2005
Polonsky W: *Diabetes Burnout: What to Do When You Can't Take It Anymore* (book and audiotape). Alexandria, VA, American Diabetes Association, 1999

Ms. Rhiley is an Adjunct Supervisor, Marriage and Family Therapy Program, at Friends University, Wichita, KS, and works in marriage and family therapy in a private practice.

22. Depression, Anxiety, and Eating Disorders

ANN GOEBEL-FABBRI, PHD, AND JOHN ZREBIEC, MSW, CDE

The Diabetes Control and Complications Trial (DCCT) and the U.K. Prospective Diabetes Study demonstrated that intensive management of type 1 and type 2 diabetes improves long-term health outcomes in diabetes (1,2). However, the goal of achieving near-normal blood glucose values requires a complex set of daily behaviors and problem solving involving dietary control, exercise, blood glucose monitoring, oral hypoglycemic medications, or multiple daily insulin injections. Over the long term, it is not uncommon for patients to have difficulty sustaining the burden of these daily self-care demands and numerous lifestyle changes. It is therefore not surprising that the stress of coping with diabetes is a major risk factor for psychiatric illnesses and problems related to adhering to complex treatment recommendations.

DEPRESSION AND DIABETES

The prevalence of depression in diabetes patients is two to three times higher than that found in the general population (3). Several studies suggest that patients with depressive disorders develop worse glycemic control problems and have a heightened risk of diabetes complications such as retinopathy, nephropathy, hypertension, cardiac disease, and sexual dysfunction (4). Although depression is related to complications and disease duration, it has been found to occur relatively early in the course of diabetes, before the onset of complications (5). Therefore, the increased rate of depression and diabetes cannot be explained solely by emotional reactions to the onset of complications. Indeed, the relationship may be

Symptoms of Depression

At least five of the following symptoms have been present during the same 2-week period (including at least one of the first two):
- Depressed mood
- Loss of interest or pleasure
- Significant weight (appetite) loss or weight gain
- Insomnia or hypersomnia
- Psychomotor agitation or retardation
- Fatigue, loss of energy
- Feelings of worthlessness or guilt
- Difficulty concentrating or indecisiveness
- Thoughts of death or suicide

bidirectional because symptoms of depression, such as decreased motivation, poor energy, and hopelessness, likely interfere with adherence to diabetes treatment, leading to worse glycemic control.

In a meta-analysis of 24 studies of depression, hyperglycemia, and diabetes, Lustman et al. (6) reported a consistent, strong association between elevated glycated hemoglobin A_{1c} (A1C) values (indicating chronic hyperglycemia) and depression. However, they were unable to determine the direction of the association, so it remains unclear if hyperglycemia causes depressed mood or if hyperglycemia is a consequence of depression. Furthermore, Lustman et al. noted that the relationship might be a reciprocal one in which hyperglycemia is provoked by depression, independently contributing to the exacerbation of depression, like a feedback loop.

Studies of type 2 diabetes are less clear with regard to the development of psychiatric illness (7). In some instances, the increased rates of depression seen in patients with type 2 diabetes appear to precede the onset of illness, thereby raising an entirely different hypothesis about the etiological relationship, i.e., depressive disorders themselves may place patients at risk of developing type 2 diabetes. Depressed patients often decrease physical activity, increase cardiovascular risk factors by smoking, and eat high-calorie and fatty foods, which places them at higher risk of developing type 2 diabetes (8).

Furthermore, Jacobson et al. (9) hypothesized that the metabolic problems of diabetes (increased rates of hypoglycemia and/or hyperglycemia) could themselves play a causal role in the development of depression. Preliminary evidence suggests that diabetes may lead to changes in white matter in the brain and that these white matter abnormalities (if present in regions of the brain involved in affect regulation, e.g., the limbic system) may play a causal role in the development of depression. More recent data show differences in gray matter density in the brains of type 1 diabetes patients with histories of depression compared with those of patients without depression (10). These early studies

PRACTICAL POINT

Emerging evidence concludes that depression may be a risk factor for the development of type 2 diabetes (8).

implicate an association between brain structural changes (in both white and gray matter) and depression in patients with diabetes, which may be related to underlying metabolic fluctuations of diabetes.

Evidence indicates that treatment for depression can lead to improvements in diabetes regimen adherence and improved glycemic control. The combination of high rates of depression in patients with diabetes and the known effectiveness of treatments for depression reinforces how critical it is to identify and treat depression early in its onset. Attention to the possibility of comorbid depression should also be considered when treating patients with worsening glycemic control and who have trouble adapting to diabetes. A small number of studies have demonstrated that treatment of depression, including cognitive behavior therapy and antidepressants (particularly selective serotonin reuptake inhibitors [SSRIs]), has equivalent efficacy in depressed patients with diabetes versus patients with depression alone.

The mutual identification, support, and problem solving offered by other people with diabetes makes group therapy an increasingly popular option for treatment of depression. Thus, whatever the causal links between depression and diabetes, psychiatric treatment can improve glycemic control and reduce depressive symptomatology (6,11).

PRACTICAL POINT

Treatment of depression will help people with diabetes have longer, more enjoyable, healthier lives.

ANXIETY DISORDERS AND DIABETES

All patients are anxious about their diabetes at one time or another. Whether anxiety is normal or abnormal depends on its intensity and on the duration, consequences, and circumstances that caused it. Anxiety can have negative effects on regimen adherence and glycemic control.

Diagnostically, anxiety disorders encompass generalized anxiety disorder, panic disorder, obsessive-compulsive disorder, posttraumatic stress disorder, and various phobias. In addition to depression, they are some of the most disabling of psychiatric illnesses and often coexist with depression. These illnesses are notorious for their chronicity, negative impact on quality of life, and interference with receiving medical care. In a review of 18 studies, Grigsby et al. (12) reported that generalized anxiety disorder was present in 14% of patients with diabetes compared with 4% for the general population. Elevated anxiety levels were present in 40% of subjects, with no difference in prevalence between individuals with type 1 diabetes and those with type 2 diabetes. Women with diabetes were more likely to have higher levels of anxiety than men with diabetes.

Anxiety commonly focuses on fears of hyperglycemia and complications or fears of hypoglycemia and feeling out of control. Less frequently, there may be phobic avoidance of needles and fingersticks or compulsive monitoring of blood glucose levels. Ordinarily, chronic anxiety (commonly called *stress*) is created simply by the effects of diabetes on day-to-day life. The demands of self-care are complex, never ending, and often frustrating. Patients can feel overwhelmed, guilty, angry, fearful, or unmotivated, particularly when blood glucose levels are high or unpredictable despite their best efforts.

The psychophysiological effects of stress on blood glucose levels have also been studied. Although most people with diabetes report that stress affects their

Symptoms of Anxiety

Excessive worry associated with at least three of the following symptoms, with some symptoms present for more days than not in the past 6 months:
- Restless, keyed-up, on edge
- Easily fatigued
- Difficulty concentrating
- Irritability
- Muscle tension
- Sleep disturbance

PRACTICAL POINT

Anxiety about diabetes tends to peak at distinct periods of stress, which can include the initial crisis of diagnosis, the onset of major complications, and failure to achieve the desired therapeutic response (13). These crises give the nurse a unique opportunity to have an enormous impact on patients and their families, who are likely to be more receptive to outside support at these times.

blood glucose levels, the results of research have been inconsistent, with some studies reporting blood glucose responses (usually hyperglycemic) to stress, whereas others have found no response (14). Thus, while there is no conclusive evidence reporting the effects of stress on blood glucose, its potential as a factor influencing the achievement of self-care goals in diabetes should be considered in the treatment of diabetes patients.

Diabetes is a disease that affects the family, and the behavior of the family can have an effect on the person with diabetes. Family members may add stress by being too overprotective, accusatory, unrealistic, or uninvolved with diabetes care. The person with diabetes may complicate these family dynamics by rejecting family support or becoming overly dependent, leaving family members feeling frustrated and worried. Once again, the nurse plays a crucial role in helping families find effective ways to communicate about diabetes management.

Treatment Recommendations

Psychopharmacological treatments for anxiety, including the SSRIs, appear to be effective for patients with diabetes, although they have not been closely studied with either type of diabetes. Likewise, while there has been little formal research done on other forms of psychotherapeutic intervention and diabetes per se, it is reasonable to assume that other accepted forms of psychotherapy would be equally effective with diabetes (15). Stress management training holds promise as a cost-effective treatment for improving glycemic control (16). Cognitive behavioral treatments are being used successfully with a range of anxiety disorders. In general, this approach identifies maladaptive thought patterns and troublesome behaviors and instructs patients in developing more adaptive substitute thoughts and behaviors. Relaxation training and hypnotic suggestion have potential for individuals suffering from needle phobias. (See CHAPTER 21 for more on helping the patient deal with his or her diabetes.)

EATING DISORDERS AND DIABETES

> **PRACTICAL POINT**
>
> Researchers estimate that 10–20% of girls in their mid-teen years and 30–40% of late teenaged girls and young adult women skip or alter their insulin doses to control their weight (see "Diabetes and Eating Disorders" in RESOURCES).

Despite the promise of risk reduction for the long-term complications of type 1 diabetes, the negative side effect of intensive diabetes management is weight gain. For example, during the first 6 years of follow-up in the DCCT, the patients in the intensively treated group gained an average of 10.45 lb more than patients in the standard treatment cohort (17). The most recent follow-up of these patients, 9 years after the completion of the DCCT, indicated that once patients on intensive treatment gained weight, this weight was difficult to lose (18). A survey of patients' responses to the recommendations of the DCCT documented that women with type 1 diabetes were especially concerned about tight glucose control causing weight gain (19,20). Researchers and clinicians have argued that the attention to food portions, blood glucose levels, and risk of weight gain associated with intensive diabetes management parallels the rigid thinking about food and body image characteristic of women with eating disorders and may place women with diabetes at heightened risk of developing eating disorders. Women with type 1 diabetes may use insulin manipulation (i.e., administering reduced insulin doses or omitting necessary doses altogether) as a means of caloric purging. Intentionally induced glycosuria is a powerful weight loss behavior and a symptom of eating disorders unique to people with type 1 diabetes. This behavior is more common in women but can also occur in men, especially during adolescence (see also "Diabetes and Eating Disorders," a patient handout in RESOURCES).

The most recent controlled studies suggest an increased risk of eating disorders among female patients with type 1 diabetes. Jones et al. (21) report that young women with type 1 diabetes have 2.4 times the risk of developing an eating disorder and 1.9 times the risk for subclinical eating disorders (i.e., when symptoms of disordered eating do not meet the level of severity to warrant a formal diagnosis) than age-matched women without diabetes (21). Intermittent insulin omission

Symptoms of Anorexia

- Refusal to maintain normal body weight
- Intense fear of becoming fat, even though underweight
- Disturbance in the way weight or shape is experienced
- Absence of at least three consecutive menstrual cycles

Symptoms of Bulimia

- Recurrent episodes of binge eating
- Recurrent inappropriate compensatory behavior to prevent weight gain
- Binge eating or compensatory behaviors occur at least twice per week for 3 months
- Self-evaluation is unduly influenced by body shape and weight

and reduction for weight loss purposes has been found to be a common practice among women with type 1 diabetes. For example, in women with type 1 diabetes between the ages of 13 and 60 years, Polonsky et al. (22) found that 31% reported intentional insulin omission. Rates of omission peaked in late adolescence and early adulthood, with 40% of women between the ages of 15 and 30 years reporting intentional omission. Additionally, studies show that this behavior, even at a subclinical level of severity, places women at heightened risk for the medical complications of diabetes. Women reporting intentional insulin misuse had higher A1C levels, higher rates of hospital and emergency room visits, and higher rates of neuropathy and retinopathy than women who did not report insulin omission (22). In a longitudinal study, Rydall et al. (23) reported that after 4 years of eating disordered behavior, 86% of patients classified as highly eating disordered had retinopathy compared with 43 and 24% of women with moderate or no reported eating disturbance, respectively. Women with diabetes and eating disorders are in poorer glycemic control, with A1C levels approximately two or more percentage points higher than those of similarly aged women without eating disorders (23). The chronic hyperglycemia found in women with diabetes who intentionally omit or reduce their insulin doses places these women at much greater risk for frequent episodes of diabetic ketoacidosis and the long-term onset of macro- and microvascular complications of diabetes.

Disordered eating behaviors are often well hidden, and because these patients may not use other means of purging (such as self-induced vomiting or laxative abuse), their eating disorders may go undiagnosed. Once established as a long-standing behavior pattern, the problem of frequent insulin omission may be particularly difficult to treat. For this reason, early detection and intervention appears to be crucial. Questions such as "Do you ever change your insulin dose or skip insulin doses to influence your weight?" or "Tell me about your weight issues and how you feel insulin affects them" can be helpful in screening for insulin omission, especially when patients present with persistently elevated A1C levels or unexplained diabetic ketoacidosis.

Because obesity is a significant risk factor in type 2 diabetes, recurrent binge eating may increase the chances of developing this form of diabetes. Research indicates that among obese adults, there is a distinct subgroup (20–46%) who report engaging in recurrent binge eating, defined as consumption of a large amount of food while feeling out of control of the behavior (24).

The literature on binge eating in type 2 diabetes is still in its infancy, with initial studies relying on small, nonrepresentative samples. Kenardy et al. (25) found that 14% of the patients with newly diagnosed type 2 diabetes experienced problems with binge eating compared with 4% of the age-, sex-, and weight-matched control subjects. Recurrent binge eating may make it more difficult to control blood glucose levels, thereby increasing the likelihood of developing the medical complications associated with diabetes.

Treatment Recommendations

A multidisciplinary team approach is considered the optimal treatment for both eating disorders and diabetes. When designed to treat a patient with both diabetes and an eating disorder, such a team should include an endocrinologist/diabetologist, nurse educator, nutritionist with eating disorder and/or diabetes training, and a psychologist or social worker to provide weekly individual therapy. Depending on the level of comorbid depression, anxiety, and frequency of binge eating, a psychiatrist may also be needed for psychopharmacological evaluation and treatment. At this time, little research has examined treatment efficacy for eating disorders in the context of diabetes; however, a large volume of research on treatment outcomes in bulimia nervosa supports the use of cognitive behavioral therapy in combination with antidepressant medications as the most effective treatment (26). These approaches would need to be adapted slightly in order to directly address the role of insulin omission as the means of caloric purging.

Weekly psychotherapy is strongly recommended. Early in the treatment, monthly appointments with the endocrinologist, nurse educator, and nutritionist may be necessary to maintain medical stability. Laboratory tests (especially A1C and electrolytes) and weigh-ins should occur at each of the medical appointments. Some patients may require a medical or psychiatric inpatient hospitalization until they are medically stable and emotionally ready to engage in treatment as outpatients.

With regard to diabetes management, the treatment team must be willing to set incremental goals that the patient feels ready to achieve. Early in treatment, intensive glycemic management of diabetes is not an appropriate target for a person with diabetes and an eating disorder. The first goal must be to establish medical safety for the patient. Gradually, the team can build toward increasing doses of insulin, increases in food intake, greater flexibility in meal plans, regularity of eating routines, and more frequent blood glucose monitoring.

SUMMARY

Nursing takes a holistic approach to chronic care, seeing the physical, emotional, and spiritual issues that contribute to the health problems of an individual. Many times, a patient will see the nurse as the safest person to talk with to share feelings of anger, depression, or anxiety. The role of the nurse can be pivotal in helping patients

---

PRACTICAL POINT

Helpful questions to ask:
- Do you feel sad or blue?
- What part of diabetes management is the hardest for you?
- What aspects of diabetes do you worry about most?
- Do you ever change your insulin dose or skip insulin doses to influence your weight?

For more on eating disorders, the Spring 2002 (volume 15) issue of *Diabetes Spectrum* can be reviewed (available from http://spectrum. diabetesjournals.org).

to seek treatment (medication and/or counseling) to address these mental health problems.

When psychiatric problems are suspected by the nurse, it can be helpful to remind the patient, the family, and the treatment team that diabetes management is burdensome and requires support. This support can come from family members, friends, coworkers, and a multidisciplinary diabetes treatment team. Both the patient and treatment team must be encouraged to work collaboratively to set small, attainable diabetes treatment goals that can increase in complexity over time. Because of the interplay of psychological factors and diabetes control, it is crucial to include mental health treatment in the multidisciplinary treatment approach, especially when adherence problems arise.

REFERENCES

1. Diabetes Control and Complications Trial Research Group: The effect of intensive treatment of diabetes on the development and progression of long-term complications in insulin-dependent diabetes mellitus. *N Engl J Med* 329:977–986, 1993
2. Krentz AJ: UKPDS and beyond: into the next millennium: United Kingdom Prospective Diabetes Study. *Diabetes Obes Metab* 1:13–22, 1999
3. Anderson R, Freedland KE, Clouse RE, Lustman PJ: The prevalence of comorbid depression in adults with diabetes. *Diabetes Care* 24:1069–1078, 2001
4. de Groot M, Anderson R, Freedland KE, Clouse RE, Lustman PJ: Association of depression and diabetes complications: a meta-analysis. *Psychosom Med* 63:619–630, 2001
5. Jacobson AM, Samson JA, Weinger K, Ryan CM: Diabetes, the brain, and behavior: is there a biological mechanism underlying the association between diabetes and depression? *Int Rev Neurobiol* 51:455–479, 2002
6. Lustman PJ, Anderson RJ, Freedland KE, de Groot M, Carney RM, Clouse RE: Depression and poor glycemic control: a meta-analytic review of the literature. *Diabetes Care* 23:934–942, 2000
7. Talbot F, Nouwen A: A review of the relationship between depression and diabetes in adults: is there a link? *Diabetes Care* 23:1556–1562, 2000
8. Freedland KF: Hypothesis 1: depression is a risk factor for the development of type 2 diabetes. *Diabetes Spectrum* 17:150–152, 2004
9. Jacobson AM, Weinger K, Hill TC, Parker JA, Suojanen JN, Jimerson DC, Soroko DJ: Brain functioning, cognition and psychiatric disorders in patients with type 1 diabetes (Abstract). *Diabetes* 49 (Suppl. 1):A132, 2000
10. Sparks C, Musen G, Lyoo I, Weinger K, Renshaw PF, Hwang J, Ryan CM, Jimerson DC, Jacobson AM: Brain structure changes in type 1 diabetes patients with past depression [online]. Program No. 114.14. *2004 Abstract Viewer and Itinerary Planner.* Washington, DC, Society for Neuroscience, 2004.
11. Lustman PJ, Griffith LS, Freedland KE, Kissel SS, Clouse RE: Cognitive behavior therapy for depression in type 2 diabetes mellitus: a randomized, controlled trial. *Ann Intern Med* 129:613–621, 1998
12. Grigsby AB, Anderson RJ, Freedland KE, Clouse RE, Lustman PJ: Prevalence of anxiety in adults with diabetes: a systematic review. *J Psychosom Res* 53:1053–1060, 2002
13. Hamburg BA, Inoff GE: Coping with predictable crises of diabetes. *Diabetes Care* 6:409–416, 1983

14. Rubin RR, Peyrot M: Psychological issues and treatments for people with diabetes. *J Clin Psychol* 57:457–478, 2001
15. Anderson BJ, Rubin RR: *Practical Psychology for Diabetes Clinicians.* 2nd ed. Alexandria, VA, American Diabetes Association, 2002
16. Surwit RS, Bauman A: *The Mind-Body Diabetes Revolution: A Proven New Program for Better Blood Sugar Control.* New York, Free Press, 2004
17. Diabetes Control and Complications Trial Research Group: Weight gain associated with intensive therapy in the Diabetes Control and Complications Trial. *Diabetes Care* 11:567–573, 1988
18. Diabetes Control and Complications Trial Research Group: Influence of intensive diabetes treatment on body weight and composition of adults with type 1 diabetes in the Diabetes Control and Complications Trial. *Diabetes Care* 24:1711–1721, 2001
19. Thompson CJ, Cummings JF, Chalmers J, Gould C, Newton RW: How have patients reacted to the implications of the DCCT? *Diabetes Care* 19:876–879, 1996
20. Jones J, Colton P: Prevalence of eating disorders in girls with type 1 diabetes. *Diabetes Spectrum* 15:86–89, 2002
21. Jones JM, Lawson ML, Daneman D, Olmsted MP, Rodin G: Eating disorders in adolescent females with and without type 1 diabetes: cross sectional study. *BMJ* 320:1563–1566, 2000
22. Polonsky WH, Anderson BJ, Lohrer PA, Aponte JE, Jacobson AM, Cole CF: Insulin omission in women with IDDM. *Diabetes Care* 17:1178–1185, 1994
23. Rydall AC, Rodin GM, Olmsted MP, Devenyi RG, Daneman D: Disordered eating behavior and microvascular complications in young women with insulin-dependent diabetes mellitus. *N Engl J Med* 336:1849–1854, 1997
24. de Zwaan M, Mitchell JE, Seim HC, Specker SM, Pyle RL, Raymond NC, Crosby RB: Eating related and general psychopathology in obese females with binge eating disorder. *Int J Eat Disord* 15:43–52, 1994
25. Kenardy J, Mensch M, Bowen K, Pearson SA: A comparison of eating behaviors in newly diagnosed NIDDM patients and case-matched control subjects. *Diabetes Care* 17:1197–1199, 1994
26. Peterson CB, Mitchell JE: Psychosocial and pharmacological treatment of eating disorders: a review of research findings. *J Clin Psychol* 55:685–697, 1999

Dr. Goebel-Fabbri is a Psychologist at Joslin Diabetes Center, Boston, MA, and an Instructor in Psychiatry at Harvard Medical School, Boston, MA. Mr. Zrebiec is Associate Director, Behavioral and Mental Health Unit, at Joslin Diabetes Center, Boston, MA, and a Lecturer in Psychiatry at Harvard Medical School, Boston, MA.

23. Polypharmacy

Barbara McCloskey, PharmD, BC-PS, CDE

Polypharmacy, the use of multiple medications, can be associated with increased costs, poorer compliance, and increased risk of side effects and drug interactions. Having diabetes and its associated comorbidities increases the risk of polypharmacy complications, particularly in the elderly (1) (Table 23.1). The use of two medications puts a person at a 6% risk of having an adverse reaction. This risk increases to 100% with eight medications (1). In patients with diabetes, polypharmacy is often a necessity to achieve optimal blood glucose, blood pressure, and lipid control and to manage other diabetes-related complications and comorbidities.

PRACTICAL POINT

Polypharmacy is common and often necessary when a patient has diabetes and multiple comorbidities. Frequent review of medications will help decrease the risk of harmful interactions and reduce cost to the patient (see also "Keeping Medicine Costs Under Control," a patient handout in RESOURCES).

POLYPHARMACY AND ADHERENCE

Studies evaluating adherence to polypharmacy in diabetes have had mixed results (2,3). Unfortunately, self-reporting of medication adherence is often overestimated, making it difficult for the patient and health care professional to effectively and safely manage diabetes and its comorbidities. In addition, people do not want to be labeled the "bad patient," so they may not admit to difficulties with taking medication in terms of cost, effectiveness of the drug, and adverse effects. Some may take medications every other day to make the pills last longer or take them inconsistently. Others simply do not like to take "too many pills" and may decide to discontinue some medications without reporting it. Studies of the issues surrounding polypharmacy are difficult because of the problems with self-reporting and the use of electronic medication caps (caps that record the number of times the cap is removed) or pill counts that may improve adherence to medications in the short term, but not in the long term.

Table 23.1 Factors Contributing to Polypharmacy in Patients with Diabetes

- Need for tight blood glucose control, often requiring multidrug therapy
- Frequent comorbidities requiring drug therapy:
  - Hypertension
  - Dyslipidemia
  - Coronary artery disease
  - Renal disease
  - Congestive heart failure
  - Neuropathy
  - Glaucoma
  - Peripheral arterial disease, lower-extremity ulcers
  - Gastrointestinal problems

Adapted from Good (9).

Suggestions for Appropriate Medication Use in the Elderly

- Attempt nonpharmacological measures when feasible.
- Before starting a new drug, consider the possibility that the patient's symptoms are related to an adverse drug reaction.
- When a new drug is started, provide education about indications for use, taking the medication, common side effects, and potential serious adverse effects, as well as what to do when these side effects occur.
- Regularly review all medications, including over-the-counter drugs, herbal products, and vitamin and mineral supplements. Encourage patients to maintain and carry an up-to-date medication list.
- Coordinate care with all providers to eliminate the chances of duplicate prescriptions.
- Identify indications for each medication.
- Regularly assess therapeutic responses to medication.
- Drugs without a clear indication for use should be discontinued or tapered and then discontinued, if appropriate.
- Drugs that have not achieved their therapeutic goal should be discontinued.
- Medications with a high incidence of adverse outcomes in the elderly should be avoided.
- When possible, combine indications with a single drug.
- Regularly assess patient compliance, especially before a drug dosage is changed or a new drug is added.

Adapted from Good (9).

Adherence to medication schedules decreases as the medication regimen becomes more complex, in terms of both numbers of pills to be taken and frequency of dosages.

ADVERSE EFFECTS OF POLYPHARMACY

Polypharmacy in diabetes can result in drug-to-drug interactions between prescription and over-the-counter drugs (Tables 23.2 and 23.3). Also, there are over-the-counter drug–to–disease interactions (Table 23.4) that may cause problems.

Some medications can affect glucose levels themselves. Glucocorticoids commonly cause an increase in blood glucose levels (see CHAPTER 28 for a discussion of the impact of glucocorticoids on glucose levels and management issues). Other medications that are known to raise blood glucose levels are thiazide diuretics, phenytoin (Dilantin), estrogen compounds, and atypical antipsychotics (e.g., clozapine, olanzapine, risperidone). Individuals on these medications should monitor their blood glucose levels when initiating these medications. If the patient is taking atypical antipsychotics, he or she should routinely be monitored for the development of hyperglycemia. Some medications may decrease blood glucose levels, including some antibiotics (e.g., Levaquin, Biaxin) and large doses of salicylates. It is prudent to frequently monitor blood glucose levels when treating any infection with an antibiotic (4–7).

Doing the following helps ensure safe and appropriate medication use by patients (8):

- Encourage patients to keep an up-to-date list of all of their medications, including vitamins, over-the-counter medications, and herbal products. Patients can obtain a list of their current prescription medications from their pharmacy, a good place to start.
- Be aware of both the brand and generic names of medications. It is not uncommon for patients to be taking the same medication two ways, with one prescription vial dispensed and labeled as the brand name and the other vial dispensed and labeled as the generic name. Usually this

Table 23.2 Significance Rating Scales

Source A[4]		Assigned Rating A & B	Source B[5]
Severity of Consequences	Support from Literature		Avoidance Risk
Major	Probable or Suspected	1	Avoid combination
Moderate	Probable or Suspected	2	Avoid combination if possible
Minor	Probable or Suspected	3	Monitor and take action if necessary
Major/Moderate	Possible	4	No action necessary
Minor	Unlikely or Possible	5	No interaction

Adapted from Rhoades (10).

Table 23.3 Prescription Drug and Over the Counter (OTC) Interactions

Prescription Drug	OTC	Significance Rating		Description and Management
		A[4]	B[5]	
Antihypertensive Agents				
ACE INHIBITORS				
Benazepril (Lotensin), *captopril (Capoten),** enalapril (Vasotec), fosinopril (Monopril), lisinopril (Prinivil, Zestril), ramipril (Altace), quinapril (Accupril)	Antacids (*aluminum hydroxide, magnesium hydroxide*)	5	Not rated	Antacids may reduce the absorption and effectiveness of captopril. Separate the administration of each by 2 hours.
Benazepril, *captopril,* enalapril, fosinopril, lisinopril, ramipril, quinapril	*Capsaicin*	5	Not rated	Capsaicin may exacerbate the ACE inhibitor–related cough. Case reports have occurred with topical application as well as inhaled capsaicin.
Benazepril, *captopril, enalapril,* fosinopril, *lisinopril,* moexipril (Univasc), ramipril, quinapril, trandolapril (Tarka)	Salicylates (*aspirin,* bismuth subsalicylate, magnesium salicylate, sodium salicylate)	4	3	High-dose salicylates inhibit prostacyclin synthesis, which may decrease the hypotensive and vasodilator effects of ACE inhibitors. Monitor blood pressure and either reduce the dosage of aspirin or change to an alternative agent.
β-BLOCKERS				
Acebutolol (Sectral), *atenolol (Tenormin),* betaxolol (Kerlone), bisoprolol (Zebeta), carteolol (Cartrol), *metoprolol (Lopressor, Toprol),* nadolol (Corgard), penbutolol (Levatol), pindolol (Visken), *propranolol (Inderal),* timolol (Blocadren), *sotalol (Betapace)*	Aluminum salts (aluminum carbonate, *aluminum hydroxide,* aluminum phosphate, attapulgite, kaolin, magaldrate)	3	4	Reduced absorption and delayed gastric emptying may alter the effect of β-blockers. Separate the administration of each by 2 hours.
Acebutolol, *atenolol,* betaxolol, bisoprolol, carteolol, metoprolol, nadolol, penbutolol,	Calcium salts (*calcium carbonate, calcium citrate, calcium*	4	3	Calcium salts may impair the absorption of β-blockers. Monitor for signs of decreased

(continued)

Table 23.3 Prescription Drug and Over the Counter (OTC) Interactions (*Continued*)

Prescription Drug	OTC	Significance Rating		Description and Management
		A[4]	B[5]	
pindolol, propranolol, timolol, sotalol	*gluconate, calcium lactate,* dibasic calcium phosphate)			efficacy and adjust dosage if necessary.
Acebutolol, atenolol, betaxolol, bisoprolol, carteolol, *metoprolol,* nadolol, penbutolol, pindolol, *propranolol, timolol,* sotalol	Cimetidine	2	4	Cimetidine may reduce hepatic clearance of β-blockers, creating an increased effect. Monitor for signs of toxicity and adjust dosage if necessary or change to alternative histamine2-blocker.
Acebutolol, *atenolol,* betaxolol, bisoprolol, carteolol, metoprolol, nadolol, penbutolol, *pindolol, propranolol,* timolol	NSAIDs (*ibuprofen, indomethacin, naproxen, piroxicam*)	2	3	NSAIDs may decrease the antihypertensive effect of β-blockers by inhibiting prostaglandin synthesis. Monitor blood pressure and adjust β-blocker dosage if necessary.
Acebutolol, atenolol, betaxolol, bisoprolol, carteolol, metoprolol, nadolol, penbutolol, *pindolol, propranolol,* timolol	Salicylates (*aspirin,* bismuth subsalicylate, magnesium salicylate, sodium salicylate)	4	4	High-dose salicylates may alter the effect of β-blockers by inhibition of prostaglandins. Monitor blood pressure and adjust dosage if necessary or change to alternative agent.

CALCIUM-CHANNEL BLOCKERS

Prescription Drug	OTC	A[4]	B[5]	Description and Management
Diltiazem (Cardizem, Cartia XL, Dilacor, Tiazac), nifedipine (Adalat, Procardia), nisoldipine (Sular), *verapamil (Calan, Covera, Isoptin, Verelan)*	Calcium salts (calcium carbonate, calcium citrate, *calcium gluconate,* calcium lactate, dibasic calcium phosphate)	2	3	When large doses of calcium salts are given, a reduction of the hypotensive effects of calcium-channel blockers may be seen. Monitor vital signs and adjust dosages if necessary.
Diltiazem, *nifedipine,* nisoldipine, verapamil	Histamine2 antagonists (*cimetidine,* ranitidine, famotidine)	2	3	Cimetidine may increase the plasma concentration of calcium-channel blockers, creating an

Table 23.3 Prescription Drug and Over the Counter (OTC) Interactions (*Continued*)

Prescription Drug	OTC	Significance Rating		Description and Management
		A[4]	B[5]	
				increase in hypotensive effects. Monitor blood pressure and adjust dosage if necessary or change to alternative agent.
LOOP DIURETICS				
Bumetanide (Bumex), ethacrynic acid (Edecrin), *furosemide (Lasix),* torsemide (Demadex)	NSAIDs *(diclofenac, ibuprofen, indomethacin,* ketoprofen, naproxen, *sulindac,* oxaprozin, piroxicam)	3	3	NSAIDs may decrease the effectiveness of loop diuretics. Monitor for reduction of efficacy and adjust loop diuretic dosage if necessary or change to alternative NSAID.
Bumetanide, ethacryinic acid, *furosemide,* torsemide	Salicylates *(aspirin,* bismuth subsalicylate, magnesium salicylate, sodium salicylate)	5	4	A decreased diuretic response may be possible in patients with cirrhosis and ascites. Monitor these patients for decreased effect and adjust dosage if necessary.
THIAZIDE DIURETICS				
Chlorothiazide (Diuril), chlorthalidone (Hygroton), *hydrochlorothiazide (Esidrix, HydroDiuril, Oretic),* indapamide (Lozol), metolazone (Zaroxolyn)	Calcium salts *(calcium carbonate,* calcium citrate, calcium gluconate, calcium lactate, dibasic calcium phosphate)	4	3	Hypercalcemia may result from this combination. Monitor serum calcium and for signs of hypercalcemia. Avoid excessive or prolonged administration of calcium salts.
Chlorothiazide, *chlorthalidone, hydrochlorothiazide,* indapamide, *metolazone*	NSAIDs *(diclofenac,* ibuprofen, *indomethacin,* ketoprofen, naproxen, *sulindac,* oxaprozin, piroxicam)	5	4	NSAIDs may cause a mild reduction in antihypertensive effects of thiazide-type diuretics by induction of sodium/ water retention and inhibition of renal prostaglandin. Monitor blood pressure and adjust dosage if necessary.

(continued)

**Table 23.3 Prescription Drug and Over the Counter (OTC)
Interactions (*Continued*)**

Prescription Drug	OTC	Significance Rating		Description and Management
		A[4]	B[5]	
Antidiabetic Agents				
INSULINS AND SULFONYLUREAS				
Insulin, chlorpropamide (Diabenese), glipizide (Glucotrol), glyburide (DiaBeta, Micronase), tolbutamide (Orinase)	Salicylates (aspirin, magnesium salicylate, sodium salicylate)	2	3	Salicylates may enhance insulin secretion and may increase the effectiveness of sulfonylureas. Monitor blood glucose and adjust medications if necessary.
Chlorpropamide, glipizide, glyburide, tolbutamide	Magnesium salts (magnesium-aluminum hydroxide, magnesium hydroxide)	5	3	Magnesium salts may enhance absorption of sulfonylureas, therefore increasing the hypoglycemic effect. Monitor blood glucose and adjust dosage if necessary.
Acetohexamide (Dymelor), chlorpropamide, glipizide, glyburide, tolazamide (Tolinase), tolbutamide	Histamine2 antagonists (cimetidine, ranitidine, famotidine)	4	3	Reduced hepatic metabolism of sulfonylureas may occur, and changes in gastric pH may lead to increases in efficacy of sulfonylureas. Monitor blood glucose levels and adjust dosage if necessary.
Metformin (Glucophage)	Cimetidine	2	3	Cimetidine increases metformin concentrations by reducing renal clearance, thereby increasing the blood glucose–lowering effect. Monitor blood glucose and adjust dosage if necessary or change to alternative histamine2 antagonist.
Antihyperlipemic Agents				
BILE AND SEQUESTRANTS				
Cholestyramine (Questran, Prevalite), colestipol (Colestid), colesevelam (Welchol)	NSAIDs (ibuprofen, ketoprofen, naproxen sodium)	3	3	Bile acid sequestrants may decrease the effectiveness of NSAIDs. Take the NSAID either 2 hours before or 6 hours after the administra-

Table 23.3 Prescription Drug and Over the Counter (OTC) Interactions (*Continued*)

Prescription Drug	OTC	Significance Rating		Description and Management
		A[4]	B[5]	
				tion of the bile acid sequestrant.
OTHERS				
Niacin (Niacor, Niaspan)	Salicylates (*aspirin*)	5	4	Aspirin reduces the cutaneous flushing and increases the plasma concentration of niacin.

*Italics indicate medications specifically reported in the literature. NSAIDs, nonsteroidal anti-inflammatory drugs.

Adapted from Rhoades (10).

Table 23.4 OTC Drug-Disease Interactions

Medication	Effect on Disease State
ANTIHISTAMINES	
Brompheniramine, chlorpheniramine, clemastine, dexbrompheniramine, diphenhydramine, triprolidine	Typically this class of medication causes no detrimental effect on the disease state.
ANTITUSSIVES	
Dextromethorphan, diphenhydramine	Typically this class of medication has no effect on blood glucose. However, there are two pediatric case reports in which high doses of dextromethorphan caused a reversible type 1 diabetes.
ANTIHYPERLIPEMICS	
Niacin	Niacin may increase blood glucose levels. Monitor blood glucose and make appropriate adjustments if necessary or change to alternative agent.
DECONGESTANTS	
Ephedrine, naphazoline,* oxymetazoline, phenylephrine, pseudoephedrine, xylometazoline	Decongestants may increase blood pressure secondary to vasoconstrictive properties. Monitor blood pressure and adjust dosage if necessary.
EXPECTORANTS	
Guaifenesin	Typically this medication causes no detrimental effect on the disease state.

*The products underlined represent the topical nasal decongestants. Systemic effects are less likely to occur with topical use.

Adapted from Rhoades (10).

problem can be avoided if patients have all of their prescriptions filled at the same pharmacy.

- Help patients simplify their medication regimens by suggesting that they use pillboxes, calendars, watch alarms, or some other system that will help them remember when to take their medications.
- Assess patient beliefs regarding the use of medications. Cultural groups have differing beliefs regarding the use of medications or certain herbs or have incorrect perceptions about what different medications can do. Patients may not understand the chronic nature of diabetes and may see the medication as a temporary measure. Or patients may discontinue medications once they have achieved blood pressure or cholesterol level goals. In addition, patients may add cultural or folk remedies that may interact or cause side effects when combined with prescription medications. Patients may seek care from nontraditional sources that prohibit the use of allopathic medications and may resist adding medications to the treatment program.

There are additional strategies useful in decreasing the risks of polypharmacy.

- Interview patients individually about medication use to assess their beliefs, adherence, and problems related to the medication. Ask questions in a nonjudgmental manner, such as, "Sometimes it can be difficult to take all of these medications. How often does that happen to you?"
- Review all medications with the patient and identify which medication is being used for which health problem.
- Determine whether any of the medications are in the same class; using more than one medication in the same class of drug is probably ineffective.
- Determine whether the medication dosages and the manner in which the patient is taking them are safe and effective. Sometimes patients will take more medication than has been prescribed, thinking "more is better."
- If specific medications require periodic safety laboratory monitoring, make sure this is being performed.
- Ask the patient about the presence of symptoms that could be adverse effects from the medications.
- Ask a pharmacist about potential drug-to-drug interactions when questions arise.
- Discuss polypharmacy issues with the health care team, such as simplifying the medication regimen, using generic drugs if cost is an issue, decreasing the number of medications needed, using modified-release medications that can be taken once a day, or using fixed-combination drugs.

SUMMARY

Improved understanding regarding the importance of good glucose, lipid, and blood pressure control has led us to an age of polypharmacy. It is important for the nurse to assist the patient in understanding the purpose, benefits, and potential risks of the medications and the importance of consistent dosing. The nurse should also encourage the patient to always tell the prescribing health care provider about any side effects experienced. Patient use of multiple medications highlights the need for the nurse to be knowledgeable about multiple medications, both prescription and over the counter, as well as nutritional supplements, herbal products, and other complementary therapies. With the rapid change in therapies, it will be imperative that the nurse have a strong resource on prescription medications as well as over-the-counter medications and supplements.

REFERENCES

1. Shaughnessay AF: Common drug reactions in the elderly. *Emerg Med* 24:21–32, 1992
2. Grant DW, Devita NG, Singer DE, Meiges JB: Polypharmacy and medication adherence in patients with type 2 diabetes. *Diabetes Care* 26:1408–1412, 2003
3. Kuo YF, Raji MA, Markides KS, Ray LA, Espino DV, Goodwin JS: Inconsistent use of diabetes medications, diabetes complications and mortality in older Mexican Americans over a 7-year period. *Diabetes Care* 26:3054–3060, 2003
4. Harmel AP, Mathur R: *Davidson's Diabetes Mellitus: Diagnosis and Treatment.* 5th ed. Philadelphia, W. B. Saunders, 2004
5. Citrome LL, Jaffe AB: Relationship of atypical antipsychotics with development of diabetes mellitus. *Ann Pharmacother* 37:1849–1857, 2003
6. Hedenmalm K, Hagg S, Stahl M, Mortimer O, Spigset O: Glucose intolerance with atypical antipsychotics. *Drug Saf* 25:1107–1116, 2002
7. American Diabetes Association, American Psychiatric Association, American Association of Clinical Endocrinologists, North American Association for the Study of Obesity: Consensus development conference on antipsychotic drugs and obesity and diabetes. *Diabetes Care* 27:596–601, 2004
8. McCloskey BA: Polypharmacy: boon or bane for health care providers? *Diabetes Spectrum* 15:237–238, 2002
9. Good CB: Polypharmacy in elderly patients with diabetes. *Diabetes Spectrum* 15:240–248, 2002
10. Rhoades KR: Prescribed medications and OTCs: interactions and timing issues. *Diabetes Spectrum* 15:256–261, 2002

Dr. McCloskey is the Diabetes Education Coordinator at Baylor Health Care Diabetes Services, Irving, TX.

24. Continuous Subcutaneous Insulin Infusion (Insulin Pump Therapy)

Donna Tomky, MSN, RN, C-ANP, CDE

In search of optimal insulin delivery, technological advances have led to the development of small portable devices that mimic physiological insulin replacement. These portable devices continuously infuse insulin under the subcutaneous tissue through a pumping mechanism. Continuous subcutaneous insulin infusion (CSII) via an insulin pump has allowed people with diabetes to attain improved blood glucose control. Attaining and maintaining blood glucose control on a sustained basis requires habitual and frequent monitoring of blood glucose levels by the pump wearer because these devices do not continuously monitor blood glucose. CSII therapy gives people with diabetes the ability to make sensible alterations to their insulin regimen to attain targeted blood glucose levels. Successful CSII therapy requires appropriate candidate selection, intense diabetes education, skill building, and training by a knowledgeable diabetes care team that results in consistent attention to details and competent self-care behaviors.

An insulin pump is a small battery-operated mechanical device containing a reservoir or syringe of fast- or rapid-acting insulin. The reservoir is attached to plastic tubing called an infusion set. At the end of the infusion set is a detachable 25- or 27-gauge needle or soft Teflon catheter. The catheter (needle) is inserted into the subcutaneous tissue and stays in place with self-adhesive tape or a bioclusive dressing. The pump wearer changes the infusion site every 24–72 h using an aseptic technique. Insulin pumps became available for clinical use in the early 1980s and weighed slightly less than 1 lb, with simple delivery of basal and bolus insulin. Current models weigh as little as 3 oz and can be worn discreetly under clothing or on a belt like a pager or cell phone. The newer models contain miniature computers that provide an array of basal and bolus functions.

Pump therapy requires a professional staff knowledgeable about the unique and special requirements of diabetes patients who wear pumps. Ideally, CSII therapy should be prescribed, implemented, and followed by a skilled professional team familiar with CSII therapy and capable of supporting the patient (1). Pump therapy is considered a subspecialty in the milieu of diabetes care. Typically, the pump therapy team consists of at least an endocrinologist, a nurse, and a dietitian familiar with CSII therapy. Before initiating pump therapy, potential pump candidates must have basic and advanced knowledge and skills regarding intensive insulin therapy. They must also demonstrate safe and consistent behavior in the regular tasks of diabetes self-management, including frequent blood glucose monitoring, injection of insulin, carbohydrate counting, problem solving for high and low blood glucose levels, and sick-day management.

PRINCIPLES OF PUMP THERAPY

CSII therapy is the modality that most closely duplicates the fully functioning pancreas. The Diabetes Control and Complications Trial conclusively demonstrated the beneficial effects and impact of optimal glycemic control (2). Insulin is needed to use food for fueling the body and storing energy for future needs. During the fasting state, insulin is released at a slow and steady rate (basal), with larger amounts (bolus) released during the fed state (Fig. 24.1). Only rapid- or fast-acting insulin (insulins lispro or aspart or regular insulin) is used in the pump, and intermediate- and long-acting insulins are never used. Insulin is delivered by either the basal rate or a bolus.

The benefits of CSII therapy are derived from the pharmacological advantage of using rapid-acting insulin that is delivered as a continuous infusion with incremental bolus administration at meals. Rapid-acting insulin is associated with the least amount of variation in day-to-day absorption. Bolus insulin activated by the wearer is given in anticipation of food or to correct an elevated blood glucose level. Meals can be skipped, delayed, or altered without loss of glycemic control. Bolus insulin activated by the pump user is given just before eating food or as needed to correct high blood glucose levels (Fig. 24.2). The bolus can be given all at once to cover carbohydrate intake or over time to mimic the insulin release for a more slowly digested meal.

Basal insulin, or metabolic/background insulin, supplies the body's continuous fasting or basic body insulin needs. The basal delivery mode is preprogrammed with a continuous infusion of insulin for 24 h/day. Usually, the basal rate approximates 50% of the total daily insulin needs. If basal rates are set appropriately,

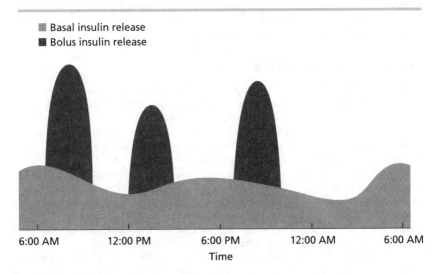

Figure 24.1 Normal insulin secretion in nondiabetic individuals.

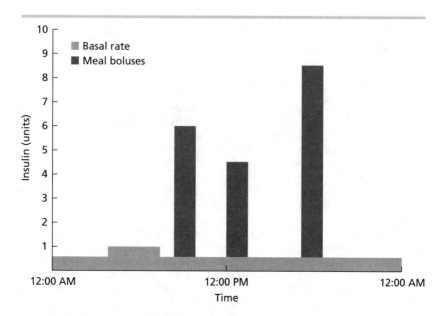

Figure 24.2 Pump insulin delivery.

the pump wearer can fast and does not need to eat to maintain fairly level blood glucose values. The basal rate is prescribed by the pump therapy team and can be set or changed by the pump wearer. Basal infusion can be programmed to coincide with the diurnal variation of insulin sensitivity and the requirements at different times of day. Programmed basal rates can vary throughout the day and are usually determined after wearing the pump for a few days. Temporary basal rate adjustments can be made during exercise, after exercise, during stress, or during illness, when lower or higher insulin requirements may exist.

WHO IS A PUMP CANDIDATE?

Successful CSII therapy depends in part on appropriate candidate selection and preparation for initiating pump therapy. It is generally accepted that highly motivated patients who use insulin and have well-established diabetes self-care behaviors, including problem-solving skills and frequent self-monitoring of blood glucose, are most successful at insulin pump therapy. Some pump therapy teams believe a structured screening protocol (with a trial pump that infuses saline) increases safety while initiating therapy in an outpatient setting and lowers discontinuation rates (3). A saline pump trial before initiating insulin pump therapy allows the candidate to understand the challenges of being continuously tethered to the pump before going forward with CSII. Many pump therapy teams would agree on the identified candidate selection criteria in Table 24.1 (3–5) (see also "Is an Insulin Pump Right for Your Child and Family?", a patient handout in RESOURCES).

Most individuals using CSII have type 1 diabetes. Although less common, it is sometimes used in individuals with insulin-treated type 2 diabetes. Criteria set forth by most health insurance plans require that the individual have type 1 diabetes

Table 24.1 Candidate Selection Criteria for CSII

Medical/metabolic indications	■ Suboptimal glycemic control ■ Wide blood glucose excursions ■ Dawn phenomenon with elevated fasting blood glucose levels ■ Frequent severe hypoglycemia ■ Nocturnal hypoglycemia ■ Pregnant or planning conception ■ Inconsistent daily schedule not well managed with injections ■ Insulin sensitivity and requirement of low doses of insulin
Cognitive/psychomotor criteria	■ Has sound rationale for pursuing and realistic expectations of CSII therapy ■ Capacity to learn the technical and cognitive components of the pump ■ Has appropriate problem-solving skills for troubleshooting hyper- and hypo-glycemic events and sick days ■ Able to match insulin with food using carbohydrate-counting skills ■ Adaptability of behavior or aspects of the regimen in response to outcome evaluation
Motivational ability	■ Perform frequent blood glucose monitoring as a lifetime behavior ■ Comply with recommendations for safe insulin pump use ■ Pay attention to details regarding the insulin regimen and the needed adjustments ■ Anticipate insulin needs as situations change
Technical/physical ability	■ Perform blood glucose monitoring accurately and frequently, up to 6–10 times daily ■ Perform the technical components of insulin pump use or have necessary support if visually impaired ■ Absence of serious disease that could impair technical performance
Financial resources	■ Can obtain adequate financial resources to cover the initial and ongoing costs of CSII therapy (approximately $6,400 for setup and $1,500–3,000 for yearly supplies) (6)

Data are from Refs. 3–6 and 9.

or require insulin treatment. Medicare ensures the pump candidate's insulin dependency by requesting verification of low C-peptide levels or presence of GAD or insulin antibodies (7).

CSII therapy has not been fully evaluated in patients with type 2 diabetes. A limited number of clinical studies show that CSII therapy can safely improve glycemic control and β-cell function in a relatively short period. Pump therapy may be particularly useful in treating patients with type 2 diabetes who do not satisfactorily respond to more conventional insulin treatment strategies (8). Usually, higher insulin doses are required for individuals with type 2 diabetes because both insulin deficiency and insulin resistance are common.

Characteristics of Pump Therapy in Type 2 Diabetes Compared With Type 1 Diabetes

- Patients with type 2 diabetes usually need a higher basal rate
- Meal-related boluses are larger in type 2 diabetes
- The time between reservoir refills is shorter in type 2 diabetes
- Battery life may be shorter in type 2 diabetes
- Pump therapy may improve endogenous insulin secretion and resistance in type 2 diabetes
- Patient acceptance and satisfaction are similar in type 2 diabetes (8)

Benefits of Pump Therapy

Research has shown that using pump therapy to maintain normal or near-normal blood glucose levels can improve health and reduce the long-term complications of diabetes (1).

- Improvement in blood glucose levels is possible with pumps.
  - Pumps do not use long-acting insulin, but instead only use rapid or short-acting insulin, which is more predictable and can be delivered more physiologically.
  - Pump wearers often experience fewer and less severe hypoglycemic events.
  - Insulin dosing can be precise, to within one-hundredth of a unit.
  - There is more predictable insulin absorption from a continuous insulin depot.
  - Dawn phenomenon effects are easier to manage with the basal rate and can be set to accommodate the rise in insulin requirements overnight.
  - Basal rates can be quickly changed to accommodate growth spurts in children or increased insulin needs during pregnancy.
- Improvement in the safety profile is possible.
  - Reducing the basal rate during periods of low physiological requirements can minimize nocturnal or daytime hypoglycemia.

Benefits of Pump Therapy (Continued)

> - Using a temporary basal rate that meets short-term physiological needs can accommodate the patient when sick.
> - Improvement in lifestyle flexibility and patient satisfaction is possible.
>   - Meals and food can be customized to fit the individual's schedule and preference in timing, size of meal, and type of food.
>   - Carbohydrate counting using an insulin-to-carbohydrate ratio is one method of matching appropriate amounts of (bolus) insulin to the food consumed.
>   - Weight loss may be more easily achieved in motivated patients, although initial improved glycemia may promote weight gain.
>   - Pumps can deliver insulin to coincide with travel or work schedules.

Limitations of Pump Therapy

> - The risks or drawbacks of pump therapy must be fully understood by the wearer and the health care team.
>   - Pumps are not for everyone, and patients must maintain a high degree of motivation before and throughout pump therapy.
>   - Patients must be willing to maintain habitual and frequent self-monitoring of blood glucose.
>   - The learning curve is steep, and some patients struggle with the concepts and problem-solving skills required for CSII.
>   - Being connected to a pump is a visual reminder of having diabetes.
>   - Technical or mechanical failure is possible with a pump and, if not corrected in a timely manner, can quickly lead to diabetic ketoacidosis in individuals with type 1 diabetes.
>   - Skin irritations and infections are possible.
>   - Weight gain is possible with improved glycemic control.
>   - Some patient populations, such as children or the visually impaired, may require assistance from a caregiver.
> - Many physicians and health care providers are unfamiliar with pump therapy and may not provide the necessary training and support.
> - The cost of insulin pumps is usually over $5,000, and supplies (not including blood glucose monitoring items) cost $1,500–3,000 per year. Insurance companies typically cover only 80% of pump expenses, and coverage varies from state to state and plan to plan. Reimbursement for diabetes education to support the patient also varies (6).

Contraindications to Pump Therapy

- Some individuals have unrealistic expectations that pump therapy will cure their diabetes and automatically control it.
- Severe depression or other serious mental health disorders may distract patients from paying attention to details that are critical to successful pump therapy.
- A history of poor self-care behaviors and health care practices, such as failure to perform self-monitoring of blood glucose, keep appointments, weigh and estimate portions of food to appropriately match food with insulin, and apply problem-solving skills, will signal failure.
- Financial resources are needed for initiating and maintaining optimal pump therapy practices.

CONSIDERATIONS FOR PROBLEM SOLVING

Hyperglycemia

Because the insulin pump only uses short- or rapid-acting insulin, even a partial interruption of insulin flow can result in hyperglycemia in patients with absence of endogenous insulin. Complete interruption can result in ketosis or ketoacidosis

PRACTICAL POINT

Troubleshooting Hyperglycemia in Insulin Pump Therapy
- Red, tender, and swollen catheter site (the insulin is not being absorbed correctly and leads to high blood glucose levels, which indicates that the site needs to be changed.)
- Leakage, breakage, or kinking of tubing
- Battery failure
- Empty reservoir or cartridge
- Improper positioning of reservoir or piston rod
- Improper basal rate programming
- Air in tubing
- Illness
- Menstrual cycle fluctuations
- Omitted bolus or improper amount given
- Ineffective insulin (expired date, exposure to heat or cold)
- Crimped catheter or needle not penetrating skin
- Change in usual routine
- Suspect site not absorbing, if no other apparent reason for high blood glucose

CAUTION: Any of these can occur even though the infusion site/set was recently changed.

PRACTICAL POINT

When assessing a patient on pump therapy:
- Correct known problems immediately.
- Advise the patient to change infusion sites with each new reservoir or cartridge, infusion set, and catheter.
- Check urine for ketones.
- Check serum for bicarbonate to determine the severity of diabetic ketoacidosis.
- Advise the patient to take supplemental insulin with a conventional insulin syringe.
- Provide nursing support for symptoms of nausea, dehydration, or infection.

---

within a few short hours. High blood glucose can occur for various reasons, including infection, illness, stress, menstrual cycle in women, battery failure, infusion set or catheter occlusion, leaking connection, inadequate or missed meal bolus, or poorly absorbing insulin from the site.

Hypoglycemia

Hypoglycemia is the main side effect of insulin, regardless of delivery method. Insulin pump therapy does not seem to have a higher rate of hypoglycemia than multiple daily injections. In fact, pump therapy has been shown to reduce severe hypoglycemia due to pumping small amounts of insulin, particularly in children (10).

There is a danger of losing consciousness with severe hypoglycemia. Not everyone gets warning signs of low blood glucose, i.e., hypoglycemia unawareness; therefore, reinforcing frequent blood glucose monitoring to pump wearers, especially before driving or when operating equipment, is essential. Testing blood glucose is the only dependable way to verify blood glucose levels at any time. Significant others, including family members, friends, or coworkers, need education and training on how to administer intramuscular glucagon in the event that the pump wearer experiences a severe hypoglycemic event.

Safety Concerns

Insulin dosages vary from person to person and can be significantly altered by changes in diet, exercise, stress levels, and many other variables. Performing frequent blood glucose testing is necessary to safely use a pump. Blood glucose levels can be maintained near the normal range after individualized basal rate and bolus requirements have been determined based on blood glucose results. A basic rule is to always check blood glucose before providing insulin.

Reimbursement Issues

Most insurance plans provide reimbursement for insulin pump therapy because physicians prescribe pumps in response to specific clinical issues, e.g., the inability to safely achieve adequate blood glucose control, low glucose levels during sleep, work/shift schedules that require flexible insulin delivery.

Some insurance companies are beginning to apply Medicare's rules for reimbursing insulin pumps. These rules were updated in 2005 and state that under certain criteria in some patients, the administration will cover the costs of an external insulin infusion pump and related items for treating diabetes. Under this provision, patients must be *1*) insulinopenic as verified by fasting C-peptide testing or *2*) positive for β-cell autoantibodies. The requirement to meet these criteria is a fasting serum C-peptide level ≤110% of the lower limit of normal of the laboratory's measurement method. For patients with renal insufficiency and a creatinine clearance ≤50 ml/min, this level is ≤200% of the same limit. Additionally, fasting C-peptide measurements are only valid if a simultaneously obtained fasting blood glucose measurement is ≤225 mg/dl (7). Thus, if the normal range for C-peptide in a laboratory is 0.9–4.0 ng/ml, a C-peptide level of ≤0.99 ng/ml (i.e., 0.9 × 1.10) would qualify for coverage. If the patient has renal insufficiency and a qualifying creatinine clearance, the level would be ≤1.80 ng/ml (i.e., 0.9 × 2.00).

MANAGING CSII DURING TESTS, PROCEDURES, AND HOSPITALIZATIONS

The insulin pump may be continued in the hospital if the staff is competent in insulin pump therapy or the patient and family are able to safely operate the insulin pump. The insulin pump should be discontinued during x-rays, MRIs, and other procedures that might affect a pump's reliability of insulin delivery. If a person is going to be off of the insulin pump for >1 h, compensatory insulin should be administered. For short surgical procedures, the pump can be left on, infusing at the basal rate. Each hospital should establish a policy for use of the insulin pump depending on the expertise of the staff within the facility.

SUMMARY

In general practice, nurses, unless they are diabetes pump specialists, will likely not be trained in operating CSII pumps. However, they should be able to access resources for the patient in any health care setting to assist with pump management. Nurses should recognize that most patients on CSII are very knowledgeable and that the patient's expertise should be acknowledged. When feasible, the pump therapy should be maintained. It is paramount that each institution or setting has a policy on insulin pump therapy. Interrupted CSII therapy can disrupt the glucose control of the patient and lead to rapid deterioration in metabolic status. Continuing pump therapy during hospitalization helps to maintain target glucose levels and reduce risk factors for infection and increased length of stay.

REFERENCES

1. American Diabetes Association: Continuous subcutaneous insulin infusion (Position Statement). *Diabetes Care* 27 (Suppl. 1):S110, 2004
2. Diabetes Control and Complications Trial Research Group: The effect of intensive treatment of diabetes on the development and progression of long-term complications in insulin dependent diabetes mellitus. *N Engl J Med* 329:977–985, 1993

3. Sanfield JA, Hegstad M, Hanna RS: Protocol for outpatient screening and initiation of continuous subcutaneous insulin infusion therapy: impact on cost and quality. *Diabetes Educ* 28:599–607, 2002
4. Klingensmith GJ (Ed.): *Intensive Diabetes Management.* 3rd ed. Alexandria, VA, American Diabetes Association, 2003
5. Brooks AM, Kulkarni K: Insulin pump therapy and carbohydrate counting for pump therapy: carbohydrate-to-insulin ratios. In *A Core Curriculum for Diabetes Education: Diabetes Management Therapies.* Franz MJ, McCloskey BA, Nath CR, Polonsky W, Eds. Chicago, IL, American Association of Diabetes Educators, 2001, p. 249–278
6. Kanakis SJ, Watts C, Leichter SB: The business of insulin pumps in diabetes care: clinical and economic considerations. *Clinical Diabetes* 20:214–216, 2002
7. Department of Health and Human Services, Centers for Medicare & Medicaid Services: Infusion pumps: C-peptide levels as a criterion for use [Internet], 2005. Available from www.cms.hhs.gov/medlearn/matters/mmarticles/2005/MM3705.pdf. Accessed 24 March 2005
8. Mudaliar S: Insulin therapy in type 2 diabetes. *Endocrinol Metab Clin North Am* 30:935–982, 2001
9. Lenhard MJ, Reeves GD: Continuous subcutaneous insulin infusion: a comprehensive review of insulin pump therapy. *Arch Intern Med* 161:2293–3000, 2001
10. Litton J: Insulin pump therapy in toddlers and preschool children with type 1 diabetes mellitus. *J Pediatr* 141:490–495, 2002

ADDITIONAL READING

American Diabetes Association, American Dietetic Association: *Basic Carbohydrate Counting.* Alexandria, VA, American Diabetes Association, 2003

Bode BW, Tamborlane WV, Davidson PC: Insulin pump therapy in the 21st century: strategies for successful use in adults, adolescents, and children with diabetes. *Postgrad Med* 111:69–77, 2002

Bolderman KM: *Putting Your Patients on the Pump.* Alexandria, VA, American Diabetes Association, 2002

Fredrickson L, Rubin RR, Rubin S: *Optimal Pumping: A Guide to Good Health with Diabetes.* Northridge, CA, Medtronic MiniMed, 2001

McCarren M: *Counting Carbs Made Easy for People with Diabetes (Fast Fact Series).* Alexandria, VA, American Diabetes Association, 2002

Walsh J, Roberts R: *Pumping Insulin: Everything You Need for Success With an Insulin Pump.* 3rd ed. San Diego, CA, Torrey Pines Press, 2000

Warshaw HS, Bolderman KM: *Practical Carbohydrate Counting: A How-to-Teach Guide for Health Professionals.* Alexandria, VA, American Diabetes Association, 2001

Ms. Tomky is a Certified Adult Nurse Practitioner and Diabetes Educator at Lovelace Sandia Health Systems, Albuquerque, NM.

SPECIAL POPULATIONS

25. Women and Diabetes

CAROL J. HOMKO, RN, PhD, CDE

D iabetes is a serious chronic illness that affects ~18 million people in the U.S. Although men and women are equally affected by type 1 diabetes, the prevalence of type 2 diabetes is higher in women than in men. More women die each year from diabetes and its complications than from breast cancer, making diabetes a significant "women's health issue" (1). Women with diabetes face special health challenges throughout their lives (see "Making Time for Diabetes Care in a Woman's Busy Life," a patient handout in RESOURCES). This chapter examines the available data concerning the impact of diabetes on women, beginning with the implications for childbearing and ending with its effects in later life on the risks of cardiovascular disease (CVD) and osteoporosis.

PREGNANCY IN DIABETES

Preconception Counseling and Pregnancy

Diabetes is generally classified into the following categories: type 1 diabetes, type 2 diabetes, and gestational diabetes mellitus (GDM). It is estimated that 150,000 pregnancies are complicated by diabetes each year in the U.S. GDM accounts for 135,000 of these pregnancies, type 2 diabetes for 12,000, and type 1 diabetes for 7,000 (2). Additional data from the 2002 edition of *Diabetes in America* estimate that maternal diabetes complicates 2–3% of all pregnancies (3). White's classification remains the most commonly accepted system for categorizing diabetes during pregnancy (Table 25.1). This system relates the onset of disease, disease duration, and presence of vascular complications to pregnancy outcome. Women in the highest categories and their offspring are at the greatest risk of diabetes-related adverse pregnancy outcomes (Table 25.2) (i.e., a Class A pregnancy is at least risk, whereas Class T is at highest risk).

Fuel Metabolism

Pregnancy is recognized as having a profound effect on maternal carbohydrate metabolism. These pregnancy-related alterations are necessary to meet the demands of the developing fetus. Early pregnancy is characterized by greater-than-

Table 25.1 White's Classification of Diabetes in Pregnancy

Class A	GDM
Class B	Onset at ≥20 years of age and <10 years' duration
Class C	Onset between 10 and 19 years of age or 10–19 years' duration
Class D	Onset <10 years of age or >20 years' duration
Class F	Diabetic nephropathy
Class R	Proliferative retinopathy
Class FR	Nephropathy and proliferative retinopathy
Class H	Coronary artery disease
Class T	Renal transplantation

normal insulin sensitivity, which produces a milieu that favors maternal fat accumulation in preparation for the increasing energy requirements of late gestation and lactation. Late pregnancy is characterized by accelerated growth of the fetoplacental unit, increasing plasma concentrations of several diabetogenic hormones, including human placental lactogen and estrogens, and increasing insulin resistance. Studies have demonstrated that insulin sensitivity is reduced by 33–50% by the third trimester of pregnancy (4,5). The cause or causes of this decline in insulin sensitivity are not entirely clear. However, the parallel development of insulin resistance and increases in blood levels of human placental lactogen and other diabetogenic hormones, including cortisol, progesterone, and estrogens, suggest that these hormones are responsible for much of the observed insulin resistance. In healthy pregnant women, insulin secretion must be increased by 200–300% in late gestation to overcome the resistance and maintain euglycemia. Women who are unable to increase their insulin secretion to compensate for the physiological changes of advancing gestation go on to develop impaired glucose tolerance (IGT) and GDM.

Diabetes-Related Congenital Malformations

Congenital malformations continue to complicate between 6 and 10% of all diabetic pregnancies and account for ~40% of the perinatal mortality among these infants (6). The malformations associated with diabetes can involve multiple organ systems, but the cardiovascular and nervous systems are most frequently involved. The defects most often associated with diabetes occur before the seventh week of gestation. Both animal and human studies have demonstrated that diabetes-associated

Table 25.2 Pregnancy Complications

Maternal	Fetal/Neonatal
Preterm labor	Stillbirth
Infectious morbidities	Congenital malformations
Polyhydramnios	Altered fetal growth
Pregnancy-induced hypertension	Metabolic abnormalities
Worsening of diabetic retinopathy, nephropathy	Cardiomyopathy
Hypoglycemia, ketoacidosis	Respiratory distress syndrome

malformations are related to hyperglycemia during the period of organogenesis (6–9). In addition, numerous clinical trials in humans have demonstrated that strict glycemic control before and during early pregnancy can, in most cases, reduce the rate of structural defects to the background level (10,11). Despite this evidence, ~60% of women with diabetes still only seek medical care after they learn that they are pregnant (12).

Preconception Care

Care of women with type 1 or type 2 diabetes ideally begins 3–6 months before conception to allow sufficient time to evaluate the mother's heath status and to maximize glycemic control. The prepregnancy assessment includes a careful history and thorough physical examination to assess the patient's vascular status. Baseline creatinine clearance and protein excretion levels are evaluated, and an electrocardiogram is performed. Ideally, these women are referred for an ophthalmologic consultation. Care should include counseling about the risks associated with hyperglycemia. Achieving low-risk glycemia requires a plan for reaching glycated hemoglobin A_{1c} (A1C) levels <1% above the normal range of 4–6%, and lower if possible (13). This level of blood glucose control needs to be achieved before the woman is advised to become pregnant, and women need to receive appropriate contraceptive therapy while they are preparing for pregnancy. For patients who have not met treatment goals, an extensive period of education and the initiation of self-blood glucose monitoring are also necessary (14). Women with type 2 diabetes controlled with oral antiglycemic agents that are classified as teratogenic need to begin insulin therapy.

Gestational Diabetes

GDM is a common problem, complicating ~2–5% of all pregnancies in the U.S. (15). The likelihood of developing GDM is significantly increased among certain subgroups, including individuals with a family history of type 2 diabetes, advancing maternal age, obesity, and non-white ethnicity. Excess risks for both GDM and IGT have been demonstrated in African-American, Hispanic, and Native American women, as well as women from the Indian subcontinent and the Middle East (16).

Glucose testing is recommended for women in all high-risk groups and should be done as early as feasible. However, there are certain populations of low-risk women in whom it may not be cost-effective to routinely screen for GDM. This low-risk group includes women who are not members of the previously highlighted ethnic groups and have all of the following characteristics: age <25 years,

Preconception Assessment

- Maximize glucose control
- History and physical examination for vascular status
- Electrocardiogram
- Baseline creatinine clearance
- Baseline urine total protein
- Fundoscopic examination

normal body weight, and no family history of diabetes (15). Screening should be performed between the 24th and 28th week of gestation for those of average risk and in women at high risk whose initial screening did not lead to diagnosis of GDM (see CHAPTER 1).

The presence of fasting hyperglycemia (>105 mg/dl [>5.8 mmol/l]) may be associated with an increase in the risk of intrauterine fetal death during the last 4–8 weeks of gestation. GDM is also associated with an increased incidence of maternal hypertensive disorders (17).

Management of Pregnancy Complicated by Diabetes

The main goal of management for pregnancies complicated by diabetes is to achieve and/or maintain euglycemia throughout gestation. The treatment approach requires a combination of medical nutrition therapy, exercise, insulin therapy, and daily multiple blood glucose determinations. The goals of nutrition therapy are to provide adequate maternal and fetal nutrition, to achieve appropriate gestational weight gain, and to minimize glucose excursions. For women with preexisting diabetes, guidelines suggest that the composition of the meal plan be based on an individualized nutritional assessment. In GDM, it is generally accepted that carbohydrate levels should not exceed 40–45% of total calories (18).

Evidence regarding the risk and/or benefits of either periodic or regular exercise in pregnant women with preexisting diabetes is limited. However, mild exercise in the form of walking is possible for most women and has been reported to improve lipid profiles and blood glucose control (19). In regard to GDM, exercise has been recommended as an adjunct to nutritional therapy. Regular aerobic exercise has been shown to lower fasting and postprandial glucose concentrations. Several randomized controlled trials have demonstrated that upper-extremity exercise for 20 min three times a week can significantly lower blood glucose levels in women with GDM (20,21). In addition, these trials found no significant increase in either maternal or neonatal complications.

In the U.S., insulin is currently the only therapy recommended to treat diabetes during pregnancy, although a study in women with GDM found glyburide to be a safe and clinically effective alternative to insulin (22). The goal of insulin therapy is to achieve blood glucose levels that are nearly identical to those observed in healthy pregnant women. Human insulin is the least immunogenic of all insulins and is exclusively advised for use in pregnancy. There are several approaches to insulin administration that can be used during pregnancy, and the superiority of one regimen over another has never been fully demonstrated. The rapid-acting insulin analogs with peak hypoglycemic action 1–2 h after injection offer the potential for improved postprandial glucose control. Studies support their safety during pregnancy and their ability to improve glycemic control (23,24). Continuous subcutaneous insulin infusion pumps are another treatment option that has been successfully used during pregnancy (25).

Diabetes control is monitored through blood glucose levels, ketone measurements, and A1C concentrations. Although it is widely accepted that the level of metabolic control achieved in the pregnancy complicated by diabetes significantly affects perinatal outcome, what constitutes optimal control has not been established. Emerging evidence suggests that a continuum of risk exists between carbohydrate intolerance and both perinatal and neonatal morbidity. The logical approach is to achieve as near-normal glucose levels as possible without undue severe hypoglycemia. The most recent recommended plasma blood glucose goals in pregnancy are 60–90 mg/dl before breakfast, lunch, supper, and bedtime snack; <120 mg/dl after meals (1 h); and 60–90 mg/dl overnight (2:00 A.M. to 6:00 A.M.) (26).

Antepartum and Intrapartum Management

Guidelines for the antepartum management of pregnant women with diabetes can be found in Table 25.3. Early enrollment in prenatal care is encouraged for all women with preexisting diabetes. The frequency of prenatal visits will depend on the level of glycemic control. From the maternal perspective, blood pressure should be evaluated at each visit. All pregnancies complicated by diabetes require additional fetal evaluation and assessment. Fetal ultrasonography in the first trimester or early in the second trimester allows confirmation of gestational age and helps to verify the absence of any malformations. A fetal echocardiogram in midpregnancy is used to screen for congenital heart defects. Serial ultrasounds thereafter are used to assess fetal growth, measure amniotic fluid volume, and evaluate the placenta (27).

During labor and delivery, optimal blood glucose control should be maintained to prevent neonatal hypoglycemia. Maternal blood glucose levels should be maintained at a level <100 mg/dl with the use of an insulin/glucose infusion. After delivery, maternal insulin requirements tend to dramatically fall as a result of the significant decrease in the level of placental hormones.

Postpartum Management

The primary goal of the postpartum period for women with preexisting diabetes is continued maintenance of euglycemia.

An immediate decrease in insulin requirements will be noted in women with type 1 and type 2 diabetes and GDM. Typically, the woman with GDM who required insulin during pregnancy will no longer need insulin after delivery. The

---

Table 25.3 Monitoring a Pregnancy Complicated by Diabetes

Class A	■ Daily self-monitoring of blood glucose (fasting and 1–2 h after meals)
	■ Serial ultrasound examinations in third trimester
	■ Nonstress test at 34–36 weeks, then weekly
	■ A1C every 4–6 weeks
	■ No 24-h urine, ophthalmologic evaluation, or fetal electrocardiogram necessary
	■ Daily fetal movement counts
Classes B and C	■ Daily self-monitoring of blood glucose (5–7 times/day)
	■ Level II ultrasound and fetal electrocardiogram at ~20 weeks, then follow-up every 4–6 weeks
	■ A1C every 4–6 weeks
	■ Nonstress test at 32 weeks, then weekly
	■ Ophthalmologic evaluation, follow-up according to findings
	■ 24-h urine, initially and in each trimester
	■ Daily fetal movement counts (beginning at 28 weeks' gestation)
Classes D to FR	■ Above, plus electrocardiogram initially
	■ Uric acid, liver function test, fibrinogen, fibrin split products (may repeat in each trimester)

woman with type 1 diabetes may need very little insulin for up to 48 h after the delivery. No reduction in insulin may signal an underlying infection.

In some instances, it is difficult to determine whether the woman had underlying type 2 diabetes that was diagnosed during pregnancy or whether the change in glucose metabolism experienced during pregnancy was related to GDM. If type 2 diabetes is present, hyperglycemia will persist after the delivery of the infant and the mother will continue to need medication/insulin to maintain euglycemic levels.

Women who breast-feed are more likely to need less insulin than mothers who do not breast-feed. Mothers should be encouraged to monitor blood glucose regularly. Breast-feeding mothers expend more energy and require more calories than non–breast-feeding mothers. Education on the prevention of hypoglycemia should be provided. Additional blood glucose testing and snacks may be required before, during, or after breast-feeding (28).

> **PRACTICAL POINT**
>
> Because of the high risk of developing type 2 diabetes after GDM, women should have their glycemic status retested at least 6 weeks after delivery according to the diagnostic criteria (17).

For women with GDM, the goal is to prevent subsequent diabetes. An individualized reproductive health plan will need to be developed that addresses contraception, the importance of planning future pregnancies, and lifestyle changes aimed at preventing diabetes or its long-term complications. The risk of GDM occurring in subsequent pregnancies has been reported to be 60–90%, depending on the woman's weight in the first trimester (29).

The use of contraception in all women with diabetes or a prior history of GDM cannot be emphasized strongly enough. Contraception is the only way to ensure that preconception care can be provided. A variety of family planning methods are currently available. Natural family planning is a contraceptive method that requires that women abstain from intercourse during the fertile phase of the menstrual cycle. Barrier methods of contraception create mechanical and/or chemical barriers to fertilization and include diaphragms, male and female condoms, spermicidal foam, jelly or foam, and cervical caps. Although both of these methods pose no health risks to women with diabetes, they are user dependent and therefore have a high failure rate, particularly in the first year.

Oral contraceptives remain the most popular form of birth control despite controversy over potential side effects. The main reasons for their popularity are their failure rate of generally <1% and ease of use. Low-dose formulations are preferred and are recommended only for patients without vascular complications or additional risk factors such as smoking or a strong family history of myocardial disease. Their effects on carbohydrate and lipid metabolism are minimal. Progestin only ("minipill") oral contraceptives are an option for women with contraindications to the estrogen component, such as hypertension or thrombosis (30,31).

An intrauterine device (IUD) is the most effective nonhormonal device. It should only be offered to women with diabetes who have a low risk of sexually transmitted diseases because any infection might place the patient with diabetes at risk for sepsis and ketoacidosis. Patient education should include the early signs of sexually transmitted diseases, such as increased and abnormal vaginal discharge; dyspareunia; heavy, painful menses; lower abdominal pain; and fever (30,31).

Depo-Provera is a long-acting progestin that provides highly effective pregnancy prevention. It is administered intramuscularly every 3 months and works by inhibiting ovulation. The high efficiency and long period of action of Depo-Provera makes it an attractive option for women with a history of poor medication compliance (30,31). Unfortunately, this long-acting progestin has not been studied in women with diabetes.

Permanent sterilization, including tubal ligation or vasectomy, may be considered by the patient or her partner when they desire no more children.

INFANTS OF WOMEN WITH DIABETES

The offspring of women with diabetes have an increased risk for perinatal mortality and morbidity. The two major causes of perinatal mortality are unexplained fetal death and congenital malformations (32). The causes of unexpected death are not well understood. In animal models, sustained hyperglycemia has been associated with increased insulin secretion, elevated fetal oxygen consumption, acidosis, and death. It has been postulated that fetal polycythemia and increased platelet aggregation could explain the increased incidence of intravascular thrombosis in infants of diabetic mothers and that thrombotic episodes could be the underlying cause for late unexplained intrauterine deaths (32–35).

Macrosomia is a hallmark of the pregnancy complicated by diabetes and is reported to occur in 20–25% of pregnancies complicated by diabetes. Macrosomia is defined as excessive birth weight (>90%) for gestational age or as birth weight >4,000 g. Increased adiposity is the primary cause of the increased birth weight seen in offspring of women with diabetes. Numerous studies have established a relationship between macrosomia and the level of maternal glucose control achieved during pregnancy. Other factors associated with an increased risk for fetal macrosomia include increased maternal weight, increased parity, previous delivery of a macrosomic infant, and insulin requirements >80 units/day (32,33). Perinatal mortality is associated with macrosomic infants. These infants also have an increased demand for oxygen and asphyxia can occur, which may account for the increased death rate for macrosomic infants.

Hypoglycemia occurs in infants when plasma glucose levels fall below 40–45 mg/dl (34). Infants of mothers with diabetes can develop hypoglycemia during the first few hours of life, particularly in cases of poor glycemic control. Macrosomic infants and infants with elevated cord blood C-peptide or immunoreactive insulin levels are also at increased risk. The incidence of hypoglycemia is reported to range from 25 to 40% in infants of mothers with diabetes. Both poor glycemic control during pregnancy and elevated maternal plasma glucose levels at the time of delivery increase the risk of its occurrence.

The incidence of hypocalcemia is also significantly increased in infants of women with diabetes. Hypocalcemia generally occurs in association with hyperphosphatemia and occasionally with hypomagnesemia. Neonatal hypocalcemia is defined as a calcium level <7 mg/dl. Serum calcium levels are usually lowest on the second or third day of life.

Polycythemia is defined as a venous hematocrit that exceeds 65% and is reported to occur in one-third of neonates born to women with diabetes. Polycythemia is believed to occur as a result of chronic intrauterine hypoxia, which leads to an increase in erythropoietin and consequently results in an increase in red blood cell production. Neonates born to women with diabetes also have a higher incidence of hyperbilirubinemia compared with nondiabetic control subjects (32–35).

Offspring born to women with diabetes are also at increased risk of developing various hypertrophic types of cardiomyopathies and congestive heart failure. The exact incidence is not known, but one study reported that 10% of infants born to women with diabetes might have evidence of myocardial and septal hypertrophy. Thickening of the interventricular septum as well as the left or right ventricular wall can occur and is felt to be a result of the fetal hyperinsulinemic state. In most cases, these infants are asymptomatic and the myocardial abnormalities regress by 6 months of age.

Respiratory distress syndrome (RDS) is another common complication associated with diabetes. In the past, offspring born to women with diabetes had a four- to sixfold greater incidence of RDS, but this incidence has dramatically decreased with the initiation of strict metabolic control. More recent studies, in fact, seem to indicate that stringent metabolic control may reduce the incidence of RDS in neonates of women with diabetes to near background level in the population (32–35). Last, there may be long-term consequences of diabetic pregnancies, including childhood obesity, neuropsychological deficits, and an increased tendency to develop overt diabetes.

OTHER WOMEN'S HEALTH ISSUES

Effects of the Menstrual Cycle on Glucose Control

Menstrual cycle–related alterations in blood glucose control have been reported in some women with type 1 diabetes. Most of these women describe deterioration in glycemic control around the time of menstruation, although some women have reported improvements (36). As a result, both diabetic ketoacidosis as well as mild and severe hypoglycemia have been noted to occur more frequently at this time. The exact mechanism of these changes in glucose homeostasis in women with diabetes is unknown, but it is presumed to be related to changes in levels of estrogen, progesterone, and other reproductive hormones.

Studies examining this phenomenon have yielded controversial results. Some studies have demonstrated decreased insulin sensitivity during the luteal phase compared with the follicular phase, whereas other studies have not found these differences (36–38). Data from Widom, Diamond, and Simonson (39) suggest that there is a subgroup of women with type 1 diabetes who exhibit worsening premenstrual (luteal phase) hyperglycemia and a decline in insulin sensitivity. In these studies, this deterioration in glucose utilization was associated with greater increments in estradiol levels from the follicular to the luteal phase. From a clinical perspective, women with diabetes need to be counseled regarding the possibility of altered glucose control at various points in the menstrual cycle. They will need to monitor blood glucose levels more frequently and adjust insulin dosages accordingly. In some women, increases in food cravings for high-carbohydrate food during the premenstrual phase may further accentuate the loss of glucose control. Therefore, attention to dietary changes is also important.

Polycystic Ovary Syndrome

Polycystic ovary syndrome (PCOS) is an endocrine disorder that affects 4–6% of all women and is the leading cause of infertility in the U.S. There is no firm consensus as to the definition of PCOS. However, the diagnosis is based on the findings of the presence of hyperandrogenism and ovulatory dysfunction after all other known causes of androgen excess or ovulatory dysfunction are excluded. The presence of polycystic ovaries on sonography is suggestive of PCOS but not diagnostic because these can be present in women without PCOS. The vast majority of women with PCOS will demonstrate frank elevations in circulating androgens, particularly free testosterone, and ~60% of these women are obese (40). Although not part of the diagnostic criteria, many women with PCOS are also insulin resistant and exhibit secondary hyperinsulinemia.

PCOS should be suspected in women who present with infertility, amenorrhea or irregular menses, hirsutism, acne, and obesity. Acanthosis nigricans may be present as well as dyslipidemia (41). PCOS tends to develop shortly after menarche and persists throughout most of the woman's reproductive life. The menstrual irregularities and hyperandrogenism appear to normalize as women approach perimenopause. However, the associated metabolic abnormalities, especially glucose intolerance, actually worsen with age. The inherent insulin resistance present in PCOS that is aggravated by the high prevalence of obesity places these women at increased risk of IGT. Approximately 40% of individuals with PCOS develop either type 2 diabetes or IGT (42).

The most common reason that women with PCOS present to the gynecologist is infertility, secondary to chronic anovulation. Treatment with thiazolidinediones has been shown to decrease both androgen and insulin levels. Resumption of ovulation has been reported to occur in ~60% of women (42). Other approaches to improve insulin sensitivity and restore ovulation have included weight reduction and metformin therapy. Women with PCOS are at increased risk for the development of GDM during pregnancy. Treatment of PCOS with metformin throughout pregnancy in one study was associated with a 10-fold reduction in the incidence of GDM

> **PRACTICAL POINT**
>
> Women who are anovulatory may ovulate when metformin and/or glitazone are prescribed. Premenopausal women without appropriate contraception may be at risk for pregnancy. All premenopausal women should be counseled regarding the risk for pregnancy and provided guidance regarding appropriate contraception.

(43); however, metformin in pregnancy is not currently recommended. Counseling for women with PCOS should emphasize the importance of lifestyle interventions to prevent diabetes.

DIABETES IN OLDER WOMEN

Cardiovascular Disease

CVD is the leading cause of death in women with diabetes, surpassing both breast and ovarian cancers (1). Women without diabetes are generally protected from heart disease before menopause. However, for women with diabetes, this protective effect is absent. Studies have found that individuals with diabetes are at greater risk for CVD than individuals without diabetes and that the risk for women with diabetes actually exceeds that of men with diabetes. In a population-based study of ~2,500 men and women, Lundberg et al. (44) found that the relative risk for CVD was 2.9 in men with diabetes but 5.0 in women with diabetes. In addition, the mortality rate from myocardial infarction was four times higher in men with diabetes and seven times higher in women with diabetes compared with healthy individuals. Both the Strong Heart Study (45) and Rancho Bernardo Study (46) reported similar increases in mortality.

Not only are women with diabetes at increased risk for CVD compared with their nondiabetic female counterparts, but they also appear to fare worse in terms of morbidity and mortality compared with men with diabetes (47,48). Other sex-based differences have been found in the presentation and treatment of coronary heart disease in women. Studies have found that women are more likely to have their initial manifestation as angina pectoris, are more likely to be referred for diagnostic tests at a more advanced stage of disease, and are less likely than men to have corrective invasive procedures (47). Early and ongoing assessment of cardiovascular risk factors coupled with intense intervention and education is needed for all women with diabetes.

Osteoporosis

Osteoporosis is the most prevalent metabolic bone disease in the U.S. Although more common in white women, it does affect both sexes and all ethnic groups. Whether there is an increased risk of osteoporosis in individuals with type 1 or type 2 diabetes remains controversial. Most studies in women with type 1 diabetes have reported lower bone mineral density (BMD) levels than in either nondiabetic control subjects or women with type 2 diabetes (49). Why these differences occur is not well understood. Moreover, it is not clear whether the low BMD in type 1 diabetes is the result of reduced peak bone mass or of increased bone loss. All women with diabetes should be evaluated for the risk of osteoporosis and related fractures. Consensus is lacking on when to begin BMD testing, but screening is recommended for all postmenopausal women >65 years of age or those who are considered at high risk (50). In addition, they should be counseled regarding appropriate preventive measures, which include adequate dietary calcium and vitamin D intake, regular exercise, and avoidance of smoking and other potential risk factors (see also "Are You at Risk for Osteoporosis?", a patient handout in RESOURCES).

Hormone Replacement Therapy

Conventional wisdom based on cross-sectional data is to prescribe hormone replacement therapy (HRT) for postmenopausal women with the goal of reducing CVD, preventing osteoporosis, preserving memory, promoting sexual well-being, and maintaining overall health and vitality. Data specific to HRT in women with diabetes are scarce but of potential interest because these women are at high risk of developing CVD. The Third National Health and Nutrition Examination Survey (51) found that postmenopausal women with diabetes had increased dyslipidemia compared with nondiabetic counterparts. Among women with diabetes in that trial, individuals using HRT had significantly better lipoprotein profiles and glycemic control than women with diabetes who had never used or previously used HRT. However, recent trials in women without diabetes have not supported the safety or benefits of HRT. The Heart and Estrogen/Progestin Replacement Study (HERS), published in 1998 (52), demonstrated that HRT had an early adverse effect in women with preexisting coronary disease. Most recently, the Woman's Health Initiative (53), which investigated the health risks and benefits of combined estrogen and progestin replacement therapy in healthy postmenopausal women, was concluded early because the risk of breast cancer as well as increases in the risk of coronary heart disease, stroke, and pulmonary embolism outweigh the evidence for benefits in the rates of fracture and possibly colon cancer. Unequivocally, the conclusion from the Women's Health Initiative is that HRT should not be recommended for primary prevention of CVD or fractures in women with or without diabetes. HRT may still be appropriate for short-term therapy for menopausal symptoms including vasomotor instability with hot flushes, sleep disturbance, night sweats, and mood lability.

Key Points

- Diabetes is a significant health problem that affects women throughout their life cycles.
- Strict blood glucose control before conception and throughout gestation can reduce and/or eliminate the excess risk for both mother and baby.
- All women with diabetes of childbearing age should be counseled regarding the importance of preconception glycemic control and planning their pregnancies.
- All pregnant women except for those deemed at low risk should be screened for GDM between 24 and 28 weeks' gestation.
- Women with PCOS are at increased risk for developing IGT and diabetes.
- Not only are women with diabetes at increased risk for CVD compared with their nondiabetic female counterparts, but they also appear to fare worse in terms of morbidity and mortality compared with men with diabetes.

SUMMARY

Nursing plays a key role in the education and care of women throughout the life cycle. In women with diabetes, health concerns begin at puberty and continue through preconception and pregnancy, culminating in menopause-related issues. Anticipatory guidance and education in each phase of development can help avoid health care problems and achieve desired outcomes.

Frequently, women who see specialists for health care management do not have primary care providers. As a consequence, they may not receive routine screenings such as Pap smears and mammograms. As practitioners of preventive care, nurses need to remind women of the need for these screening tests.

Future nursing research is needed in the treatment of women with diabetes.

- Identification of the modifiable barriers to preconception care and strategies to increase the proportion of women with diabetes who plan their pregnancies is needed.
- The development and testing of innovative programs and strategies to prevent CVD and reduce excessive risk for poor outcomes among women with diabetes should be explored.

- The effects of various treatment modalities on the psychosocial impact of high-risk pregnancy require investigation.
- The impact of the patient-provider relationship on compliance and self-care behaviors in women with diabetes is important to determine the success of any treatment regimen.

REFERENCES

1. Giardina EG: Call to action: cardiovascular disease in women. *J Womens Health* 7:37–43, 1998
2. Engelgau NM, Herman WH, Smith PJ, German RR Aubert: The epidemiology of diabetes and pregnancy in the U.S., 1988. *Diabetes Care* 18: 1029–1033, 1995
3. Buchanan TA: Pregnancy in preexisting diabetes. In *Diabetes in America*. 2nd ed. Harris MI, Cowie CC, Stern MP, Boyko EJ, Reiber GE, Bennett PH, Eds. Available from http://diabetes.niddk.nih.gov/dm/pubs/america/pdf/chapter36.pdf. Accessed 16 October 2004
4. Homko CJ, Sivan E, Reece EA, Boden G: Fuel metabolism during pregnancy. *Semin Reprod Endocrinol* 17:119–125, 1999
5. Catalano PM, Tyzbir ED, Roman NM, Amini SB, Sims EAH: Longitudinal changes in insulin release and insulin resistance in nonobese pregnant women. *Am J Obstet Gynecol* 165:1667–1672, 1991
6. Reece EA, Homko CJ, Wu YK: Multifactorial basis of the syndrome of diabetic embryopathy. *Teratology* 54:171–182, 1997
7. Eriksson UJ: Congenital malformations in diabetic animal models: a review. *Diabetes Res* 1:57–61, 1984
8. Rose BI, Graff S, Spencer R, Hensleigh P, Fainstat T: Major congenital anomalies in infants and glycosylated hemoglobin levels in insulin-requiring diabetic mothers. *J Perinatol* 8:309–311, 1998
9. Ylinen K, Aula P, Stenman UH, Kesaniemi-Kuokkanen T, Teramo K: Risk of minor and major fetal malformations in diabetics with high hemoglobin A1c values in early pregnancy. *Br Med J* 289:345–346, 1984
10. Fuhrmann K, Reiher H, Semmler K, Fischer F, Fischer M, Glockner E: Prevention of congenital malformations in infants of insulin-dependent diabetic mothers. *Diabetes Care* 6:219–223, 1983
11. Kitzmiller JL, Gavin LA, Gin GD, Jovanovic-Peterson L, Main EK, Zigrang WD: Preconception care of diabetes: glycemic control prevents congenital anomalies. *JAMA* 265:731–736, 1991
12. Janz NK, Herman WH, Becker MP, Charron-Prochownik D, Shayna VL, Lesnick TG, Jacober SJ, Fachnie JD, Kruger DF, Sanfield JA, Rosenblatt SI, Lorenz RP: Diabetes and pregnancy: factors associated with seeking pre-conception care. *Diabetes Care* 18:157–165, 1995
13. American Diabetes Association: Preconception care of women with diabetes (Position Statement). *Diabetes Care* 27 (Suppl. 1):S76–S78, 2004
14. Kitzmiller JL, Buchanan TA, Kjos S, Combs CA, Ratner RE: Pre-conception care of diabetes, congenital malformations, and spontaneous abortions. *Diabetes Care* 19:514–541, 1996
15. Metzger BE, Coustan DR: Summary and recommendations of the Fourth International Workshop-Conference on Gestational Diabetes. *Diabetes Care* 21 (Suppl. 2):B161–B167, 1998
16. Marshall JA, Hamman RF, Baxter J, Mayer EJ, Fulton DL, Orleans M, Rewers M, Jones RH: Ethnic differences in risk factors associated with

prevalence of non-insulin dependent diabetes mellitus: the San Luis Valley Diabetes Study. *Am J Epidemiol* 137:706–718, 1993

17. American Diabetes Association: Gestational diabetes mellitus (Position Statement). *Diabetes Care* 27 (Suppl. 1):S88–S90, 2004
18. Major CA, Henry J, deVeciana M, Morgan MA: The effects of carbohydrate restriction in patients with diet-controlled gestational diabetes. *Obstet Gynecol* 91:600–604, 1998
19. Hollingsworth DR, Moore TR: Postprandial walking exercise in pregnant insulin dependent (type I) diabetic women: reduction of plasma lipid levels but absence of a significant effect on glycemic control. *Am J Obstet Gynecol* 157:1359–1363, 1987
20. Jovanovic-Peterson L, Peterson CM: Exercise and the nutritional management of diabetes during pregnancy. *Obstet Gynecol Clin North Am* 23:75–86, 1996
21. Bung P, Artal R, Khodiguian N, Kjos S: Exercise in gestational diabetes: an optional therapeutic approach? *Diabetes* 40 (Suppl. 2):182–185, 1991
22. Langer O, Conway DL, Berkus M, Elly M, Xenakis J, Gonzales O: A comparison of glyburide and insulin in women with GDM. *N Engl J Med* 343: 1134–1138, 2000
23. Bhattacharyya A, Brown S, Hughes S, Vice PA: Insulin lispro and regular insulin in pregnancy. *QJM* 94:255–260, 2001
24. Jovanovic L, Ilic S, Pettitt DJ, Hugo K, Gutierrez M, Bowsher RR, Bastyr EJ 3rd: Metabolic and immunologic effects of insulin lispro in gestational diabetes. *Diabetes Care* 22:1422–1427, 1999
25. Jornsay DL: Pregnancy and continuous insulin infusion therapy. *Diabetes Spectrum* 11:26–32, 1998
26. American Diabetes Association: Pregnancy. In *Medical Management of Type 1 Diabetes.* 4th ed. Bode BW, Ed. Alexandria, VA, American Diabetes Association, 2004, p. 146–157
27. Jornsay D: Fetal monitoring: how's your baby doing in there? *Diabetes Self-Management* 13:40–44, 1996
28. Riordan J: Women's health and breastfeeding. In *Breastfeeding and Human Lactation.* Sudbury, MA, Jones and Bartlett, 2005, p. 459–461
29. Jovanovic L, Pettitt D: Gestational diabetes mellitus. *JAMA* 286:2516–2518, 2001
30. Kjos SL: Contraception in women with diabetes mellitus. *Diabetes Spectrum* 6:80–86, 1993
31. Kjos SL: Postpartum care of women with diabetes. *Clin Obstet Gynecol* 43:46–55, 2000
32. Weintrob N, Karp M, Hod M: Short- and long-range complications in offspring of diabetic mothers. *J Diabetes Complications* 10:294–301, 1996
33. Schwarz R, Teramo KA: Effects of diabetic pregnancy on the fetus and newborn. *Semin Perinatol* 24:120–135, 2000
34. Kalhan S, Peter-Wohl S: Hypoglycemia: what is it for the neonate? *Am J Perinatol* 17:11–18, 2000
35. Reece EA, Homko CJ: Infant of the diabetic mother. *Semin Perinatol* 18:459–469, 1994
36. Case A, Reid RL: Effects of the menstrual cycle on medical disorders. *Arch Intern Med* 158:1405–1412, 1998
37. Jarrett RJ, Graver HJ: Changes in oral glucose tolerance during the menstrual cycle. *BMJ* 2:528–529, 1968

38. Moberg E, Kollind M, Lins PE, Adamson U: Day-to-day variation of insulin sensitivity in patients with type 1 diabetes: role of gender and menstrual cycle. *Diabet Med* 12:224–228, 1995
39. Widom B, Diamond MP, Simonson DC: Alterations in glucose metabolism during menstrual cycle in women with IDDM. *Diabetes Care* 15:213–220, 1992
40. Legro RS, Azziz R: Androgen excess disorders. In *Danforth's Obstetrics and Gynecology.* 9th ed. Scott JR, Gibbs RS, Kaplan BY, Haney AF, Eds. Philadelphia, Lippincott Williams & Wilkins, 2003, p. 669–672
41. Hill KM: Update: the pathogenesis and treatment of PCOS. *Nurse Pract* 28:8–23, 2003
42. Bloomgarden ZT: Diabetes issues in women and children. *Diabetes Care* 26:2457–2463, 2003
43. Glueck CJ, Wang P, Kobayashi S, Phillips H, Sieve-Smith L: Metformin therapy throughout pregnancy reduces the development of gestational diabetes in women with polycystic ovary syndrome. *Fertil Steril* 77:520–525, 2002
44. Lundberg V, Stegmayr B, Asplund K, Eliasson M, Huhtasaari F: Diabetes as a risk factor for myocardial infarction: population and gender perspectives. *J Intern Med* 241:485–492, 1997
45. Howard BV, Cowan LD, Go O, Welty TK, Robbins DC, Lee ET: Adverse effects of diabetes on multiple cardiovascular disease risk factors in women: the Strong Heart Study. *Diabetes Care* 18:1258–1265, 1998
46. Barrett-Connor E, Ferrara A: Isolated postchallenge hyperglycemia and the risk of fatal cardiovascular disease in older women and men. *Diabetes Care* 21:1236–1239, 1998
47. Kaseta JR, Skafar DF, Ram JL, Jacober SJ, Sowers JR: Cardiovascular disease in the diabetic woman. *J Clin Endocrinol Metab* 84:1835–1838, 1999
48. Berra K: Women, coronary heart disease and dyslipidemia: does gender alter detection, evaluation or therapy? *J Cardiovasc Nurs* 14:59–78, 2000
49. Tuominen JT, Impivaara L, Puukka P, Ronnemaa T: Bone mineral density in patients with type 1 and type 2 diabetes. *Diabetes Care* 22:1196–1200, 1999
50. Chau DL, Goldstein-Fuchs J, Edleman S: Clinical decision making: osteoporosis among patients with diabetes: an overlooked disease. *Diabetes Spectrum* 16:176–182, 2003
51. Crespo CJ, Smit E, Snelling A, Sempos CT, Anderson RE: Hormone replacement therapy and its relationship to lipid and glucose metabolism in diabetic and nondiabetic postmenopausal women: results from the Third National Health and Nutrition Examination Survey (NHANES III). *Diabetes Care* 25:1675–1168, 2002
52. Hulley S, Grady D, Bush T, Furberg C, Herrington D, Riggs B, Vittinghoff E: Randomized trial of estrogen plus progestin for secondary prevention of coronary heart disease in postmenopausal women: Heart and Estrogen/Progestin Replacement Study (HERS) research group. *JAMA* 280:605–613, 1998
53. Women's Health Initiative Investigators Writers' Group: Risks and benefits of estrogen plus progestin in healthy postmenopausal women: principal results from the Women's Health Initiative randomized controlled trial. *JAMA* 288:321–333, 2002

Dr. Homko is an Assistant Research Professor at the General Clinical Research Center, Temple University School of Medicine, Philadelphia, PA.

26. Children with Diabetes

Barbara Schreiner, RN, MN, CDE, BC-ADM

Having diabetes during childhood and adolescence poses distinct challenges and requires unique solutions. Although the child with diabetes will typically have type 1 diabetes, increasing numbers of children and teens are developing type 2 diabetes.

Children with type 1 diabetes typically present with the classic symptoms of diabetes: polyuria, polydipsia, ketonuria, and weight loss. In the very young child, early symptoms of diabetes such as lethargy, irritability, and dehydration are often mistaken for flu or gastroenteritis. The child with type 2 diabetes will classically have a BMI >85th percentile and have a strong family history of diabetes, display features of insulin resistance, and/or belong to a high-risk population, i.e., Latino, African American, Native American, or Pacific Islander (1). Overweight children should be screened for type 2 diabetes with fasting plasma glucose every 2 years if they meet these criteria (2). In addition to type 1 and type 2 diabetes, there are other metabolic disturbances of glucose metabolism in children. Cystic fibrosis–related diabetes (see CHAPTER 29) and maturity-onset diabetes of the young (MODY) are two types seen in children. Cystic fibrosis–related diabetes is neither an autoimmune disease nor a disease of insulin resistance. Rather, it results from β-cell dysfunction due to pancreatic fibrosis and fatty infiltration. MODY is also a distinct type of metabolic disorder. Occurring mostly in children, it is a type of familial diabetes characterized by autosomal-dominant inheritance. MODY results in an insulin-secretion defect leading to hyperglycemia. The child has neither insulin resistance nor insulin antibodies. Children with MODY have mild hyperglycemia with no ketones and generally are lean. The term MODY has often been incorrectly used to label type 2 diabetes in children. A comparison of type 1 and type 2 diabetes is presented in Table 26.1.

INITIATING TREATMENT

When managing diabetes in children, a health care professional must consider a number of issues unique to the pediatric population.

Goals of Care

Managing diabetes for the child and family includes goals for achieving normal physical growth and psychosocial development. These goals are in addition to

Table 26.1 Comparison of Type 1 Diabetes, Type 2 Diabetes, and the Metabolic Syndrome in Children

	Type 1 Diabetes	Type 2 Diabetes	Pre-Diabetes/ Metabolic Syndrome
Mean age at onset (yr)	10	13.5	Unknown
Ethnicity	Caucasian	African American Latino Native American Pacific Islander	African American Latino Native American Pacific Islander
Fasting plasma glucose	≥126 mg/dl (≥7.0 mmol/l)	≥126 mg/dl (≥7.0 mmol/l)	>100 and <126 mg/dl (>5.6 and <7.0 mmol/l)
Random plasma glucose	≥200 mg/dl (≥11.1 mmol/l)	≥200 mg/dl (≥11.1 mmol/l)	>140 and <200 mg/dl (>7.8 and <11.1 mmol/l)
Body shape	Lean	Obese, often central	Obese, often central
Acanthosis nigricans	None	Possible	Probable
Genetics	Possible	Probable	Probable
Primary treatment	Insulin	Diet and exercise	Diet, exercise (≥150 min/week), and weight loss (7–10%)
Additional treatment	Diet and exercise	Metformin and insulin	No currently approved medications
Underlying pathophysiology	Autoimmune destruction of β-cells	Insulin resistance, β-cell exhaustion, and excess hepatic glucose production	Insulin resistance and hyper-insulinemia
Progression of disease	From honeymoon period (remission) in the first year, for some, to β-cell destruction	From β-cell hypertrophy to β-cell exhaustion	Unclear, hyper-insulinemia may present as any of the comorbid diseases
Comorbidity	Other autoimmune diseases	Other insulin-resistance diseases	Hyperlipidemia, hypertension, hyper-glycemia, obesity, polycystic ovary syndrome, and other endocrine disorders

Adapted from Cook et al. (56) and Rosenbloom and Silverstein (2).

the typical objectives for gaining glycemic control, delaying and preventing chronic complications, and minimizing acute complications.

The Honeymoon Period and Type 1 Diabetes

As many as 62% of children with type 1 diabetes experience a partial remission of their disease (3). Known as the "honeymoon period," this is a time of decreased demand for injected insulin because the child's pancreas produces some insulin. Insulin doses decrease, and the patient's diabetes may be a bit easier to manage (4). The honeymoon period may last 6 weeks to 2 years (5). Some children never seem to have a remission. Once the honeymoon period is finished, the β-cells stop producing insulin, and the child's need for injected insulin increases. Families must be prepared for the beginning and end of the honeymoon because many believe their child's diabetes has been cured.

Linear Growth

Monitoring height and weight and pubertal development are necessary components to pediatric care. Although now rare, Mauriac syndrome, a diabetes-related growth disorder, may affect children who have long-term suboptimal control (6). Features of this condition include delayed linear growth and sexual maturity, joint contractures, and hepatomegaly.

Children should be weighed and measured quarterly. Their growth should be plotted not only on age-appropriate standardized height and weight charts, but also on BMI charts, which are available from the Centers for Disease Control and Prevention at www.cdc.gov. BMI is used differently in assessing children versus adults. Body fat differs in girls and boys as they mature. BMI charts are thus based on sex and age. Percentile cutoffs are used to identify overweight children (Table 26.2).

The growing child who has diabetes requires an ongoing source of nutrients. Parents of the child with type 1 diabetes will sometimes try to limit carbohydrate intake to control blood glucose or limit insulin doses. But appropriate calories are necessary for linear growth. The more reasonable approach is to adjust (increase) insulin doses as the child grows. The growing child may require an insulin dose adjustment every 3–4 days during growth spurts.

Growth of Specific Organs

In addition to linear growth, the young child experiences rapid development of organs, such as the central nervous system (CNS) and the gastrointestinal system. The CNS requires a constant supply of glucose, with the brain requiring about 6 g glucose per hour. Because glycogen stores are limited in the young child, this

Table 26.2 Classification of Children Based on BMI

Classification	BMI for Age
Underweight	<5th percentile
At risk of overweight	85th to 95th percentile
Overweight	>95th percentile

From www.cdc.gov/nccdphp/dnpa/bmi/bmi-for-age.htm.

glucose requirement must be met by consumed calories. Having limited glycogen stores also means that young children using insulin are at increased risk of hypoglycemia. Such physiological changes have implications for the child's meal plan. Meals and snacks must be spaced throughout the day, especially for the infant, toddler, and preschooler.

Cognitive Development

The growing child is also in the process of developing cognitive skills. This process will affect the child's health beliefs and problem-solving skills. For the very young child, illness is often viewed as punishment and temporary. A young child hospitalized at onset might believe that his or her diabetes will go away once he or she returns home. Preschoolers might believe that they will lose all of their blood through a fingerstick. The infant responds to the parent's anxiety and sadness during injection time. Abstract concepts such as causes of hyperglycemia are not understood until later childhood, and the math skills required for dose changing and carbohydrate counting are not honed until young adolescence.

Psychosocial Development

Another difference for the child with diabetes involves developing psychological and social skills. As the child matures, his or her psychosocial focus changes. The infant, for example, depends on his or her parents, whereas the school-aged child begins to form relationships with peers and other adults, such as teachers and school nurses. Adolescents focus on individuation while maintaining a peer-group relationship. Diabetes will affect each developmental stage (7,8). Table 26.3 summarizes the issues pertinent to each age and stage of development.

MEDICAL NUTRITION THERAPY

Medical nutrition therapy for the infant with type 1 diabetes focuses on providing adequate calories for rapid growth. The infant will need to feed every 3–4 h. Parents eventually learn how to coordinate meals with insulin and naps. The toddler with type 1 diabetes poses particular meal-planning challenges. Typical behaviors include food jags (eating only one or a few foods rather than a variety) and negativity. A young child may prefer to eat only one food for the whole week and refuse to eat anything else. The preschooler's appetite will often increase immediately before a growth spurt. The toddler and preschooler will need morning, afternoon, and bedtime snacks to build and maintain an available source of glycogen. Toddlers and preschoolers are easily distracted by other activities and often do not complete a meal or snack. Parents may find it nearly impossible to predict what the child will eat, making it difficult to plan a safe insulin dose. Fortunately, the rapid-acting insulin analogs make it possible to give the insulin dose after a meal. Parents can then more safely decide a dose based on what is truly consumed.

For the school-aged child, medical nutrition therapy challenges include school lunches, snacks, parties, and eating out. Parents begin to have less control over their child's food choices and less knowledge about what the child is eating. School-aged children must begin to develop their own meal-planning skills, including carbohydrate counting, food choices, and portion control. Planning and schedules become increasingly important as these children participate in more

Table 26.3 Impact of Diabetes at Different Ages

Characteristics	Impact of Diabetes	Approaches
Infants		
Developing trust	Parents must perform invasive procedures; leads to parental anxiety, tension, guilt	Coaching and counseling parents: diabetes is not their fault; anticipatory guidance for parents; parents should cuddle and comfort child after each procedure; parents must interact with child outside of times for diabetes care
Interactions with caregivers around food	Mealtime may become a battleground; parents fear giving insulin and baby not eating; difficult to quantify carbohydrate intake in breast-fed infants	Loosen overall blood glucose control goals (100–200 mg/dl [5.5–11.1 mmol/l] is more safe); injections after meals
Immunizations	May have high blood glucose with or without ketones	More frequent monitoring for 24 h after immunizations
Physical development	Activity and exercise are inconsistent and unpredictable; hypoglycemia is dangerous to the developing CNS; small stomach; small liver glycogen stores (must be replenished frequently); limited tissue for subcutaneous injections	Loosen blood glucose target; frequent feedings; use legs, arms, and hips for injection sites; watch sites carefully; use short, fine (31-gauge) insulin syringes; do not reuse needles, use a fresh, sharp needle each time
Parenting issues	Symptoms of diabetes may have been ignored or misdiagnosed (diabetes is rare in infants); parents feel guilty about delay in treatment; parents are overwhelmed and lonely, with added responsibility and tasks	Counseling for parents: focus on parents' success in controlling diabetes; simplify the treatment plan as much as possible; parent support groups
Developing motor, speech, and social skills	Difficulty differentiating hypoglycemia from normal distress	Use blood glucose testing to learn infant's symptoms; feed before naps

Toddlers

Developing autonomy	Balkiness or stubborn around shots, testing, and food; regressive behaviors (speech, toilet training); temper tantrums may be symptom of hypoglycemia	Be matter-of-fact with tasks; use blood glucose tests to distinguish hypoglycemia from behavior; use usual behavior management approaches
Exploring environment	Caregivers may be overprotective of toddler; excitement may result in hypoglycemia (rather than hyperglycemia)	Counseling/coaching parents; watch for signs of low blood glucose at parties, holidays, etc.
Food jags and rituals are common	Picky eaters may result in parents becoming "short-order" cooks, doing anything to get the child to eat; parental anxiety about hypoglycemia; illness may result in poor appetite and hypoglycemia (rather than hyperglycemia)	Three meals/three snacks; use nutrient-dense foods (raisins instead of an apple); injections after the meal; creative insulin programs, minidose glucagon; do not focus on "cheating," instead say, "Did you want that extra cookie because you were hungry?"
Rapid physical growth	Frequent, routine insulin and food adjustments are needed; limited liver glycogen stores; activity and exercise are inconsistent and unpredictable	Parents should be taught to adjust insulin doses; snacks are important; record in a log book particularly active or inactive days—such notes may help in interpreting blood glucose patterns

Preschoolers

Concerned about body integrity and strength, fear of body mutilation	Invasive aspects of care become a problem; child may use procrastination to avoid injections and fingersticks	Use injection devices and lots of Band-Aids; needle/medical play; behavioral charts
Moody	May mimic hypoglycemia	Blood glucose tests to help distinguish
Imitation and symbolic play	May want to participate in aspects of self-care	Gradually add portions of the tasks, e.g., pick and wipe the injection site, turn on meter
Limited attention span; gets easily distracted	May not finish meals and snacks	Behavioral approaches to limit mealtime; use carbohydrate-dense foods
Needs to feel in control	Diabetes increases dependence	Create a log book for the child to keep, with stickers to identify blood glucose within target; encourage child in aspects of self-care; offer reasonable choices with diet

(continued)

Table 26.3 Impact of Diabetes at Different Ages (*Continued*)

Characteristics	Impact of Diabetes	Approaches
Preschoolers (continued)		
Egocentrism and absolutism	Reasoning with the child about the need for testing and shots will not work; in the child's mind, injections either hurt or don't hurt (nothing in between)	Perform skills quickly with assistance from child if possible; recognize that shots hurt; try comments such as, "It's time for your insulin—insulin will keep you healthy."
Magical thinking	May believe that diabetes goes away when you leave the hospital or clinic; views illness as the result of misdeeds or as being transferred magically	Use care with phrases such as "taking your blood glucose" or "taking a test"
Parenting issues	Parents view child as vulnerable or endangered because of diabetes; daycare/preschool/babysitting challenges	Counseling and guidance from diabetes care team; support groups; mentoring from other parents; educate parents about the rights of children in daycare and schools
School-Aged Children		
Development of motor, intellectual, and social skills	Involved in athletics, PE, sports—requires planning/ adjustment of food and/or insulin; may become sedentary after school, with TV, computers, increased snacking; lack of activity has impact on blood glucose control; has appropriate psychomotor skills to perform self-care skills, but needs supervision	Keep records of impact of activity on blood glucose patterns; child should learn injections and blood glucose testing skills; parents cannot abdicate their diabetes care roles yet; encourage family to engage in exercise
Attachment shifts from family to peers	Food choices may be difficult at parties; diabetes care may interfere with sleepovers; child may have trouble telling friends, teachers, coaches, etc., about diabetes; parents may become overprotective	Snack lists are helpful; encourage self-care skills; explore options for increasing the child's independence; science fair projects are a good way to share knowledge about diabetes
Sensitive to feeling adequate	Child may feel different, especially if care is required at school; hypoglycemia may happen in front of friends; childhood depression; may be more aware of genetic factors of diabetes	Simplify the care program; role-play managing hypoglycemia; educate about the causes of diabetes

Physical growth	Needs frequent food and insulin adjustments	Parents should know how to use blood glucose data to make dose and food adjustments
Development of concrete thought; understands cause and effect	Can recognize and treat hypoglycemia; typically receptive to diabetes education, but will be bored with didactic approaches	Diabetes education; role-play anticipated problems and solutions; use interactive approaches to diabetes education
School demands	Lunch and snack schedule may be variable (timing and amount of carbohydrate); testing at lunch may be a hassle; need for knowledgeable school personnel; PE schedule and diabetes knowledge of coach	Diabetes education; encourage problem solving; educate school personnel; educate parents about the rights of children with diabetes in schools; decrease care required at school
11- to 14-Year-Old Adolescents		
Worries about appearance, self-consciousness	Doesn't want fingersticks to show; won't wear medical ID tag; self-conscious about injection sites; worries that hypoglycemia will happen with friends or during sports	Alternatives to traditional ID tags; use self-consciousness as a motivator to rotate sites; use hypoglycemia worry to motivate blood glucose testing; understand that such concern may motivate the teen to keep blood glucose high
Hormonal changes	Blood glucose fluctuations; insulin resistance of puberty; mood changes may mimic hypoglycemia	Creative medical management; modify sick-day rules
Asserts independence from family	Experiments with diabetes management; may skip insulin; ignores diet/meal plan; choices and decisions may not always be best; may not be ready for diabetes care independence; deals with overprotective parents	"Personal scientist" approach—use personal experimentation in a safe way; see diabetes team alone at office visits; modify diabetes plan; work with parents on their changing roles; if teen was diagnosed as infant or child, complete reeducation about diabetes care is important
Rebellious, defiant	Refuses diabetes self-care; hates reminders	Counseling; communication skills; how to deal with anger
Peers are more important	Peers have priority over diabetes care; may want to hide diabetes or use it to establish role within a group	Talk about priority setting and how priorities change over time; talk about when diabetes care will take precedence
Strong sense of justice; hard to compromise	"Why me?" questioning; adolescent depression	Support groups; peer support; assess for depression and intervene

(continued)

Table 26.3 Impact of Diabetes at Different Ages (*Continued*)

Characteristics	Impact of Diabetes	Approaches
11- to 14-Year-Old Adolescents (continued)		
Oriented to the present	Little thought to long-term complications	Scare tactics have little value; focus on immediate concerns
Emerging sexuality	Wonders if more at risk for sexually transmitted diseases and AIDS because of diabetes	Education
15- to 16-Year-Old Adolescents		
Increased ability to compromise	Can make more choices about diabetes care	Include the teen more fully in management decisions; use negotiation; use behavioral contracting
Increased independence and decision making	Can begin to adjust all aspects of management: exercise, diet, insulin; understands the relationship of exercise, diet, and insulin; increased stress from social, school, and family responsibilities	Diabetes education can be more sophisticated; stress management; assertive communication training
Experiments to determine self-image	Begins to define self as an individual with diabetes, not as a "diabetic"	Support positive self-image and ways to integrate self-care into active lifestyle
Tests boundaries, takes risks; sense of invulnerability	May try drugs, alcohol, smoking, unprotected sex, etc.; skips doses; may not take risks because of diabetes (too scared to try)	Educate about teen issues; discuss logical consequences
Builds set of values, personal sense of morality	Determines how diabetes fits into life	Values clarification
Starts to make more lasting friendships	Determines who and when to tell about diabetes	Role-playing; communication skills

Accepts own sexuality	May become sexually active; worries how diabetes may affect sexual performance	Sexuality education; decision making
Wider interests; abstract thinking	Can participate in intensive management protocols	Diabetes education; interact directly with teen
Increased mobility	Obtaining driver's license: telling motor vehicle department about diabetes; driving safely with diabetes	Diabetes education: focus on driving responsibly
17- to 18-Year-Old Adolescents		
Idealistic	May be interested in political side of health care; may wish to participate in diabetes research; "If I do everything right, it won't happen to me"	Involve in support groups, camps, American Diabetes Association activities
Increased involvement with work and relationships; preparing to set off on own	Diabetes may cause career goals to change; what to tell employers; preparing for college life: dorm living/roommate, cafeteria food, erratic schedules, "all-nighters," etc.	Vocational counseling; role-play college issues; values clarification; diabetes education with focus on transitioning to adult care
Set course for financial or emotional independence	Health insurance; obtaining supplies	Diabetes education
Increased self-reliance	Finding an adult doctor; doctor visits on own	Diabetes education: standards of care

activities away from home. As the school-aged child begins to participate in activities outside of the home, parents will need to plan more carefully and consider

- whether the child eats a school lunch or packs a lunch from home
- changes in the child's overall schedule with each new school year
- the types of food that are provided to the child at school

Planning the school-aged child's day means considering the schedule for lunchtime, physical education and exercise time, after-school snacks, and after-school athletics. Timing of meals and snacks may vary considerably from weekday to weekend. Schedules become particularly important when the child's insulin program uses a split-mixed regimen (for example, two injections per day of NPH with Humalog). Snacks should be planned if meals are >4 h apart.

The adolescent with diabetes also finds meal planning demanding. Teens desperately want to be part of the crowd, and their nutrition habits may include frequent fast food meals, attempts at a vegetarian diet, or disordered eating behaviors. Regular soft drinks and sports drinks are favorites in this age-group and must be limited to maintain glycemic control. Teens typically do not get enough calcium or other important nutrients in their diet. At this age, boys are interested in building muscle and bulk, whereas girls are concerned about weight gain. The focus, therefore, for the teen with diabetes is portion sizes, consuming fewer calorie-dense foods, and increasing fruits, vegetables, and calcium in the meal plan. Eating disorders are more common in adolescents with diabetes than in other teens (9,10). Warning signs of such problems include binge eating, skipping insulin doses, family stress, frequent hypoglycemia or diabetic ketoacidosis (DKA), and concerns about being weighed.

Medical nutrition therapy for the child with type 2 diabetes focuses on calorie reduction in the context of a healthy diet. Simple ways to decrease calories are to eliminate sugar-filled drinks such as soda and sports drinks and limit fruit juice portions. The family should limit weekly or daily visits to fast food restaurants and avoid super-sizing servings. The food-guide pyramid and the plate method are helpful teaching tools (11).

EXERCISE

As the young child with diabetes becomes more active and mobile, insulin and nutrition plans must be adjusted. For the toddler, play and erratic activity patterns are the norm. While encouraging the child's physical activity, it is important to monitor blood glucose carefully to avoid hypoglycemia. School-aged children have more predictable activity patterns, including school physical education and sports. For the child with type 1 diabetes, a snack will be necessary before exercise if his or her blood glucose level is ≤100 mg/dl (≤5.6 mmol/l). For the child with type 2 diabetes, pre-exercise snacks are usually not necessary. For the athletic child using insulin, adjusting meals, snacks, and insulin doses is required to accommodate practice days versus game days.

Despite the importance of sports and after-school exercise, more children are leading inactive, sedentary lives. Computer games and television have replaced softball games and bike riding. The prevalence of childhood obesity is highest in children who watch ≥4 h of television per day (12), and obesity risk increases 6% for each additional hour of television viewing per day (13). Diabetes self-management education includes recommendations to limit such sedentary activities.

Case Study

Jerry is a 12-year-old who takes two injections a day with NPH and Humalog at breakfast and supper. He has swim practice 4 days a week immediately after school. On Fridays, he has a swim meet from 6:00 to 8:00 P.M. His afternoon snack is at 3:00 P.M., and his supper is at 6:00 P.M. On Fridays, he does not want to eat a meal before swimming. After discussing his concerns with his diabetes team, he and his parents made the following adjustments for swim meet days:

- *6:00 P.M.:* Have a snack (equivalent of bedtime amount of carbohydrate).
- *Go to swim meet:* Take blood glucose meter, insulin, and glucose gel.
- *After swim meet:* Dinner with the team, taking usual supper insulin dose before eating.
- *Before bed:* Check blood glucose. If <100 mg/dl (<5.6 mmol/l), eat a 30-g carbohydrate snack.

MEDICATIONS

There are distinct issues concerning insulin injections for the infant with diabetes. First, the infant has less surface area and thus fewer potential injection sites. Site rotation is important, with the arms, legs, and buttocks as preferred sites. There are now syringes and insulin pens that have half-unit markings, allowing for much more precise dosing for the young child. Parents need to receive instruction in the use of half-unit syringes because the unit and half-unit markings are opposite each other on the syringe barrel. Some infants require very small amount of insulin, necessitating dilution of the insulin. Most insulin manufacturers have diluting fluid specific to the brand and type of insulin; a pharmacist is a great resource for help with diluting insulin to U10 or U25. For example, to dilute U100 insulin to U10 insulin, 0.9 cc of diluting fluid would be added to 0.1 cc of U100 insulin in a sterile mixing bottle. To administer 1 unit of insulin, 10 units (0.1 cc) is drawn into the syringe, i.e., 10 units/cc insulin.

The young child's insulin requirement will vary considerably as he or she grows. At onset, most children with type 1 diabetes require between 0.5 and 0.8 units/kg/day. During the honeymoon phase, insulin requirements may drop to near zero. As the child enters puberty, insulin needs may soar to 1.0–1.5 units/kg/day. Parents need to be aware that their child may require two or three dose changes per week during growth spurts. Most children will need ~50–60% of their daily dose as basal insulin. Because of the need for flexibility in dosing, commercially premixed insulins are not recommended for the child with type 1 diabetes.

Young children may be exquisitely sensitive to fast-acting insulins. Some insulin programs use only intermediate-acting insulin given several times during the day, thus providing basal requirements only. Insulin glargine may also be used as the basal insulin. For young children, rapid-acting insulin is often given after meals. This allows the parent to determine a correct dose based on what the child actually ate.

Knowing when to transfer self-care is another issue for parents and is unique to pediatric diabetes. Most children can begin to help with injections at an early age (as young as 4 years old) (14). They can select the injection site, wipe the skin with an alcohol swab, and push in the plunger after the parent has given the injection. Many 8- to 10-year-old children have the skills to completely give an injection. Some can even accurately draw a mixed dose of insulin. How quickly a child gains these skills is highly individual. Parents can facilitate self-care by encouraging the child to participate in some small way. By the age of 10–12 years, children with diabetes are able to draw the insulin, mix doses, and inject without assistance (15). However, parental supervision is still required throughout childhood.

For the older child and adolescent, multiple daily injections and insulin pumps are becoming more common forms of insulin delivery (see CHAPTER 24 and "Is an Insulin Pump Right for Your Child and Family?", a patient handout in RESOURCES). Both systems require more involvement, skill, and knowledge from the child. Math skills become important, for instance. Even though the children may demonstrate these skills, they commonly forget meal boluses or guess at a dose. Newer pumps have reminder alarms and are able to communicate directly with blood glucose meters to calculate recommended doses for the child based on a preprogrammed algorithm.

Insulin pumps have also been successfully implemented in toddlers and preschoolers. In these children, pump therapy provides a more consistent delivery of insulin and has been associated with less hypoglycemia. Parents who are conscientious and have a strong health care team knowledgeable in pump therapy are those whose children are most successful (16).

For the child with type 2 diabetes, there are limited medication choices. Currently, only metformin is approved for children ≥10 years of age (17). Most pediatric diabetes centers are using this drug as initial therapy and adding insulin as required later.

MONITORING

Blood glucose monitoring for the young child requires some adaptation. Very fine–gauge lancets and adjustable tips on the lancing devices are important tools. The young child's body has less surface area for fingersticks. Parents should use shallow-depth settings on the lancet devices, rotate fingerstick sites, inspect the sites for soreness, and consider alternate site testing. Alternate site testing is a good option for children but has some limitations. Blood glucose from a site other than the fingertip can vary as much as 10–15% if proper technique is not used. Testing from the forearm or other site should not be used if blood glucose is rapidly changing, if the child is having hypoglycemia, or during illness (18,19).

Blood glucose monitoring is generally recommended before each meal and at bedtime for the child with type 1 diabetes. This means that the child will be checking blood glucose at school or at daycare. Parents, school or daycare personnel, and the diabetes team will need to develop a plan that addresses *1*) location of testing, *2*) frequency of testing, *3*) management of glucose level, and *4*) safe disposal of sharps (20,21).

Additional glucose checks are needed overnight at times when the child has been unusually active in the evening, did not eat a bedtime snack, required extra insulin at bedtime, has been ill, or had hypoglycemia at bedtime. Overnight testing is also helpful when evening insulin doses are being adjusted. Parents may also check a young child's blood glucose to determine the cause of behaviors such as sleepiness, crankiness, or crying. Parents want to discipline unacceptable behaviors but need to distinguish these behaviors from hypoglycemia. Postprandial blood glucose level may need to be tested to determine the adequacy of the insulin-to-carbohydrate ratio.

Goals for blood glucose levels are not standardized for children. Most diabetes teams will loosen blood glucose control in the infant or very young child. This avoids undetected hypoglycemia in the child and protects the developing CNS. On the other hand, an adolescent using an insulin pump will often have fairly tight blood glucose targets. Because blood glucose goals may be more liberal for the child with diabetes, so will the glycated hemoglobin A_{1c} (A1C) goals. An example of modifying blood glucose and A1C targets based on age is given in Table 26.4. These goals are adjusted if the child begins to have frequent or severe hypoglycemia.

There are distinct psychosocial issues related to monitoring in children. The preschooler, for example, relies on magical thinking to explain his or her world and may, for example, believe that all of his or her blood will be lost with a fingerstick. Children this age will often insist on a Band-Aid for every fingerstick and insulin injection. School-aged children may find that peers confuse blood glucose monitoring with HIV or AIDS. Teens may avoid monitoring altogether or falsify

Table 26.4 Plasma Blood Glucose and A1C Goals for Type 1 Diabetes by Age-Group

Values by age (years)	Plasma blood glucose goal range (mg/dl)		A1C	Rationale
	Before meals	Bedtime/ overnight		
Toddlers and preschoolers (0–6)	100–180	110–200	≤8.5 (but ≥7.5%)	High risk and vulnerability to hypoglycemia
School age (6–12)	90–180	100–180	<8%	Risks of hypo-glycemia and relatively low risk of complications prior to puberty
Adolescents and young adults (13–19)	90–130	90–150	<8%	▪ Risk of severe hypoglycemia ▪ Developmental and psychological issues ▪ A lower goal (<7.0%) is reasonable if it can be achieved without excessive hypoglycemia

Key concepts in setting glycemic goals:
• Goals should be individualized and lower goals may be reasonable based on benefit:risk assessment.
• Blood glucose goals should be higher than those listed above in children with frequent hypoglycemia or hypoglycemia unawareness
• Postprandial blood glucose values should be measured when there is a disparity between preprandial blood glucose values and A1C levels
From American Diabetes Association: Standards of medical care in diabetes (Position Statement). *Diabetes Care* 28 (Suppl. 1):S4–S36, 2005.

their record books. Table 26.5 lists suggestions for assessing the child whose blood glucose logs do not match his or her A1C values.

Some parents are so anxious about their child's blood glucose that they check levels seven or eight times a day. This behavior especially occurs after a child has severe hypoglycemia (22). These parents need time to build self-confidence and to feel less scared. Strategies for helping these families include ongoing reassurance, frequent contact with the diabetes team, and adjusting glucose targets to avoid further severe hypoglycemia (23,24).

MANAGING ROUTINE PROBLEMS

Hypoglycemia

The mechanisms for hypoglycemia in children with diabetes are similar to those in adults. However, in the very young child, limited glycogen stores or unrecognized hypoglycemia can lead to more severe or frequent episodes. For the toddler, excitement may lead to hypoglycemia. Illness may also be a cause of hypoglycemia in the child who is not eating well when sick. The longer a child has diabetes, the more risk for severe hypoglycemia, possibly due to defects in glucagon secretion (25).

Parents and children fear hypoglycemia, particularly overnight. They worry that the hypoglycemia will be undetected and result in seizures or death. The incidence of mild-to-moderate nocturnal hypoglycemia in children has been reported to be 14–35% (26), whereas 6.6–22% of pediatric patients will experience a hypoglycemic seizure (27). The mortality associated with hypoglycemia in children with diabetes is not well documented but may be as low as one-tenth of the mortality associated with DKA (28). Predictors of nighttime hypoglycemia include younger age and lower A1C levels. More recent studies using continuous glucose monitoring in children have found that nocturnal hypoglycemia is a common occurrence, can be prolonged, tends to happen in the early part of the night, and is associated with bedtime glucose values of <150 mg/dl (<8.3 mmol/l) (29).

There is controversy about the impact of hypoglycemia on the child's later cognitive functioning. Kaufman et al. (27) in general found no association between severe hypoglycemia and decrease in memory skills, except in children who had a

---

Table 26.5 Troubleshooting When the Blood Glucose Log and A1C Value Do Not Correlate

Meter factors	■ Meter coded improperly ■ Strips outdated ■ Battery low ■ Control solution outdated
User factors	■ Errors recording in log book ■ Not testing when blood glucose may be high ■ Technique errors in meter use ■ Avoiding negative responses from parents and health care professionals for having high blood glucose readings ■ Fabricating log book entries
Physiological factor	■ High postprandial or nocturnal blood glucose levels occur when testing is not done

PRACTICAL POINT
Hypoglycemia in the child is treated with 10–15 g carbohydrate, with the dose repeated every 15 min as needed; this is known as the rule of 15. This treatment often needs to be followed with a snack if the next meal or snack is >1 h away. Insulin regimen, however, primarily determines the need for a snack, e.g., a child using insulin glargine likely will not need follow-up calories.

history of hypoglycemic seizures. Wysocki et al. (30) also found no adverse effects on cognitive function after severe hypoglycemia.

For the adolescent who is driving, assessing and treating hypoglycemia is particularly important. Adults with type 1 diabetes have reported driving even when their blood glucose level was <40 mg/dl (31). Adolescents may make similar errors in judgment. Thus, patient education should include a discussion about responsible self-care when driving: checking blood glucose before driving, having testing supplies in the vehicle, wearing a medical identification tag, and having snacks available.

For the ill child who refuses to eat or drink and is having hypoglycemia, small doses of glucagon may be given (32). This minidose glucagon treatment is outlined in Table 26.6. Glucagon is mixed according to the package insert. The parent then uses a standard insulin syringe to withdraw an amount of glucagon appropriate for the child's age. The dose may be repeated if blood glucose does not improve.

Parents and caregivers must also know how to administer glucagon for severe hypoglycemia. The dose of glucagon for adults and children >20 kg is 1.0 mg. For children <20 kg, the glucagon dose is 0.5 mg or the equivalent of 20–30 µg/kg (33). The American Diabetes Association sells an educational video titled *Managing Diabetic Hypoglycemia* that is appropriate for parents, relatives, and caregivers (http://store.diabetes.org).

Hyperglycemia and Sick Days

Management for the child with type 1 diabetes during illness involves fluid replacement and glucose control. When ill, infants and young children are at increased risk of dehydration, so fluid replacement is crucial to preventing DKA. Illness, colds, and infections are the main causes of hyperglycemia. But, in the infant, hyperglycemia may follow routine immunizations or even teething. For the adolescent, hyperglycemia and ketosis may result from missed insulin doses (34), emotional stress, or the impact of insulin resistance due to pubertal hormones (35).

Although urine glucose testing is no longer used, urine ketone testing is still the most common tool for monitoring sick days. When blood glucose is >300 mg/dl (>16.7 mmol/l), urine ketones should be checked. Oral fluids are important at this point. The child should be encouraged to drink 0.5–1.0 cup sugar-free liquid every hour. If ketones are moderate or large, the child will also need additional fast-acting insulin. The child will need as much as 10% of the total daily dose or 0.1 units/kg of additional fast-acting insulin. This dose is repeated every 2–4 h until the blood glucose level is <300 mg/dl (16.7 mmol/l) and/or ketones fall below moderate levels. If the child is not eating, sugar-containing liquids may be needed with the frequent fast-acting insulin injections.

Table 26.6 Using Minidose Glucagon

Step 1: Assess Dose Amount

Age	Initial Minidose of Glucagon
0–3 years	3 "units" (amount drawn on syringe) of glucagon (i.e., 30 µg glucagon/year of age)
>3 years	1 "unit" (amount drawn in syringe) per year of age, i.e., 10 µg glucagon/year of age. The initial dose is not to exceed 15 "units."

Step 2: Observe

Check blood glucose and record values immediately before the injection and at 30 and 60 min postinjection.	The glucagon dose may be repeated every 30–60 min as long as the child is at risk of hypoglycemia and blood glucose is <60 mg/dl (3.3 mmol/l).

Step 3: Respond

Blood Glucose at 30 or 60 min After Initial Injection	Immediate Action	Follow-Up
Blood glucose >60 mg/dl (>3.3 mmol/l) and taking carbohydrate	Observe	Repeat dose if blood glucose decreases again
Blood glucose <60 mg/dl (<3.3 mmol/l), but has increased >15 mg/dl (>0.8 mmol/l)	Repeat initial dose	Measure blood glucose every 30–60 min and treat as needed
Blood glucose <60 mg/dl (<3.3 mmol/l), has increased <15 mg/dl (<0.8 mmol/l), and no severe symptoms	Double the previous dose	Measure blood glucose every 30–60 min and treat as needed
Blood glucose <60 mg/dl (<3.3 mmol/l) and severe symptoms, e.g., coma or seizure	Give 500–1,000 µg subcutaneously or intramuscularly	Call diabetes center for further instructions or call Emergency Medical Services for transport to local emergency room

---

PRACTICAL POINT

An easy way to collect enough urine from an infant or toddler is to place several cotton balls in the child's diaper. This will prevent the sample from being wicked into the diaper. Serum ketones provide a measurement of the more abundant β-hydroxybutyrate and may be useful in managing ketosis in the child.

Parents need to know when to call for help during a sick-day episode. DKA is a medical emergency and may be avoided with early and aggressive management (36). Signs that the child will need medical attention include prolonged vomiting or diarrhea, refusing to drink, lethargy, rapid and deep (Kussmaul) breathing, signs of moderate to severe dehydration, or persistent hyperglycemia and ketosis.

Repeated episodes of DKA, often seen during adolescence, merit further assessment. These children may be depressed and often live in chaotic or stress-filled families. Family counseling and close follow-up by the diabetes team are important interventions for these children (37).

Chronic Complications

When do chronic complications happen in the child with type 1 diabetes? Some believe that the clock begins to tick at puberty. One longitudinal study found that children diagnosed with type 1 diabetes before puberty, and especially those diagnosed before age 5 years, have a longer time free from complications such as retinopathy and albuminuria (38). Elevated A1C values during adolescence seem to accelerate the onset of complications.

For children with type 2 diabetes, however, cardiovascular risk factors and comorbidities may be present at diagnosis (39). The child with type 2 diabetes, therefore, should be assessed for hypertension and dyslipidemia.

Diabetes education for both children with type 1 diabetes and those with type 2 diabetes must include information about complications, especially detection and prevention. The nurse should provide information in a nonthreatening way and avoid scare tactics. A good approach is to focus on the positive impact of maintaining near-target blood glucose and A1C values. Having near-normal blood glucose levels may avoid future complications, but will also give the child energy to play and participate in sports. Having near-normal A1C levels will allow the child to reach maximal height potential. Maintaining euglycemia may allow parents to feel more confident and thus allow the child more independence.

SPECIAL ISSUES FOR THE CHILD WITH DIABETES

Parents and Other Caregivers

Parents of a newly diagnosed child will grapple with confusion and guilt. They will wonder if they were responsible for their child's diabetes and how they could

Threatening Versus Nonthreatening Approaches

Threatening
"Do you want to end up on dialysis or have your leg amputated? Because that's going to happen if you don't do what the doctor tells you."

Nonthreatening
"Lowering your overall blood glucose levels will help prevent the complications from diabetes. What is the hardest thing to do when taking care of your diabetes?" Give them time to answer. "Maybe together we can find a way to make that a little easier."

have prevented it (40). The parents of a child newly diagnosed with diabetes will be confused and concerned. A hundred questions will arise: How did this happen? Where did it come from? What did I do or not do? Is it my fault? What about my other children? What is going to happen? They will deal with family members who have the same questions. They will find themselves explaining to and, eventually, educating anyone who comes into contact with their child. They will fear hypoglycemia and other complications. They will fear making mistakes. They will have to learn to trust other caregivers. Their parenting skills will be tested.

The diabetes team can best help parents by providing consistent, accurate information and encouraging hope and optimism. Parents need to have their efforts and successes recognized. They need role models and support from other families. They need accurate information about the risk of diabetes for their other children (41).

Families that are most successful in raising a child with diabetes are highly cohesive and organized. The parents share open communication and provide consistent guidance and problem solving. Successful parents must be warm and nurturing (42–44).

The sibling's response to diabetes may range from feeling guilty and responsible to being fearful of also developing the disease. Some nondiabetic children hope they do get diabetes so they will get as much attention as their sibling with diabetes. Older siblings often feel extraordinarily responsible for the care of their brother or sister. They worry about hypoglycemia and monitor the child's food choices. Siblings are often forgotten in the care plans and teaching sessions. It is important to prepare families for the typical reactions of siblings to the child's diabetes.

Diabetes is also a concern for others outside of the child's immediate family. As the child grows, he or she will be in the care of many other adults: teachers, school nurses, daycare workers, babysitters, and so forth. Any care plan or teaching plan must include these other individuals. Babysitters in particular must be educated about basic diabetes care. Instructions should include how and when to prepare meals and snacks, how to detect and treat hypoglycemia, and how to check blood glucose and urine ketones. Other instructions may include who to call and when to call for help.

A valuable resource for the school nurse and other school personnel, titled "Helping the Student with Diabetes Succeed: A Guide for School Personnel," has been developed by the National Diabetes Education Program, in partnership with over 200 other organizations. This guide is available online at http://diabetes.org/for-parents-and-kids/for-schools.jsp (accessed 29 January 2005) and provides valuable information for the school nurse in guiding others in understanding diabetes and in providing a safe environment for all children with diabetes.

Diabetes Camps

One of the best places for peer support for the child with diabetes is a summer camping program or weekend retreat. Diabetes camps expose the child to other children with diabetes in a nonthreatening way. The focus of the camp will vary from an educational agenda to a purely recreational one. Children will often learn to give their first injections or may try a new injection site at camp. Both the American Camping Association and the American Diabetes Association maintain lists of recommended camps for children with diabetes.

Diabetes and Discrimination

Children with diabetes are protected from discrimination in daycare settings and schools. However, parents will have to educate each new school or babysitter about the particular needs of their child. For the school-aged child, a "504 Plan" (a plan for services under Section 504 of the Rehabilitation Act) or an Individualized Education Program (a plan for services under the Individuals with Disabilities Education Act) can delineate the medical and educational needs of the child (21,45). Templates for these plans may be found at the American Diabetes Association's Advocacy & Legal Resources web page at http://www.diabetes.org/advocacy-and-legalresources/discrimination/school/scrights.jsp.

Transferring Care to the Child

Parents must maintain a role in their child's care through adolescence. But that role changes from caregiver to coach as the child matures. Gradually, the child will need to take over his or her own care. The speed of the transfer and the skills to be transferred will vary with each child. Tips to keep in mind when transferring care to the child are included in Table 26.7.

Generally, school-aged children are ready to begin drawing and injecting insulin. Older school children and adolescents have the math skills necessary to make insulin dose decisions (15,46,47).

Adolescent Issues

For the adolescent with diabetes, there are unique and complicating factors. Puberty creates an insulin-resistant state in the adolescent, making glycemic control more challenging (48). On the other hand, chronic, suboptimal glycemic control can delay puberty. The teen's self-esteem and body image can be affected by the diagnosis of diabetes and its daily demands. The seemingly constant attention to food,

---

Table 26.7 Transferring Responsibility of Diabetes Care to the Child

- Consider each child individually.
  - Is the child ready and eager to assume self-care?
  - What is motivating the child to take on self-care tasks?
  - Does the child have the physical dexterity or cognitive ability to take on the self-care task?
- Consider the parents' assessment of the child's readiness.
- Assess the parents' willingness to "let go."
  - How comfortable is the parent in allowing mistakes?
  - How much supervision will the parent continue to provide?
- Transfer care in small, manageable steps.
- Expect lapses in self-care, at any age.
  - The parent still has an important role in supervision and guidance.

nutrition, and blood glucose may contribute to eating disorders in some teens. Omitting insulin doses to control weight is common (49). Also, normal developmental tasks, which may include experimentation with drugs, smoking, or alcohol, can be particularly risky for the adolescent with diabetes.

In addition, at a time when the young person is seeking differentiation and independence, parents may feel more overprotective and concerned (50). When parents most need to understand what is happening with the teen's diabetes management, communication may be the most strained. Parents are often not prepared for their changing role from caretaker to coach and supporter.

Adolescents with diabetes may also suffer from depression or diabetes burnout. Sometimes the signs of these problems are mistaken for typical adolescent behavior. Depression, for example, is two to three times more prevalent in youth with diabetes than in their nondiabetic peers (51). Depression in the adolescent may display as withdrawal, dramatic changes in sleeping or eating patterns, lack of goals, or suicidal ideation. Further clinical evaluation and management is needed for the teen with depression.

Diabetes burnout in the adolescent, however, may appear as feelings of failure or hopelessness, omission of insulin treatment or blood glucose monitoring, or loss of motivation (52). These teens typically have high A1C values and suboptimal self-care behavior. Management for these adolescents may include more flexible, less complex insulin programs, such as the use of commercially premixed insulin pens twice a day. Other strategies include setting realistic goals for self-care behavior, acknowledging the teen's feelings, and reinforcing the adolescent's efforts at self-care. Helping parents provide further guidance and support is also important. Teaching the teen social skills, problem-solving skills, effective communication, and stress management skills can increase the young person's self-efficacy and sense of control (53,54).

Transition to Adult Care

When the adolescent approaches adulthood, he or she will transition from pediatric to adult diabetes care. Many young adults will make this change between 17 and 20 years of age. Such transitions can be fraught with problems. The adolescent/young adult may still be living at home with some parental input or may be dealing with the stress of school, choosing a career, and evolving personal relationships. Poor transition to adult care may result in years of unsupervised medical management and limited complication prevention (55). In addition to the adolescent's concerns, parents may be anxious about moving to a more formal, less supportive environment that encourages the teen's independence. The health care professional should help the family through this transition by introducing the topic in early adolescence and by aiding in gradually transferring care and independence to the emerging young adult.

SUMMARY

The challenges posed by diabetes during childhood require the nurse to find creative solutions based on knowledge of normal growth and development. Such innovative strategies will help the growing child and adolescent emerge with the emotional and technical skills necessary for a lifetime of successful diabetes self-care. Nurses play a key role in the support of children with diabetes and their families by providing support and appropriate resources, including referral to child specialists, diabetes camps, and other local resources. Establishing healthy lifestyle behaviors as a child will carry into adulthood.

REFERENCES

1. Kaufman F: Type 2 diabetes in children and youth: a new epidemic. *J Pediatr Endocrinol Metab* 15 (Suppl. 2):737–744, 2002
2. Rosenbloom A, Silverstein J: *Type 2 Diabetes in Children and Adolescents: A Guide to Diagnosis, Epidemiology, Pathogenesis, Prevention, and Treatment.* Alexandria, VA, American Diabetes Association, 2003
3. Rewers M, Norris J, Dabelea D: Epidemiology of type 1 diabetes. In *Type 1 Diabetes: Molecular, Cellular, and Clinical Immunology.* 2nd ed. Eisenbarth G, Ed. www.uchsc.edu/misc/diabetes/eisenbook.html. Accessed 22 September 2003
4. Lombardo F, Valenzise M, Wasniewska M, Messina M, Ruggeri C, Arrigo T, DeLuca F: Two-year prospective evaluation of the factors affecting honeymoon frequency and duration in children with insulin dependent diabetes mellitus: the key-role of age at diagnosis. *Diabetes Nutr Metab* 15:246–251, 2002
5. Agner T, Damm P, Binder C: Remission in IDDM: prospective study of basal C-peptide and insulin dose in 268 consecutive patients. *Diabetes Care* 10:164–169, 1987
6. Franzese A, Iorio R, Buono M, Mascolo M, Mozzillo E: Mauriac syndrome still exists. *Diabetes Res Clin Pract* 54:219–221, 2000
7. Boland E, Grey M: Coping strategies of school-age children with diabetes mellitus. *Diabetes Educ* 22:592–597, 1996
8. Schreiner B: Disorders of pancreatic hormone secretion: diabetes mellitus. In *Wong's Nursing Care of Infants and Children.* 7th ed. Wong D, Hockenberry M, Eds. St. Louis, MO, Mosby, 2002
9. Hoffman R: Eating disorders in adolescents with type 1 diabetes: a closer look at a complicated condition. *Postgrad Med* 109:67–69, 73–74, 2001
10. Jones J: Eating disorders in adolescent females with and without type 1 diabetes: a cross sectional study. *Br Med J* 320:1563–1566, 2000
11. Brosnan C, Upchurch S, Schreiner B: Type 2 diabetes in children and adolescents: an emerging disease. *J Pediatr Health Care* 15:187–193, 2001
12. Crespo C, Smit E, Troriano R, Cartlett S, Macera C, Andersen R: Television watching, energy intake and obesity in US children: results from the Third National Health and Nutrition Examination Survey, 1984–1994. *Arch Pediatr Adolesc Med* 155:360–365, 2001
13. Dennison B, Erb T, Jenkins P: Television viewing and television in bedroom associated with overweight risk among low-income preschool children. *Pediatrics* 109:1028–1035, 2002
14. Follansbee D: Assuming responsibility for diabetes management: what age? What price? *Diabetes Educ* 15:347–353, 1989
15. Wysocki T, Meinhold P, Abrams K, Barnard M, Clark W, Bellando B, Bourgeois M: Parental and professional estimates of self-care independence of children and adolescents with IDDM. *Diabetes Care* 15:43–52, 1992
16. Litton J, Rice A, Friedman N, Oden J, Lee M, Freemark M: Insulin pump therapy in toddlers and preschool children with type 1 diabetes mellitus. *J Pediatr* 141:490–495, 2002
17. Jones K, Arslanian S, Peterokova V, Park J, Tomlinson M: Effect of metformin in pediatric patients with type 2 diabetes: a randomized controlled trial. *Diabetes Care* 25:89–94, 2002

18. Jungheim K, Koschinsky T: Glucose monitoring at the arm: risky delays of hypoglycemia and hyperglycemia detection. *Diabetes Care* 25:956–960, 2002

19. Ellison J, Stegmann J, Colner S, Michael R, Sharma M, Ervin K, Horwitz D: Rapid changes in postprandial blood glucose produce concentration differences at finger, forearm, and thigh sampling sites. *Diabetes Care* 25:961–964, 2002

20. American Diabetes Association: Diabetes care in the school and day care setting (Position Statement). *Diabetes Care* 28 (Suppl. 1):S43–S49, 2005

21. National Diabetes Education Program: *Helping the Student with Diabetes Succeed: A Guide for School Personnel.* Bethesda, MD, U.S. Department of Heath and Human Services, 2003

22. Marrero D, Guare J, Vandagriff J, Fineberg N: Fear of hypoglycemia in the parents of children and adolescents with diabetes: maladaptive or healthy response? *Diabetes Educ* 23:281–286, 1997

23. Loy V: *Real Life Parenting of Kids with Diabetes.* Alexandria, VA, American Diabetes Association, 2001

24. Sullivan-Bolyai S, Deatrick J, Gruppuso P, Tamborlane W, Grey M: Constant vigilance: mothers' work parenting young children with type 1 diabetes. *J Pediatr Nurs* 18:21–29, 2003

25. Rewers A, Chase P, Mackenzie T, Walravens P, Roback M, Rewers M, Hamman R, Klingensmith G: Predictors of acute complications in children with type 1 diabetes. *JAMA* 287:2511–2518, 2002

26. Porter P, Keating B, Byrne G, Jones T: Incidence and predictive criteria of nocturnal hypoglycemia in young children with insulin dependent diabetes mellitus. *J Pediatr* 130:366–372, 1997

27. Kaufman F, Epport K, Engilman R, Halvorson M: Neurocognitive functioning in children diagnosed with diabetes before age 10 years. *J Diabetes Complications* 13:31–38, 1999

28. Daneman D: Diabetes-related mortality: a pediatrician's view (Editorial). *Diabetes Care* 24:801–802, 2001

29. Kaufman F, Austin J, Neinstein A, Jeng L, Halvorson M, Devoe D, Pitukcheewanont P: Nocturnal hypoglycemia detected with the continuous glucose monitoring system in pediatric patients with type 1 diabetes. *J Pediatr* 141:625–630, 2002

30. Wysocki T, Harris M, Mauras N, Fox L, Taylor A, Jackson S, White N: Absence of adverse effects of severe hypoglycemia on cognitive function in school-aged children with diabetes over 18 months. *Diabetes Care* 26: 1100–1105, 2003

31. Clarke W, Cox D, Gonder-Frederick L, Kovatchev B: Hypoglycemia and the decision to drive a motor vehicle by persons with diabetes. *JAMA* 282:750–754, 1999

32. Haymond M, Schreiner B: Use of mini-dose glucagon in children with impending hypoglycemia. *Diabetes Care* 24:643–645, 2001

33. Eli Lilly: Glucagon for injection [package insert]. Indianapolis, IN, 27 April 2001

34. Bryden K: Eating habits, body weight and insulin misuse: a longitudinal study of teenagers and young adults with type 1 diabetes. *Diabetes Care* 22:1956–1960, 1999

35. Amiel S, Sherwin R, Simonson D, Lauritano A, Tamborlane W: Impaired insulin action in puberty: a contributing factor to poor glycemic control in adolescents with diabetes. *N Engl J Med* 315:215–219, 1986

36. Glaser N, Barnett P, McCaslin I, Nelson D, Trainor J, Louie J, Kaufman F, Quayle K, Roback M, Malley R, Kuppermann N, Pediatric Emergency Medicine Collaborative Research Committee of the American Academy of Pediatrics: Risk factors for cerebral edema in children with diabetic ketoacidosis. *N Engl J Med* 344:264–269, 2001

37. Betschart Roemer J, McGee T: Type 1 diabetes in youth. In *A Core Curriculum for Diabetes Education: Diabetes in the Life Cycle and Research*. Franz M, Ed. Chicago, American Association of Diabetes Educators, 2003, p. 33–62

38. Donoghue K, Fairchild J, Craig M, Chan A, Hing S, Cutler L, Howard N, Silink M: Do all prepubertal years of diabetes duration contribute equally to diabetes complications? *Diabetes Care* 26:1224–1229, 2003

39. Goran M, Beall G, Cruz M: Obesity and risk of type 2 diabetes and cardiovascular disease in children and adolescents. *J Clin Endocrinol Metab* 88:1417–1427, 2003

40. Almeida C: Grief among parents of children with diabetes. *Diabetes Educ* 21:530–532, 1995

41. Allen C, Palta M, D'Alessio DJ: Risk of diabetes in siblings and other relatives of IDDM subjects. *Diabetes* 40:831–836, 1991

42. Anderson B, Rubin R: *Practical Psychology for Diabetes Clinicians*. 2nd ed. Alexandria, VA, American Diabetes Association, 2002

43. Anderson B, Vangsness L, Connell A, Butler D, Goebel-Fabbri A, Laffel L: Family conflict, adherence, and glycaemic control in youth with short duration type 1 diabetes. *Diabet Med* 19:635–642, 2002

44. Thompson S, Auslander W, White N: Influence of family structure on health among youths with diabetes. *Health Soc Work* 26:7–14, 2001

45. Kaufman F: Diabetes at school: what a child's health care team needs to know about the federal disability law (Commentary). *Clinical Diabetes* 20:91–92, 2002

46. LaGreco A: It's "all in the family": responsibility for diabetes care. *J Pediatr Endocrinol Metab* 111 (Suppl. 2):379–385, 1998

47. Wysocki T: *The Ten Keys to Helping Your Child Grow Up with Diabetes*. 2nd ed. Alexandria, VA, American Diabetes Association, 2004

48. Hamilton J, Daneman D: Deteriorating diabetes control during adolescence: physiological or psychosocial? *J Pediatr Endocrinol Metab* 15:115–126, 2002

49. Takii M, Komaki G, Uchigata Y, Maeda M, Omori Y, Kubo C: Differences between bulimia nervosa and binge-eating disorder in females with type 1 diabetes: the important role of insulin omission. *J Psychosom Res* 47:221–231, 1999

50. Hanna K, Guthrie D: Adolescents' behavioral autonomy related to diabetes management and adolescent activities/rules. *Diabetes Educ* 29:283–291, 2003

51. Grey M, Whittemore R, Tamborlane W: Depression in type 1 diabetes in children: natural history and correlates. *J Psychosom Res* 53:907–911, 2002

52. Polonsky W: *Diabetes Burnout: What to Do When You Can't Take It Anymore* (book and audiotape). Alexandria, VA, American Diabetes Association, 1999

53. Grey M, Boland E, Davidson M, Li J, Tamborlane W: Coping skills training for youth with diabetes mellitus has long-lasting effects on metabolic control and quality of life. *J Pediatr* 137:107–113, 2000

54. Grey M, Davidson M, Boland E, Tamborlane W: Clinical and psychosocial factors associated with achievement of treatment goals in adolescents with diabetes mellitus. *J Adolesc Health* 28:377–385, 2001

55. Fleming E, Carter B, Gillibrand W: The transition of adolescents with diabetes from the children's health care service into the adult health care service: a review of the literature. *J Clin Nurs* 11:560–567, 2002
56. Cook S, Weitaman M, Auinger P, Nguyen M, Dietz W: Prevalence of a metabolic syndrome phenotype in adolescents: findings from the Third National Health and Nutrition Examination Survey, 1988–1994. *Arch Pediatr Adolesc Med* 157:821–827, 2003

Ms. Schreiner is an Adjunct Assistant Professor of Pediatrics at Baylor College of Medicine, Houston, TX.

27. Diabetes in the Elderly

Barbara McCloskey, PharmD, BC-PS, CDE

In 1889, Otto von Bismarck of Germany set the arbitrary age of 65 years as the criterion necessary to receive benefits from a Social Security system. The U.S. adopted this age for its own Social Security system in 1935, and our definition of "elderly" was born.

In 2000, there were 35 million people, or 12.4% of the U.S. population, aged ≥65 years. It is projected that by 2030, this number will increase to 70 million people, or ~20% of the U.S. population (1). Age is a risk factor for developing diabetes, and the elderly now represent an increasingly larger portion of people newly diagnosed with diabetes (2). With the rising costs of health care, lack of prescription coverage, and lower economic status of many older Americans, diabetes in the elderly will be an important health care concern in the 21st century (3). Undiagnosed and untreated diabetes is more common in the elderly than in any other age-group (4). One-half of older individuals with diabetes are unaware of their illness, which may be related to physiological changes that occur with aging, such as the increase in renal threshold for glucose (3).

CLINICAL PRACTICE GUIDELINES

The annually published American Diabetes Association Clinical Practice Recommendations set the standards of care for patients with diabetes; however, these are not specific to the elderly. In 2003, the American Geriatrics Society published "Guidelines for Improving the Care of the Older Person with Diabetes Mellitus." These guidelines provide comprehensive information regarding the elderly and diabetes care and are included in Table 27.1 (5).

SPECIAL CONSIDERATIONS IN THE ELDERLY

Successful care of older individuals with diabetes requires an understanding of the effects of the aging process in general as well as issues specific to the disease in this population.

Table 27.1 American Geriatrics Society Principles for the Care of the Elderly Adult with Diabetes

Aspirin	■ The older adult with diabetes who is not on other anticoagulant therapy and does not have any contraindications to aspirin should be offered daily aspirin therapy (81–325 mg/day).
Smoking	■ The older adult who has diabetes and smokes should be assessed for willingness to quit and should be offered counseling and pharmacological interventions to assist with smoking cessation.
Hypertension	■ If an older adult has diabetes and requires medical therapy for hypertension, the target blood pressure should be <140/80 mmHg if tolerated. Epidemiologic evidence shows that lowering blood pressure to <130/80 mmHg may provide further benefit.
	■ Because older adults may have decreased tolerance for blood pressure reduction, hypertension should be treated gradually to avoid complications.
	■ The older adult with diabetes and hypertension should be offered pharmacological and behavioral interventions to lower blood pressure within 3 months if systolic blood pressure is 140–160 mmHg or diastolic blood pressure is 90–100 mmHg or within 1 month if blood pressure is >160/100 mmHg.
Medication	■ The older adult with diabetes who is on an angiotensin-converting enzyme inhibitor or angiotensin receptor blocker should have renal function and serum potassium levels monitored within 1–2 weeks of initiation of therapy, with each dose increase, and at least annually.
	■ The older adult with diabetes on a thiazide or loop diuretic should have his or her electrolytes checked within 1–2 weeks of initiation of therapy or increase in dosage and at least annually.
Glycemic control *General recommendations*	■ For older individuals, target hemoglobin A_{1c} (A1C) level should be individualized. A reasonable goal for A1C in relatively healthy adults with good functional status is ≤7%. For frail older individuals with a life expectancy of <5 years and others for whom the risks of intensive glycemic control appear to outweigh the benefits, a less stringent target of 8% is appropriate.
Monitoring	■ The older adult who has diabetes and whose individual targets are not being met should have A1C levels measured at least every 6 months. For individuals with stable A1C levels over several years, an annual measurement may be appropriate.
	■ For the older adult with diabetes, a schedule for self-monitoring of blood glucose should be considered, depending on the individual's functional and cognitive abilities.

Table 27.1 American Geriatrics Society Principles for the Care of the Elderly Adult with Diabetes (*Continued*)

	■ The management plan for the older adult with diabetes who has severe or frequent hypoglycemic episodes should be evaluated. The patient should be offered referral to a diabetes educator or endocrinologist, and the patient and caregivers should have more frequent contacts with the health care team (e.g., physicians, certified diabetes educators, pharmacists, nurse case manager) while therapy is being adjusted.
Medications	■ If an older adult is prescribed an oral antidiabetic agent, chlorpropamide should not be used. ■ Metformin is contraindicated when serum creatinine levels are ≥1.5 mg/dl in men and ≥1.4 mg/dl in women or in anyone with decreased creatinine clearance due to increased risk of lactic acidosis. ■ The older adult with diabetes who is taking metformin should have serum creatinine measured at least annually and with any increase in dose. Individuals ≥80 years of age or those who have reduced muscle mass need a timed urine collection for measurement of creatinine clearance.
Lipids	■ For the older adult with diabetes who has dyslipidemia, efforts should be made to correct the lipid abnormalities, if feasible. ■ The older adult with diabetes and an elevated LDL cholesterol level should be managed according to the severity of elevation. – ≤100 mg/dl: Lipid status should be rechecked at least every 2 years. – 100–129 mg/dl: Medical nutrition therapy and increased physical activity are recommended, lipid status should be checked at least annually, and response to therapy should be monitored. If an LDL ≤100 mg/dl is not achieved in 6 months, then pharmacological therapy should be initiated, if feasible. – ≥130 mg/dl: Pharmacological therapy is required in addition to lifestyle modification, lipid status should be checked at least annually, and response to therapy should be monitored. ■ The older adult with diabetes who is newly prescribed or has had a dosage increase in niacin or a statin should have his or her alanine aminotransferase level measured within 12 weeks. ■ The older adult with diabetes who is taking a fibrate should have an annual evaluation of liver enzymes.
Eye care	■ The older adult with new-onset diabetes should have an initial screening dilated eye examination performed by an eye care specialist with fundoscopic training.

(continued)

Table 27.1 American Geriatrics Society Principles for the Care of the Elderly Adult with Diabetes (*Continued*)

	▪ The older adult with diabetes who is at high risk for eye disease (symptoms of eye disease present; evidence of retinopathy, glaucoma, or cataracts on an initial dilated eye examination or subsequent examinations during the prior 2 years; or A1C ≥8%, type 1 diabetes, or blood pressure ≥140/80 mmHg) should have a dilated eye examination performed by an eye care specialist with fundoscopic training at least annually. Individuals at lower risk may have a dilated eye examination at least every 2 years.
Foot care	▪ The older adult with diabetes should have a foot examination at least annually to evaluate skin integrity and check for bone deformity, sensation loss, or decreased perfusion. Examinations should be performed more frequently if there is positive evidence for any of these criteria.
Nephropathy	▪ A test for the presence of microalbumin should be performed at the time of diagnosis in patients with type 2 diabetes. After the initial screening and in the absence of previously demonstrated macro- or microalbuminuria, a test for the presence of microalbumin should be performed annually.
Diabetes education	▪ Individuals with diabetes and, if appropriate, family members and caregivers should be given written and verbal information about hypo- and hyperglycemia at diagnosis, with reassessment and reinforcement periodically as needed. Such documentation should include the following: – precipitating factors – prevention – symptoms and monitoring – treatment – when to notify a member of the health care team ▪ The monitoring technique of the older adult with diabetes who self-monitors blood glucose levels should be routinely reviewed. ▪ The older adult with diabetes should be evaluated regularly for level of physical activity and should be informed about the benefits of exercise and available resources for becoming more active. ▪ The older adult with diabetes should be evaluated regularly for diet and nutritional status, and, if appropriate, referral for culturally appropriate medical nutrition therapy should be offered. Particular attention should be focused on the intake of high-cholesterol foods, the appropriate intake of carbohydrates, and the potential benefits of weight reduction.

Table 27.1 American Geriatrics Society Principles for the Care of the Elderly Adult with Diabetes (*Continued*)

	■ The older adult with diabetes and any caregiver should receive education about the purpose of any medication, how to take it, common side effects, and important adverse reactions. All medications should be reviewed, and education should be periodically reinforced as needed.
	■ Education should be provided regarding the risk factors for foot ulcers and amputation. Physical ability to provide proper foot care should be evaluated, with periodic reassessment and reinforcement as needed.
Depression	■ The older adult with diabetes is at increased risk of major depression and should be screened for depression during the initial evaluation period (first 3 months) and when there is any unexplained decline in clinical status.
	■ Any new onset or recurrence of depression should be referred for treatment. If the patient presents a danger to him- or herself or to others, an emergency evaluation is warranted.
	■ The older adult who has received therapy for depression should be evaluated for improvement in target symptoms within 6 weeks of the initiation of therapy.
Polypharmacy (see CHAPTER 23)	■ The older adult with diabetes should be advised to maintain an updated medication list for review by the clinician.
	■ The medication list of an older adult with diabetes who presents with depression, falls, cognitive impairment, or urinary incontinence requires review.
Cognitive impairment	■ Use a standardized screening instrument at the initial visit and with any significant decline in clinical status. Increased difficulty with self-care should be considered a change in clinical status.
	■ Referrals should be made to the neurology department if there is evidence of cognitive impairment.
Urinary incontinence	■ Evaluation for symptoms of urinary incontinence should be performed during annual screening and referred to the urology department if needed.
Injurious falls	■ The older adult who has diabetes should be asked about falls.
	■ If an older adult presents with evidence of falls, the clinician should document a basic falls evaluation, including an assessment of injuries and examination of potentially reversible causes of the falls (e.g., medications, environmental factors).
Pain	■ The older adult who has diabetes should be assessed during the initial evaluation period for evidence of persistent pain.

Adapted from Brown et al. (5).

One of the concerns with achieving tight blood glucose control in the elderly is the risk of hypoglycemia. It has been suggested that the elderly are, in general, less able to detect signs of hypoglycemia and are particularly at risk for this acute complication (6). Until recently, many health care professionals believed that blood glucose levels should be higher in the elderly than in the general adult population. This has been supported by the fear that the elderly are more susceptible to oral agent–induced hypoglycemia and less sensitive to the warning signs of hypoglycemia (6). However, findings from the U.K. Prospective Diabetes Study showed that severe hypoglycemia among individuals with type 2 diabetes is a rare event (7). Tighter blood glucose control should be considered in the elderly, especially because there are now several oral diabetes medications on the market that have lower incidences of hypoglycemia. If severe or frequent hypoglycemic events do occur in an individual, the causes should be investigated and corrected. This may be an indication to change to an oral agent with a low risk of hypoglycemia.

The choice of antidiabetes medication in an elderly individual depends on several factors, including renal and liver function and the ability to purchase medications and adhere to the regimen. In general, medications should be started at the lowest dose and titrated gradually until blood glucose goals are achieved. The short-acting insulin secretagogues, such as repaglinide and nateglinide, may be a good choice for the elderly because they carry a lower risk of hypoglycemia than sulfonylureas. However, adherence may be an issue because of thrice-daily dosing. Insulin use should be considered in an elderly individual who is unable to take oral agents or has a glycated hemoglobin A_{1c} (A1C) level above target (>7%). Use of insulin requires good visual and motor skills as well as the ability to learn and perform accurate and safe administration. Specific cautions regarding antidiabetes medications in the elderly are listed in Table 27.2.

Advanced age can create special challenges in medical nutrition therapy. Food preferences may change and food consumption may decrease as age-related changes in taste and olfaction occur (4). The social and economic issues facing some elderly people may force them into poor eating habits, such as choosing to eat more canned foods, frozen foods, or fast foods. An assessment of current eating habits, as well as dentition and swallowing ability, should be conducted to establish a realistic, individualized meal plan. Older adults with diabetes in long-term care facilities are often underweight (8). Even if being overweight is a contributing factor to diabetes, weight loss should be carefully considered because a

---

Table 27.2 Antidiabetes Medication Use in the Elderly

Sulfonylureas: Increased risk of hypoglycemia and possible weight gain.
Biguanide: Contraindicated in patients with elevated serum creatinine (men >1.5 mg/dl and women >1.4 mg/dl). A baseline creatinine measurement should be obtained before starting therapy and when a possible change in renal function has occurred.
Thiazolidinediones: Use with caution in patients with congestive heart failure. Thiazolidinediones can cause fluid retention and weight gain in individuals with a history of cardiac disease, chronic obstructive pulmonary disease, or liver disease. Liver enzymes should be obtained before starting therapy and periodically thereafter.
α-Glucosidase inhibitors: Use with caution in patients with gastrointestinal disease; the adverse effects may be troublesome.
Insulins: Administration requires technical skill, visual acuity, and willingness to use.

restrictive diet in older adults may lead to nutrient deficits (8). The goal of medical nutrition therapy in the elderly with diabetes is to meet their nutritional needs and keep blood glucose, blood pressure, and blood lipids as close to normal as possible. Emphasis should be placed on the timing of meals as well as consistency in the amount eaten at each meal.

The benefits of physical activity should be discussed. An individual's exercise plan should be based on activity preferences and physical limitations, such as visual impairment and neuropathy. Cardiac status should be monitored, a treadmill test should be performed, and any symptoms suggestive of cardiac decompensation must be assessed before an exercise program is initiated and then periodically thereafter. Use of stationary bikes, walking, water aerobics, and exercise videos, such as the Armchair Fitness series, may be appropriate for recommendation.

The elderly are more prone to the effects of polypharmacy, which is the use of more medications than are clinically indicated (9). Physiological changes that occur with aging (Table 27.3) can affect how medications are handled by the body and increase susceptibility to adverse drug reactions and interactions. CHAPTER 23 discusses strategies for dealing with polypharmacy in individuals with diabetes.

SUMMARY

Nurses play a pivotal role in advocating for the elderly. Effective diabetes education gives patients the knowledge and skills needed to manage their diabetes successfully. The capacity to learn and integrate new information remains intact throughout the life cycle, although age-related changes can affect this process (4). The nurse should perform an individualized, learning-needs assessment, and educational strategies should be adjusted accordingly. A properly paced, stepwise method of teaching with the provision of practical information focused on maintaining independence and quality of life is an effective approach for older adults (4,10).

Treatment of elderly patients with diabetes is challenging due to the multiple comorbidities, social factors, and opportunities for polypharmacy that are possible,

Table 27.3 Physiological Changes that Occur with Aging

Neurological	■ Decrease in auditory acuity ■ Decreased ability to taste sweet, sour, and bitter foods (ability to taste salty foods unchanged) ■ Generalized decreased sensation, including response to pain ■ Decrease in thirst response
Ophthalmologic	■ Decrease in lens transparency and presbyopia
Body composition	■ Decreased lean body mass and increased body fat ■ Decrease in extracellular fluid volume, plasma volume, and total body water
Gastrointestinal	■ Decrease in saliva production ■ Delays in transit time ■ Achlorhydria
Hepatic	■ Decreased liver size and weight ■ Decreased phase I (oxidative) metabolism
Renal	■ Decrease in glomerular filtration rate ■ Decreased renal blood flow
Endocrine	■ Hypothyroidism occurs secondary to atrophy of the thyroid gland ■ Decreased glucose-stimulated insulin release

and their care requires a team approach (3). Multidisciplinary programs, particularly those involving family members caring for the patient, have been shown to result in improved adherence to therapy and better blood glucose control (3).

PRACTICAL POINT

Goals of Diabetes Care in the Elderly (5)

- Control of hyperglycemia and its symptoms
- Prevention, evaluation, and treatment of macro- and microvascular complications
- Self-management through education
- Maintenance or improvement of general health status

REFERENCES

1. Administration on Aging web site. Available from www.aoa.gov/prof/Statistics/ statistics.asp. Accessed 24 March 2005
2. Chau D, Edelman SV: Clinical management of diabetes in the elderly. *Clinical Diabetes* 19:172–175, 2001
3. Meneilly GS, Tessier D: Diabetes in elderly adults. *J Gerontol* 56:M5–M13, 2001
4. American Association of Diabetes Educators: Special considerations for the education and management of older adults with diabetes (Position Statement). *Diabetes Educ* 29:93–96, 2003
5. Brown AF, Mangione CM, Saliba D, Sarkisian CA: Guidelines for improving the care of the older person with diabetes mellitus. *J Am Geriatr Soc* 51 (Suppl. 5):S265–S280, 2003
6. Benjamin EM: Case study: glycemic control in the elderly: risk and benefits. *Clinical Diabetes* 20:118–122, 2002
7. U.K. Prospective Diabetes Study Group: Intensive blood glucose control with sulphonylureas or insulin compared with conventional treatment and risk of complications in patients with type 2 diabetes (UKPDS 33). *Lancet* 352:837–853, 1998
8. Yen PK: Treating diabetes with diet. *Geriatr Nurs* 23:175–176, 2002
9. Good CB: Polypharmacy in elderly patients with diabetes. *Diabetes Spectrum* 15:240–248, 2002
10. American Association of Diabetes Educators: Individualization of diabetes self-management education [Internet], 2002. Available from http://diabetes-educator.org/PublicAffairs/PositionStatements/IndivofDESelf-Manag.pdf. Accessed 16 October 2004

Dr. McCloskey is the Diabetes Education Coordinator at Baylor Health Care Diabetes Services, Irving, TX.

DISEASES AND TREATMENTS THAT AFFECT DIABETES

28. Glucocorticoid Use in Diabetes

MARJORIE CYPRESS, MSN, RN, C-ANP, CDE

The use of glucocorticoids can cause significant hyperglycemia and uncontrolled diabetes in individuals with known diabetes and can cause steroid-induced diabetes in individuals with risk factors for developing type 2 diabetes. Because glucocorticoids are used for treating numerous chronic illnesses and conditions, it is not uncommon to encounter patients with severe hyperglycemia due to their use. The mechanism by which glucocorticoids, which may be given intravenously, by injection, or orally, increase glucose levels is through insulin resistance and increased gluconeogenesis and glycogenolysis.

Treatment of resultant hyperglycemia depends on the type of glucocorticoid used; the route, amount, dosage schedule, and duration of therapy; and an individual's prior diagnosis and use of diabetes medications. Table 28.1 shows the various glucocorticoid preparations and their durations of action. The goal of treating steroid-induced hyperglycemia is to prevent diabetic ketoacidosis or hyperglycemic hyperosmolar nonketotic syndrome and, in doing so, to avoid hypoglycemia.

In patients with known diabetes, insulin is almost always indicated for treating severe hyperglycemia from glucocorticoid therapy. Although there are some reports of using oral agents effectively (1), generally this will be ineffective in controlling hyperglycemia (2). Several practitioners have advocated relaxing glycemic goals during short-term steroid therapy, due to the difficulty in managing glucose levels in both hospitalized and outpatient treatment so that fasting glucose levels are 120–140 mg/dl and 2-h postprandial levels are <200 mg/dl (3). In hospitalized patients already under significant stress from illness, intravenous glucocorticoids can raise glucose levels dangerously high, to >400–500 mg/dl. In the case of a 24-h intravenous glucocorticoid, insulin treatment should consist of a basal or intermediate-acting insulin as well as regular or rapid-acting insulin before meals or every 4–6 h, if NPO. Treating hyperglycemia with only short- or rapid-acting insulin will not maintain stable glucose levels because basal insulin is needed. As the steroid dose is reduced, it is essential to closely monitor blood glucose levels so that insulin doses can also be decreased to avoid the risk of hypoglycemia as the insulin requirements decrease.

Table 28.1 Glucocorticoid Preparations and Durations of Action

Drug	Duration (h)
Cortisone acetate	6–10
Hydrocortisone	6–10
Prednisone	16–20
Methylprednisone	16–20
Dexamethasone	24–30

PRACTICAL POINT

When glucocorticoid doses are changed, insulin requirements change at the same time. Insulin dose will need to be increased or decreased as the glucocorticoid dose is increased or decreased. Patients must be instructed in frequent blood glucose monitoring to prevent episodes of severe hyperglycemia or hypoglycemia.

For patients who receive an injection of glucocorticoids, short- or rapid-acting insulin is a good choice for managing the resultant short-term severe hyperglycemia. In patients without a prior history of diabetes, an oral agent such as glyburide may be effective in keeping blood glucose levels close to normal. It will probably become necessary to withdraw the oral agent as the blood glucose levels decrease. In this case, patients will need to be taught how to self-monitor blood glucose to be alert to changes in blood glucose levels.

Some patients are given steroid injections into joints. In individuals with diabetes, this results in hyperglycemia that may require a short-term increase in oral antihyperglycemic medications or insulin. It is important that patients be advised that these steroid injections into joints can cause increased blood glucose levels and that more frequent blood glucose monitoring is warranted. In individuals with a high risk for diabetes, a steroid injection into the joint can cause impaired glucose tolerance and progress to overt diabetes. These individuals should be counseled and monitored for symptoms of polyuria, polydipsia, polyphagia, and hyperglycemia.

Many patients are discharged from the hospital during an oral glucocorticoid therapy or are treated as outpatients with a steroid taper. Others may be on an alternate-day steroid treatment regimen. This makes glucose control more difficult. Frequent self-monitoring of blood glucose is essential because glucose levels can fluctuate widely during treatment. For patients on a short-term glucocorticoid (1–2 weeks), daily contact with the health care practitioner may be necessary to help titrate the insulin doses.

In patients whose diabetes is usually managed with insulin, it is not uncommon for their requirements to be increased by two to three times or more. However, with tapering doses of glucocorticoids, insulin requirements begin to return to normal, and hypoglycemia becomes a major risk. For patients who were previously treated with oral agents or are diet controlled and who are new to insulin during the course of glucocorticoid therapy, short- or rapid-acting insulin before meals may be a safe and appropriate therapy. Insulin algorithms can be prescribed based on blood glucose monitoring, and patients can be taught to regulate their own insulin doses based on home blood glucose readings. If long-term steroid therapy is indicated (≥4 weeks), basal or intermediate-acting insulin is often necessary to manage blood glucose levels. The most important issue for patients on insulin and a glucocorticoid is educating them about the necessity of frequent blood glucose monitoring and the risks of hyperglycemia and hypoglycemia.

Special caution must be exercised in designing insulin regimens during glucocorticoid therapy. The most common oral glucocorticoid used in the outpatient setting is prednisone, which has a duration of action of 16–20 h. If given once daily in the morning, blood glucose levels will tend to be normal or even somewhat low in the morning (fasting), but increase during the day so that predinner and bedtime glucose levels can be very high. Using morning NPH insulin may help lower late-afternoon hyperglycemia, but use of an evening NPH dose can cause hypoglycemia as the effects of prednisone wear off, insulin resistance decreases, and insulin requirements are drastically reduced. In this case, NPH and short- or rapid-acting insulin can be used in the morning, and short- or rapid-acting insulin before lunch and before dinner may be a safe and effective insulin regimen that will avoid early-morning hypoglycemia. Caution must be taken when prescribing any bedtime insulin, and using smaller doses to try to bring the glucose level into a more normal range will help in avoiding middle-of-the-night or early-morning hypoglycemia.

SUMMARY

Individualizing insulin regimens or the use of oral agents for people on glucocorticoid therapy is essential. Appetite, mealtimes, and timing of glucocorticoid treatment are all important to consider when developing a treatment regimen. Ideally, glucose control should be achieved before the initiation of glucocorticoid therapy, but this is rarely the case unless the treatment can be preplanned.

It is the role of the nurse to

- advise all individuals with diabetes that glucocorticoid therapy will result in hyperglycemia
- advise them that insulin may be needed even for short-term therapy
- caution patients that insulin requirements will increase or decrease based on the dosage of the glucocorticoid
- advise individuals with no prior history of diabetes on the possible increase in blood glucose levels related to glucocorticoid treatment and educate them regarding the signs and symptoms of hyperglycemia
- provide the telephone numbers of the health care professionals for the patient to contact in case of hyperglycemia or symptoms of hyperglycemia

REFERENCES

1. Willi SM, Kennedy A, Brant BP, Wallace P, Rogers NL, Garvey WT: Effective use of thiazolidinediones for the treatment of glucocorticoid-induced diabetes. *Diabetes Res Clin Pract* 58:87–96, 2002
2. Volgi JR, Baldwin D: Glucocorticoid therapy and diabetes management. *Nurs Clin North Am* 36:333–339, 2001
3. Braithwaite SS, Barr WG, Rahman A, Quddusi S: Managing diabetes during glucocorticoid therapy: how to avoid metabolic emergencies. *Postgrad Med* 104:163–166, 171, 175–176, 1998

Ms. Cypress is an Adult Nurse Practitioner and Certified Diabetes Educator in Albuquerque, NM.

29. Cystic Fibrosis–Related Diabetes

Geralyn Spollett, MSN, C-ANP, CDE

Cystic fibrosis (CF), one of the most common lethal genetic diseases in Caucasians, affects >30,000 Americans, with 1,000 children diagnosed each year (1). There is no cure for the disease, but with advances in research and treatment, people with CF are living longer. With the increase in survival, the number of patients with CF-related diabetes (CFRD) has also risen, becoming a leading comorbidity in this group. Approximately 40% of all adult CF patients develop diabetes (2). However, because many CF centers do not routinely screen for diabetes, the actual number of individuals with CF who are also affected by diabetes may be higher (3).

CFRD differs from both type 1 and type 2 diabetes in that it is characterized by insulinopenia, but ketoacidosis is extremely rare (3). Like type 2 diabetes, the onset is often insidious and can exist for 2–4 years before diagnosis. In CF, abnormal glucose tolerance is associated with progressive clinical deterioration (4). Research has shown that the rate of pulmonary decline is directly proportional to the magnitude of abnormal glucose tolerance and the degree of insulin deficiency (4). The diagnosis of diabetes in individuals with CF lowers survival rates. Only 25% of people with CFRD survive to 30 years of age, compared with a 60% survival rate in individuals with CF and no diabetes (5).

CF affects the tissues that produce mucus secretions and alters the properties of that mucus so that it is no longer a protective substance but rather an obstructive, damaging one. Excessive, thick, sticky mucus blocks airways, the gastrointestinal tract, the ducts of the pancreas, the bile ducts of the liver, and the male urogenital tract.

Chemical changes in the mucus proteins increase the viscosity and provide an environment ideal for bacterial growth. White blood cells are released to combat the infection but only result in complicating the problem. Genetic materials from dying white blood cells increase the stickiness of the mucus and initiate a cycle of further obstruction, infection, and inflammation.

The thick, sticky secretions can also clog the pancreatic ducts, damaging the pancreas in a variety of ways. A reduction in the amounts of pancreatic enzymes and bicarbonate alter the digestive and absorptive process. This insufficiency results in malnutrition and slowed growth and development. Stools become bulky and foul smelling. Eventually, blockage of the pancreatic ducts damages the β-cells, resulting in hyperglycemia. Fibrosis and fatty infiltrates disrupt the architecture of the islet cell and can result in islet destruction. Glucagon and pancreatic polypeptide secretion are reduced. Proinsulin levels are elevated, and first-phase insulin and C-peptide secretion in response to glucose are impaired. This results in delayed and diminished insulin secretion in response to oral stimuli (2). The pathophysiological changes associated with CF affect glucose metabolism. Malabsorption and abnormal intestinal transit time, liver dysfunction, and increased caloric need to avoid malnutrition disrupt glucose control. Chronic and acute infections and the use of steroids increase insulin resistance and cause further deterioration in glucose stability.

DIAGNOSIS AND CLASSIFICATION OF CFRD

The 1998 Cystic Fibrosis–Related Diabetes (CFRD) Consensus Conference created classification and diagnosis criteria for CF patients with glucose abnormalities based on the oral glucose tolerance test (6). Four diagnostic categories were formed: normal glucose tolerance, impaired glucose tolerance, CFRD without fasting hyperglycemia, and CRFD with fasting hyperglycemia (Table 29.1). The separation of individuals with CFRD who were with or without fasting hyperglycemia is unique to CF and was largely done to track epidemiological data for future treatment decisions (2).

The CFRD Consensus Conference committee recommended that a fasting plasma glucose (FPG) level be obtained annually in all patients ≥14 years of age. Diabetes screening should be done whenever symptoms suggestive of hyperglycemia are present: polydipsia, polyuria, weight loss, alterations in growth patterns or puberty progression, unexplained pulmonary function decline, or increased infections. During steroid therapy or at the onset of pregnancy or pulmonary exacerbations, cautious monitoring for diabetes symptoms should be increased. Glycated hemoglobin A_{1c} (A1C) testing is not used for diagnosis because it can be falsely low in this population. An elevated level may indicate the presence of hyperglycemia, but a normal A1C value does not exclude the diagnosis of diabetes. The rapid turnover rate of red blood cells in CF patients makes diagnosis through the A1C test unreliable.

Table 29.1 Glucose Tolerance Categories in CF in Response to OGTT

Category	FPG (mg/dl)	2-h PG (mg/dl)
NGT	<126	<140
IGT	<126	140–199
CFRD without FH	<126	≥200
CFRD with FH	≥126	OGTT unnecessary

FH, fasting hyperglycemia; IGT, impaired glucose tolerance; NGT, normal glucose tolerance; OGTT, oral glucose tolerance test; PG, plasma glucose.

Adapted from Brunzell and Schwarzenberg (9).

PRACTICAL POINT

Screening for CFRD

If the patient's FPG level is ≥126 mg/dl (7 mmol/l), then it must be repeated or a casual glucose level should be drawn on the following day to confirm the diagnosis. If on the next day the follow-up FPG measurement is ≥126 mg/dl (7 mmol/l) or the casual glucose level ≥200 mg/dl (11.1 mmol/l), then the diagnosis of diabetes is confirmed. An FPG level <126 mg/dl (7 mmol/l) indicates that a standard oral glucose tolerance test should be performed.

TREATMENT

In general, insulin is the treatment of choice for CFRD with fasting hyperglycemia. Depending on the level of β-cell impairment, bolus meal coverage with rapid-acting insulin may be all that is required (7). Carbohydrate counting and the use of an insulin-to-carbohydrate ratio system provide the flexible coverage needed in CFRD. Weight maintenance is critical for these patients; therefore, caloric and carbohydrate restrictions seen in the treatment of diabetes are not part of the care regimen. An outline of medical nutrition therapy recommendations for CFRD compared with type 1/type 2 diabetes illustrates the differences in approach (Table 29.2). Achieving a balance of adequate nutrition for the increased

---

Table 29.2 Medical Nutrition Therapy for Type 1/Type 2 Diabetes Versus for CFRD

	Type 1/Type 2 Diabetes	CFRD
Calories	Calculated for maintenance, growth, or reduction diets	120–150% RDA
Carbohydrate	Individualized	Individualized
Fat	Individualized; often <30% of total calories, <10% saturated fat, ≤10% of calories from polyunsaturated fat	40% of calories; no restriction on type of fat
Protein	10–20% of total calories; reduction to 0.8 g/kg with nephropathy	10–20% total calories; no reduction with nephropathy*
Sodium	<2,400 mg/day	>4,000 mg/day
Vitamins/minerals	No supplementation unless deficiency noted	Routine supplementation of vitamins A, D, E, K, and multivitamin

Adapted from Brunzell and Schwarzenberg (9).

*This is the recommendation of the consensus conference. In practice, a patient with severe nephropathy would require protein restriction to prevent azotemia. RDA, recommended dietary allowance.

metabolic needs of the person with CF and supporting the use of these calories through a matched insulin regimen is necessary for the health and survival of these patients. In some cases, basal insulin such as an evening dose of an intermediate-acting insulin or a long-acting insulin such as glargine may be needed to achieve euglycemic levels.

The use of most oral agents is not recommended in the treatment of CFRD. Metformin and the thiazolidinediones rely on clearance mechanisms that are compromised in CF. The increased potential for liver toxicity with thiazolidinediones in CF restricts their use. α-Glucosidase inhibitors affect intestinal absorption patterns in an already altered gastrointestinal tract. The side effects of the α-glucosidase inhibitors, such as nausea, flatulence, and diarrhea, may negatively affect the nutritional status of these patients. Sulfonylureas have been used but are also problematic. Higher rates of hypoglycemia have been observed before therapeutic glycemic ranges were achieved. Glyburide, 50% of which is eliminated in the bile, is not recommended because of the difficulty in drug excretion through bile ducts clogged due to CF (8).

In patients with CFRD without fasting hyperglycemia, repaglinide has been studied with some positive effect. In comparison with insulin lispro, repaglinide did not normalize glucose excursions postprandially as well as the insulin. The investigators reported that suboptimal doses may have altered the results and that further studies are needed (7).

In CFRD, patients using insulin should be seen by a diabetes team on a quarterly basis. Blood glucose targets are the same as for all other forms of diabetes and follow the recommendations set forth by the American Diabetes Association (9). A1C testing and self-monitoring of blood glucose are prescribed based on management strategies and are also used in adjusting therapy. Because microvascular complications have been reported in CFRD, annual retinopathy and microalbumin screenings are initiated at diagnosis (8).

In most patients with CFRD without fasting hyperglycemia, glucose levels are maintained through a regulation of meal timing to spread carbohydrate and calories throughout the day, thus reducing glucose excursions. Insulin therapy becomes necessary if nutritional status changes and weight is no longer maintained or if there is a decline in pulmonary function (10). Reducing consumption of regular sodas or other sweetened beverages may also help control glucose excursions. It is important to remember that food substitutions for any alteration in caloric level must be made to avoid weight loss. Helping the patient choose more nutritious replacements for the sweetened beverages is essential for the treatment of both diabetes and CF. Protein intake should be ~15–20% of the daily diet. Fat and sodium restrictions usually prescribed for individuals with diabetes are not appropriate in CFRD. These patients are frequently depleted of sodium and may require supplementation. Despite the use of pancreatic enzymes, fat malabsorption is a common component of the clinical picture. Caloric needs take precedence, with the current fat recommendation being 40% of total calories per day.

For individuals with CF and impaired glucose tolerance, increased exercise and weight loss to address glucose intolerance is not recommended. Medical nutrition therapy focuses on healthy eating and meal/snack timing. Exercise, although helpful for CF patients, should not be used as a weight loss mechanism. Individuals who choose to exercise need to replace spent calories. Appropriate glucose monitoring and the use of a portable carbohydrate snack to prevent hypoglycemia are important parts of this regimen. Yearly screening with an oral glucose tolerance test and self-monitoring of blood glucose performed during periods of infection and stress are necessary to therapeutically respond to glucose alterations.

Preconception and pregnancy care in CFRD follow the standard guidelines for glucose control. Weight maintenance takes on more significance in light of the nutritional needs of pregnancy and the caloric needs of CF. Referral to a dietitian is imperative for counseling and education to achieve positive outcomes. As with all diabetes-affected pregnancies, insulin requirements will change and the patient will need to remain in close contact with her health care providers. However, alterations in pulmonary function and its effect on both glucose control and fetal health make good communication among all members of the health care team vital.

SUMMARY

Adequate nutrition and glucose control are important components of therapy in all individuals with diabetes. However, in people with CFRD, the consequences of not meeting these basic requirements of diabetes care are life threatening. Coordination of care between the diabetes and CF health care teams is imperative for positive outcomes. Patient education and support in managing two serious chronic diseases will help the patient maintain function and increase longevity. Without proper glycemic control, the patient's nutritional status declines and weight loss occurs. Assisting the patient in analyzing glucose levels and injecting the appropriate amount of premeal insulin requires an understanding of food and insulin action. Diabetes education plays a vital role in the health maintenance of people with CFRD. In addition to the literature available from the American Diabetes Association, the Cystic Fibrosis Foundation has educational literature and an informative web site (www.cff.org) to assist both patients and health care providers in remaining current on CF treatment protocols and lifestyle interventions.

REFERENCES

1. National Institute of Diabetes and Digestive and Kidney Diseases: Cystic fibrosis research directions [Internet], 1998. Available from http://www.niddk.nih.gov/health/endo/pubs/cystic/cystic.htm. Accessed Dec 30, 2003 (NIH publ. no. 97-4200)
2. Moran A: Diagnosis, screening, and management of cystic fibrosis-related diabetes. *Curr Diabetes Rep* 2:111–115, 2002
3. Allen H, Gay AC, Klingensmith GJ, Hamman RF: Identification and treatment of cystic fibrosis–related diabetes. *Diabetes Care* 21:943–948, 1998
4. Milla CE, Warwick WJ, Moran A: Trends in pulmonary function in cystic fibrosis patients correlate with the degree of glucose intolerance at baseline. *Am J Respir Crit Care Med* 162:891–895, 2000
5. Finkelstein SM, Wielinski CL, Elliott GR, Warwick WJ, Barbosa J, Wu SC, Klein DJ: Diabetes mellitus associated with cystic fibrosis. *J Pediatr* 112:373–377, 1988
6. Moran A, Hardin D, Rodman D, Allen HF, Beall RJ, Borowitz D, Brunzell C, Campbell PW 3rd, Chesrown SE, Duchow C, Fink RJ, Fitzsimmons SC, Hamilton N, Hirsch I, Howenstine MS, Klein DJ, Madhun Z, Pencharz PB,

Quittner AL, Robbins MK, Schindler T, Schissel K, Schwarzenberg SJ, Stallings VA, Zipf WB: Diagnosis, screening and management of cystic fibrosis related diabetes mellitus: a consensus conference report. *Diabetes Res Clin Pract* 45:61–73, 1999

7. Moran A, Phillips J, Milla C: Insulin and glucose excursion following premeal insulin lispro or repaglinide in cystic fibrosis–related diabetes. *Diabetes Care* 24:1706–1710, 2001

8. Hardin DS, Moran A: Diabetes mellitus in cystic fibrosis. *Endocrinol Metab Clin North Am* 28:787–799, 1999

9. American Diabetes Association: Diagnosis and classification of diabetes mellitus (Position Statement). *Diabetes Care* 28 (Suppl. 1):S37–S42, 2005

10. Brunzell C, Schwarzenberg SJ: Cystic fibrosis-related diabetes and abnormal glucose tolerance: overview and medical nutrition therapy. *Diabetes Spectrum* 15:124–127, 2002

Ms. Spollett is an Adult Nurse Practitioner at Yale Diabetes Center, New Haven, CT.

30. Endocrinopathies and Other Disorders

MARJORIE CYPRESS, MSN, RN, C-ANP, CDE, AND
GERALYN SPOLLETT, MSN, C-ANP, CDE

Diabetes can be associated with other endocrine diseases through a shared etiological mechanism. There are three ways in which this can occur.

- In type 1 diabetes, an autoimmune process that destroys β-cells may also affect other endocrine cells, leading to adrenal, gonadal, thyroid, or parathyroid disease.
- β-Cell function may be disrupted through an infiltrative process that also damages other endocrine tissue.
- Insulin resistance and associated hyperinsulinemia may be at the root of the associated endocrinopathy (1).

The effects of the "other" endocrine diseases may cause a destabilization of diabetes control, resulting in either hypoglycemia or hyperglycemia. Most of these disorders are related to pituitary adenomas that secrete excessive amounts of counter-regulatory hormones or to the administration of exogenous hormone therapy. The main endocrinopathies associated with diabetes or glucose intolerance are acromegaly, Cushing's syndrome, pheochromocytoma, and glucagonoma (2). Autoimmune diseases associated with diabetes include thyroid disease, Addison's disease, celiac disease, and pernicious anemia. Other diseases that are sometimes associated with diabetes and/or can result in unstable diabetes control include fatty liver disease and cystic fibrosis (see CHAPTER 29).

ENDOCRINOPATHIES

Acromegaly

Acromegaly is a condition caused by excess growth hormone, usually caused by a pituitary microadenoma. Growth hormone is diabetogenic because of its effect on peripheral insulin resistance and increase in hepatic glucose production. The incidence of diabetes in acromegaly is estimated to be 13–32%, and the incidence of glucose intolerance in acromegaly is 60%. People who receive exogenous growth hormone (as in children with short stature) can also develop glucose intolerance or overt type 2 diabetes and can suffer the microvascular and neuropathic complications often associated with chronic suboptimally controlled diabetes (2).

Signs and symptoms of acromegaly in adults include excessive growth of hands and feet (with rapid increase in shoe and glove size), protruding jaw, enlarged tongue, coarse facial features, fatigue, weakness, acanthosis nigricans, hypertension, weakness, excessive growth of skin tags, and headaches (3). Sleep apnea is also noted to be very common in people with acromegaly (4).

Laboratory findings may include elevated serum growth hormone levels at fasting and after oral glucose. In healthy individuals, glucose will suppress growth hormone, but in those with acromegaly, growth hormone levels will increase (5). Other laboratory findings include elevated prolactin levels and elevated blood glucose levels. Magnetic resonance imaging (MRI) of the head may reveal a pituitary tumor in 90% of cases. Treatment consists of surgical excision of the tumor and has varying effects on glucose metabolism.

Cushing's Syndrome

Cushing's syndrome is the result of excessive cortisol secondary to either exogenous therapy or an endogenous cortisol-secreting pituitary adenoma that can be either benign or malignant. High cortisol levels can cause increased insulin resistance, increased gluconeogenesis, and decreased peripheral glucose uptake, which subsequently leads to glucose intolerance or overt type 2 diabetes. Many of the features of Cushing's syndrome closely resemble those of the metabolic syndrome. Because some of the conditions of the metabolic syndrome are reversible with treatment, it is important to evaluate patients to distinguish those who may have Cushing's syndrome versus those with metabolic syndrome. If Cushing's is suspected, there should be a thorough workup looking for a tumor if no other cause can be found. If a tumor is found, surgery may be an option.

The clinical picture of an individual with Cushing's syndrome includes truncal obesity, hypertension, glucose intolerance, facial rounding (typical moon face), osteoporosis, abdominal striae, hirsutism, acanthosis nigricans, depression or emotional lability, and menstrual irregularity (2,3,6). Individuals with Cushing's syndrome may go on to develop atherosclerosis and cardiovascular disease (CVD), which are often associated with insulin resistance or the metabolic syndrome. It is not clear to what extent Cushing's syndrome is common or uncommon. There is belief that Cushing's syndrome may be more common than previously thought because it often resembles the metabolic syndrome and further evaluation may not be performed. In addition, its features are similar to those of polycystic ovary syndrome, and the diagnoses of polycystic ovary syndrome or Cushing's syndrome can be mistaken for each other.

Laboratory evaluation is somewhat problematic in that several tests can have false-negative or some false-positive results. A current recommended laboratory evaluation, which appears to be more specific and reliable, is evening salivary cortisol level (6). Because cortisol levels peak in the early morning hours, an evening level should be lower. Other more commonly used tests include a 24-h urine-free cortisol level. This test should include a urine creatinine level to help evaluate whether the urine collection was properly done (normal urine creatinine in 24 h is ~1 g and should not fluctuate >10%). The overnight dexamethasone suppression test involves administration of 1 mg dexamethasone at 11:00 P.M., and serum levels of cortisol are drawn in the morning. In Cushing's syndrome, the cortisol level fails to be suppressed. This test, although commonly performed, can also have false-positive results, and questionable test results should be referred to an endocrinologist (6). Further evaluation may include an MRI to look for a pituitary tumor. Treatment focuses on surgical excision of the adenoma, which can result in a reversal of the metabolic abnormalities.

Pheochromocytoma

A pheochromocytoma is an adenoma that secretes excessive amounts of the catecholamines epinephrine, norepinephrine, and dopamine. Catecholamines are normally secreted in response to hypoglycemia and counter the effects of insulin by increasing glucose production through glycogenolysis. Therefore, the symptoms associated with glucose intolerance and symptoms of hypoglycemia are present and include headache, excessive diaphoresis, and palpitations.

Laboratory evaluation is conducted through urine catecholamine levels. Symptoms are controlled through α- and β-blockade, but resolution of pheochromocytoma is accomplished through tumor removal (2).

Glucagonoma

A glucagonoma is an often-malignant tumor that secretes excessive amounts of the hormone glucagon. The resulting glucose intolerance is the result of increased gluconeogenesis and glycogenolysis. Other associated symptoms are weight loss, glossitis, rash, and anemia (2). Treatment may consist of somatostatin therapy or surgical removal of the tumor.

Nonalcoholic Fatty Liver Disease

Although nonalcoholic fatty liver disease (NAFLD) does not result in diabetes, it is mentioned here because it often coexists and is associated with metabolic syndrome features, such as truncal obesity, type 2 diabetes, hyperlipidemia, and insulin resistance in adults and children (7,8). NAFLD is a common explanation for abnormal or elevated aminotransferase levels in up to 90% of cases once other causes of liver disease are excluded (7). Damage from NAFLD ranges from mild steatosis and hepatitis to cirrhosis and end-stage liver disease, but because this is a newly recognized condition, its natural history and progression require further study (9).

There are no obvious symptoms of NAFLD other than elevated liver function tests. Evaluation may include ultrasound, computed tomography, or MRI to rule out other liver pathology. People who have abnormal liver function tests, are overweight or obese, and have known diabetes or multiple risk factors for the metabolic syndrome and type 2 diabetes should be encouraged to lose weight and exercise because weight loss has been associated with improved liver function tests. Blood glucose and lipid control has also been effective in improving liver function tests and fatty liver. There is some evidence that insulin sensitizers such as metformin, thiazolidinediones, and gemfibrozil have positive effects on normalizing liver function tests (9).

AUTOIMMUNE DISEASES ASSOCIATED WITH TYPE 1 DIABETES

Autoimmune-mediated (type 1) diabetes is associated with other autoimmune diseases, most notably, thyroid disease, celiac disease, Addison's disease, and pernicious anemia. Often present in autoimmune-mediated diabetes, along with islet cell antibodies, are anti–thyroid peroxidase, adrenal, and anti–gastric parietal autoantibodies.

Diabetes and Thyroid Disease

The prevalence of thyroid disease in individuals with diabetes is much higher than in the general population (see also "Thyroid Disease and Diabetes," a patient handout in RESOURCES). Although there are no statistics for the U.S. population, a study conducted in Scotland showed that of the 13.4% of people diagnosed with thyroid disease, the highest incidence (31.4%) was found in women with type 1 diabetes and the lowest (6.8%) in men with type 2 diabetes, suggesting that those with type 1 diabetes are more susceptible to thyroid disease. In this group, the most common thyroid dysfunction was subclinical hypothyroidism (10).

Hyperthyroidism. In type 1 diabetes, Graves' disease is the most common autoimmune thyroid disease leading to hyperthyroidism. Most often diagnosed in young women, this thyroid disease has clear links to the HLA (human leukocyte antigen) markers. Thyrotoxicosis disrupts glucose control by causing an increase in glucose absorption, utilization, and production. The increased production of thyroid hormone and its subsequent effect on metabolism results in accelerated gluconeogenesis by the liver and an increase in peripheral tissue uptake of glucose. The increased glucose production and disposal stimulated by the thyroid hormones occurs independent of insulin levels. In addition to these mechanisms, thyroid hormone can also cause insulin resistance and promote an increase in insulin clearance rates. To compensate for the lack of circulating insulin, more insulin must be secreted. In previously undiagnosed patients, hyperthyroidism may unmask impaired glucose tolerance and diabetes.

For patients with type 1 diabetes with undiagnosed hyperthyroidism, the rapid disposal of insulin results in hyperglycemia and can lead to ketoacidosis. Because this is a life-threatening acute complication, the importance of screening for thyroid disease in type 1 diabetes cannot be underestimated. Conversely, if a patient has thyrotoxicosis, a screening test for latent diabetes should be done.

The presentation of clinical signs and symptoms of hyperthyroid disease warrants thyroid function evaluation. The thyroid-stimulating hormone (TSH) blood test is the best way to determine thyroid function. If the levels of TSH are suppressed, then the amount of thyroid hormone being produced is excessive, indicating a hyperthyroid state. A free thyroxine index or free T4 level will help determine the extent of the hyperthyroid problem. If the laboratory results do not match the clinical presentation, further workup by an endocrinologist may be necessary to determine the cause for the hyperthyroidism and subsequent treatment.

Symptoms of Hyperthyroidism

Tremor
Increased sweating
Heat intolerance
Nervousness and anxiety
Irritability
Muscle weakness
Palpitations and tachycardia
Fatigue
Hyperdefecation
Weight loss

In Graves' disease, therapeutic options include ablation by radioactive iodine, surgical removal of the gland, or medical control with propylthiouracil or methimazole. If the patient has tachycardia or tremors, the use of β-adrenergic blocking agents can ameliorate these symptoms, but may also decrease the patient's ability to recognize hypoglycemia and impair the counterregulatory response to hypoglycemia (1).

Lymphocytic thyroiditis, another cause of hyperthyroidism in young, usually postpartum, women, can spontaneously revert to hypothyroidism. Although the disease usually resolves, a percentage of people have permanent hypothyroidism. Careful monitoring of thyroid function must be done throughout the disease process to determine appropriate treatment. The changeable course of this condition further complicates diabetes control.

During the initial phases of treatment for hyperthyroidism, insulin needs are still increased, but as the patient becomes euthyroid, or in some cases hypothyroid, previous medication dosages may be excessive. Frequent self-monitoring of blood glucose and a flexible insulin regimen may be the best course of action to compensate for the fluctuation in the insulin requirement.

Hypothyroidism. In hypothyroidism concomitant with diabetes, the most common cause is an autoimmune thyroid dysfunction, Hashimoto's disease. It occurs in type 1 diabetes but also has an increased prevalence in type 2 diabetes unrelated to autoimmunity factors.

Hypothyroidism slows the absorption of glucose from the gastrointestinal tract, reduces glucose uptake by the peripheral tissues, and decreases gluconeogenesis. In response to prolonged insulin half-life, insulin secretion may be reduced. Although these metabolic changes in glucose may not produce clinical symptoms in a person without diabetes, the glucose control of the person with diabetes deteriorates and episodes of hypoglycemia increase. As with hyperthyroidism, TSH is the most accurate method to evaluate primary hypothyroidism. The level of TSH will be elevated in response to the decrease in thyroid hormone production. Most hypothyroidism is related to primary thyroid failure. However, in some instances, the hypothalamus or pituitary gland will be the cause of the hypothyroidism, and in such cases, the TSH may not be elevated. Further evaluation by an endocrinologist is needed to determine the cause. Regardless of etiology, the presenting clinical picture for hypothyroidism remains consistent. As hypothyroidism resolves with treatment, an increase in insulin dosage will be needed to meet the increased metabolic need (11).

Symptoms of Hypothyroidism

Dry, coarse skin and hair
Cold intolerance
Hoarseness
Facial edema
Slow speech and mentation
Poor concentration
Constipation
Weight gain
Lower-extremity edema
Depression
Weakness and lethargy
Fatigue

Treatment for hypothyroidism relies on the replacement of L-thyroxine. The usual dose of levothyroxine is 75–125 µg. In patients at risk for atherosclerotic heart disease, the initial medication dose should be reduced from the usual starting dose. Further adjustments in therapy are made based on the results of TSH testing done every 6–8 weeks. CVD is prevalent in type 2 diabetes; therefore, these therapeutic guidelines should be considered in patients with diabetes.

Dyslipidemia is prevalent in hypothyroidism. As thyroid function approaches normal levels, the lipid profile will also improve. However, with the persistence of unrecognized hypothyroidism or untreated subclinical hypothyroidism, the risk of CVD increases (12). Many patients with type 2 diabetes have the metabolic syndrome, with dyslipidemias that are slow to respond to treatment. If the underlying cause is hypothyroidism and it is not treated, there will be limited clinical improvement in lipid levels. This underlines the need for annual screening for thyroid disease in the diabetes population.

Nursing implications. The destabilization of glucose control in thyroid disease requires an intensification of diabetes management, particularly self-monitoring of blood glucose and adjustments in medication therapy. Nursing must focus on maintaining a continuity of care and coordination of therapies. Patient education regarding the interface of thyroid disease and diabetes and the ways to distinguish between the causes of clinical symptoms (for example, hypoglycemia versus hyperthyroidism) is a nursing priority (see "Thyroid Disease and Diabetes" in RESOURCES).

PRACTICAL POINT

Thyroid disease is frequently seen in individuals with both type 1 and type 2 diabetes. Thyroid function tests should be performed annually on all people with diabetes or if the patient presents with symptoms suggestive of thyroid disease. Those already diagnosed with thyroid disease need to be monitored periodically by lab tests and physical examination. It is important for nurses to advise patients of the potential for other medical and psychological complications when thyroid levels are not adequately controlled.

Celiac Disease in Type 1 Diabetes

Celiac disease is an often overlooked and underdiagnosed problem associated with type 1 diabetes. The symptoms may mimic other gastrointestinal problems and may be misdiagnosed. First noted in the late 1960s, celiac disease associated with type 1 diabetes has a prevalence rate of ~4–6% (13). Celiac disease has also been noted in other autoimmune conditions such as thyroid disease.

Pathophysiology of celiac disease. A genetically mediated disease of the small bowel, celiac disease may present in infancy and early childhood and then again later in life (>60 years of age). It is most commonly seen in people of European descent and has a 95% genetic predisposition. Viral exposures may trigger an immune response in individuals predisposed to the disease, resulting in the onset of active disease.

In celiac disease, also known as gluten-sensitive enteropathy, there is an abnormal T-cell response against gliadin, a part of wheat gluten and prolamins (derived from barley, rye, and possibly oats). An immune reaction to gluten affects the functioning of the villi of the small intestine and limits its ability to absorb nutrients. This inability to digest certain carbohydrates results in an osmotic diarrhea, hypersecretion due to crypt hyperplasia, and dysmotility due to an inflammatory reaction (14).

The usual clinical presentation is that of chronic diarrhea and failure to thrive. Weight loss, muscle tenderness, and signs of immunological illnesses such as atopic dermatitis and alopecia may also be present. A papular/vesicular rash, dermatitis herpetiformis, may appear on the base of the scalp and on the elbows, knees, and trunk. Extreme itching and burning characterize the rash. Less typical presentations may include iron-deficiency anemia, osteoporosis/osteopenia, arthritis, alteration in teeth enamel, short stature, chronic hepatitis, or neurological problems. Although some patients have profound symptoms such as abdominal cramping, flatulence, and violent diarrhea, many others are unaware of the problem or are asymptomatic. However, once a gluten-free diet is followed for a period of time, patients note improved health and an increase in energy and well-being.

Diabetes and the effect of celiac disease. Two studies in the past 5 years focused on the effect of celiac disease on blood glucose control. Acerini et al. (15) found no difference in metabolic control, as measured by glycated hemoglobin A_{1c}, in type 1 diabetes patients with or without celiac disease. No statistically significant change in insulin requirement was found. However, it was reported that after starting a gluten-free diet, some celiac patients had an increased incidence of morning hypoglycemia. The second study by Kaukinen et al. (16) found no difference in metabolic control in diabetes with treatment of celiac disease.

Before diagnosis and treatment, patients with celiac disease have hypoglycemic episodes and reduced insulin needs, which are assumed to be related to the malabsorptive state. Over time, treatment with a gluten-free diet can help reduce the incidence of hypoglycemia. Therefore, Schwarzenberg and Brunzell (17) recommend closely monitoring insulin needs and blood glucose control during the early phase of treatment with a gluten-free diet, when changes in nutritional status may influence metabolic control.

Diagnosis of celiac disease. In people with a family predisposition to the disease, serological testing, used as a screening tool, may help discover individuals with atypical or silent celiac disease. Currently, most investigators advocate a profile of three antibody assays: *1*) anti-gliadin IgG, *2*) anti-gliadin IgA, and *3*) either anti-endomysial or an anti–tissue transglutaminase assay (17). If the results of all three assays are positive or the patient has symptoms but negative results, he or she should be referred to a gastroenterologist. It is important to note that a positive serological test alone is not sufficient for diagnosis. A small-bowel biopsy is necessary to confirm the diagnosis. Although there are no guidelines for continued screening of the at-risk population, many centers have adopted a yearly testing for the first 3 years of diagnosed diabetes, then screening every 3–5 years thereafter or whenever symptoms develop (17).

Treatment of celiac disease. The current recommendation for treatment is that a gluten-free diet be maintained for life. The most important reason to adhere strictly to the diet is to reduce the risk of small-bowel lymphoma associated with celiac disease. As nutritional status improves, patients note a positive change in energy. The malabsorptive state associated with celiac disease deprives the patient of important minerals, vitamins, and micronutrients. Adherence to the diet can reverse anemia, osteopenia, and other symptoms of vitamin deficiencies such as cheilosis and neurological symptoms. After a period of time on the gluten-free diet, some patients become exquisitely sensitive to the smallest amounts of gluten, whereas others may find they can tolerate small amounts without experiencing diarrhea or cramping. Despite this diminution of symptom response to gluten, the harmful effects of ingestion have been demonstrated by small-bowel biopsies that indicated ongoing mucosal damage.

The gluten-free diet. Maintaining a gluten-free diet is difficult but not impossible. Obvious sources of gluten and prolamins such as bread, processed cheese, and various wheat-based snack foods are easily recognized and avoided (Tables 30.1 and 30.2). However, gluten is often used as a thickener, emulsifier, binder, or stabilizer in many products. Oats, amaranth, and buckwheat (18) currently appear on the list of gluten-free foods, but there is still controversy over whether these foods are safe in large amounts over time. Even certain ground spices may contain

---

Table 30.1 Starches, Grains, and Other Foods Appropriate on a Gluten-Free Diet

- Amaranth,* arrowroot, whole-bean flour, buckwheat,* corn, cornstarch, cornmeal, flax, millet,* nut flours, oats,* oat bran,* oat gum,* pea flour, potato, sweet potato and yam, potato flour, potato starch, quinoa,* rice and wild rice, rice bran, rice flour, sago, sorghum, soy, tapioca, teff*
- Fresh, frozen, or canned unprocessed fruits and vegetables
- Fresh meats, poultry, seafood, fish, game, eggs, some processed meats with gluten-free ingredients, tofu, dried peas, beans, and lentils
- Milk, yogurt, and cheese made with gluten-free ingredients
- Oils, tree nuts, seeds, natural peanut butter, and salad dressings and spreads with gluten-free ingredients
- Honey, sugar, pure maple syrup, corn syrup, jams, jellies, candy, and ice cream with gluten-free ingredients
- Pure spices and herbs, salt, wheat-free soy sauce, vinegar with gluten-free ingredients
- Coffee ground from whole beans, brewed tea, carbonated beverages, some root beer

Adapted from Schwarzenberg and Brunzell (17).
This is only a partial listing. Patients are encouraged to read all labels and to seek comprehensive food and additive lists from celiac organizations and the American Dietetic Association.
*Recommendations about acceptability are inconsistent. Many physicians restrict these grains for the first 6 months after diagnosis or until patients are in full remission.

Table 30.2　Grains and Other Foods/Ingredients Not Appropriate on a Gluten-Free Diet

- Barley, bran, bulgur, couscous, durum flour, farina, graham flour, hydrolyzed plant protein (HPP), hydrolyzed vegetable protein (HVP), kamut, malt, malt extract, malt flavoring, malt syrup, semolina, rye, spelt (dinkel), triticale, wheat, wheat bran, wheat germ, wheat starch
- Imported foods that are labeled "gluten-free" but may contain wheat starch*
- Processed meats and luncheon meats containing HVP or HPP, breaded meats, meats with sauces or gravies, casseroles
- Fruits and vegetables with sauces, breading, or thickeners
- Flavored milk, yogurt, processed cheese, and spreads made with gluten-containing ingredients
- Canned soups, soup mixes, bouillon, miso
- Candy, snack foods, desserts, frozen yogurt, and ice cream with gluten-containing ingredients
- Ground spices, condiments, and soy sauce with gluten-containing ingredients
- Margarine, salad dressing, and dips with gluten-containing ingredients
- Instant coffee, instant tea, instant cocoa mixes, some root beer, grain alcohol

Adapted from Schwarzenberg and Brunzell (17).
This is only a partial listing. Patients are encouraged to read all labels and to seek comprehensive food and additive lists from celiac organizations and the American Dietetic Association. *Food produced in the United States or Canada and labeled "gluten-free" does not contain gluten or wheat starch.

---

gluten products. Other sources of prolamins such as grain alcohol, postage stamps, cosmetics, lip balms, and mouthwashes should also be avoided. Patients must be encouraged to read the labels on all foods because sometimes ingredients on previously "safe" foods change. Foods that are gluten free may be contaminated in transport or by the cooking process. Restaurant eating can be particularly difficult, and the person with celiac disease must learn to ask many questions regarding preparation and possible kitchen contamination by gluten foods.

The addition of a gluten-free diet to the medical nutrition therapy recommended for diabetes presents a challenge and may be perceived as an additional burden. Referral to a registered dietitian can help educate and support the patient through this adaptive process. Patients who count carbohydrates need to know that gluten-free products may not contain the same number of carbohydrates as other starch products and that the digestion and glucose response may be quite different. Joining a support group or becoming active in celiac disease educational organizations will give the patient access to current information.

Psychosocial issues. Having celiac disease in addition to type 1 diabetes may present additional stress because of the nature of the symptoms, strict dietary regimen, and serious consequences if untreated. Because the disease may go unrecognized for a long period, individuals may be labeled as difficult patients. In addition, the gluten-free diet may affect individuals in social situations, making them feel uncomfortable and isolated. Education of the individual and family as well as emotional support from the health care team is important in treating this disease.

Nursing implications. Like diabetes, celiac disease is a chronic condition that requires ongoing patient self-management. Assisting the patient in achieving positive outcomes in the management of both diseases is a challenge for the nurse.

To be successful at managing both conditions, the patient must have a working knowledge of diabetes and the rudiments of medical nutrition therapy as well as a sophisticated understanding of the gluten-free diet and how it interacts with glucose control issues such as hypoglycemia. Working as a team, the nurse and dietitian can educate the patient in the initial dietary changes and support the lifelong process of adaptation and readjustment.

PRACTICAL POINT

Celiac disease is often missed as a diagnosis and its symptoms attributed to other gastrointestinal diseases or poor adherence to the treatment regimen. Patients can become frustrated with their health care team and health care system. It is important for nurses to be aware of the symptoms of this not uncommon disease and promote early detection.

Addison's Disease

The autoimmune destruction of the adrenals results in adrenal insufficiency and the absence of cortisol. Because Addison's disease can be effectively treated if diagnosed early, it is important to quickly evaluate for this disease to avoid fatalities. Clinical symptoms include weight loss; hyperpigmentation of the neck, elbows, and fingers; fatigability; muscle weakness; dehydration; increased craving for salt; and malaise. The risk of Addison's disease is 1 in 250 in individuals with immune-mediated type 1 diabetes. Therefore, individuals with immune-mediated type 1 diabetes plus the presence of thyroid autoantibodies should be tested for the presence of adrenal 21-hydroxylase autoantibodies (19). Another laboratory evaluation for Addison's disease is the adrenocorticotropic hormone cortisol stimulation test, in which adrenocorticotropic hormone is administered intravenously and a cortisol level is drawn both 30 and 60 min later. If there is no response, the diagnosis of adrenocortical insufficiency, or Addison's disease, is made. The treatment is lifelong and consists of oral hydrocortisone.

Pernicious Anemia

Another autoimmune disease associated with type 1 diabetes is anemia. Both iron deficiency anemia and pernicious anemia can be autoimmune mediated by parietal cell antibodies. The presence of antibodies to thyroid peroxidase and anti–gastric parietal cell antibodies and anti-adrenal antibodies is four to five times as frequent in individuals with type 1 diabetes than in the nondiabetic population. In a study of individuals with type 1 diabetes, 20.9% were found to be parietal cell antibody positive, and of those, 15.4% had iron deficiency anemia and 10.5% had pernicious anemia (20). Parietal cell antibodies can inhibit the secretion of the intrinsic factor necessary for the absorption of vitamin B12, leading to latent and eventually overt pernicious anemia. If laboratory tests indicate a deficiency of this vitamin, treatment typically consists of monthly injections of vitamin B12, though some elderly patients with gastric atrophy receive oral supplements in addition to the monthly injections.

SUMMARY

Many diseases can affect the level of glucose control that a person with diabetes achieves. These diseases cannot be overlooked in the treatment of diabetes. The metabolic changes that occur with the various disease states can make the self-management of diabetes more difficult. Individuals who are coping with one or more chronic disease will need nurses to provide additional patient education and psychological support to achieve positive outcomes.

REFERENCES

1. Ober K: Polyendocrine syndromes. In *Medical Management of Diabetes Mellitus.* Leahy J, Clark N, Cefalu W, Eds. New York, Marcel Dekker, 2000, p. 699–717
2. Berelowitz M, Kourides IA: Diabetes mellitus secondary to other endocrine disorders. In *Diabetes Mellitus: A Fundamental and Clinical Text.* 2nd ed. Philadelphia, Lippincott Williams & Wilkins, 2000, p. 588–594
3. Levin NA, Greer KE: Cutaneous manifestations of endocrine disorders. *Dermatol Nurs* 13:185–186, 189–196, 201–202, 2001
4. Grunstein RR, Ho KY, Sullivan CE: Sleep apnea in acromegaly. *Ann Intern Med* 115:527–532, 1991
5. Samuels MH: Growth hormone-secreting pituitary tumors. In *Endocrine Secrets.* 3rd ed. McDermott MT, Ed. Philadelphia, Hanley & Belfus, 2002, p. 189–193
6. Raff H, Findling JW: A physiologic approach to the diagnosis of the Cushing syndrome. *Ann Intern Med* 138:980–991, 2003
7. Angulo P: Nonalcoholic fatty liver disease. *N Engl J Med* 346:1221–1231, 2002
8. Jorgensen RA: Nonalcoholic fatty liver disease. *Gastroenterol Nurs* 26:150–155, 2003
9. Reid BM, Sanyal AJ: Evaluation and management of non-alcoholic steato-hepatitis. *Eur J Gastroenterol Hepatol* 16:1117–1122, 2004
10. Perros P, McCrimmon R, Shaw G, Frier B: Frequency of thyroid dysfunction in diabetic patients: value of annual screening. *Diabet Med* 7:622–627, 1995
11. Johnson J, Duick DS: Diabetes and thyroid disease: a likely combination. *Diabetes Spectrum* 15:140–142, 2002
12. Cooper D: Subclinical hyperthyroidism. *N Engl J Med* 345:260–265, 2001
13. Cronin CC, Feighery A, Ferriss JB, Liddy C, Shanahan F, Feighery C: High prevalence of celiac disease among patients with insulin-dependent (type 1) diabetes mellitus. *Am J Gastroenterol* 92:2210–2212, 1997
14. Alsace NH, Maradiegue AH: Gastrointestinal health. In *Adult Primary Care.* Meredith PV, Horan NM, Eds. Philadelphia, W. B. Saunders, 2000, p. 414–418
15. Acerini CL, Ahmed MI, Ross KM, Sullivan PB, Bird G, Dunger DB: Coeliac disease in children and adolescents with IDDM: clinical characteristics and response to gluten-free diet. *Diabet Med* 15:38–44, 1998
16. Kaukinen K, Salmi J, Lahtela J, Siljamaki-Ojansuu U, Koivisto AM, Oksa H, Colin P: No effect of gluten-free diet on the metabolic control of type 1 diabetes in patients with diabetes and celiac disease: retrospective and controlled prospective survey (Letter). *Diabetes Care* 22:1747–1748, 1999

17. Schwarzenberg SJ, Brunzell C: Type 1 diabetes and celiac disease: overview
     and medical nutrition therapy. *Diabetes Spectrum* 15:197–201, 2002
18. Thompson T: Case problem: questions regarding the acceptability of buck-
     wheat, amaranth, quinoa, and oats from a patient with celiac disease (Case
     Report). *J Am Diet Assoc* 101:586–587, 2001
19. Kukreja A, Balducci-Silano PL, Maclaren NK: Association between immune-
     mediated (type 1) diabetes mellitus and other autoimmune diseases. In *Dia-
     betes Mellitus: A Fundamental and Clinical Text*. 2nd ed. LeRoith D, Taylor
     S, Olefsky JM, Eds. Philadelphia, Lippincott Williams & Wilkins, 2000,
     p. 410–419
20. De Block CE, De Leeuw IH, van Gaal LF, the Belgium Diabetes Reg-
     istry: High prevalence of manifestations of gastric autoimmunity in parietal
     cell antibody-positive type 1 (insulin dependent) diabetic patients. *J Clin
     Endocrinol Metab* 84:4062–4067, 1999

*Ms. Cypress is an Adult Nurse Practitioner and Certified Diabetes Educator in
Albuquerque, NM. Ms. Spollett is an Adult Nurse Practitioner at Yale Diabetes
Center, New Haven, CT.*

DIABETES CARE IN COMMUNITY SETTINGS

31. Diabetes Care in the Hospital

Sylvia English, MS, RN, CDE, and Sandra Young, MSN, BCRN

Of the 3.5 million hospitalizations in the U.S. each year, patients with diabetes account for 15% (1). Most often, admission is for reasons other than diabetes (2). Regardless of whether the reason for admission is diabetes, hyperglycemia must be identified and controlled in all patients. Recent literature indicates that hyperglycemia among patients not previously diagnosed with diabetes affects morbidity and mortality (2,3). Diabetes is associated with higher incidences of preoperative morbidities, including obesity, small-vessel coronary artery disease, more severe and extensive atherosclerosis, peripheral arterial disease, renal insufficiency, hypertension, and increased rates of life-threatening postoperative infections (2). Inpatient management, regardless of the reason, requires close attention to optimal glycemic control for the best patient outcomes.

With one-third of the 18 million people with diabetes undiagnosed, a patient without a prior history of diabetes who exhibits hyperglycemia needs immediate intervention (1). Patients with new-onset hyperglycemia admitted to critical care areas or to general medicine and surgical units have significantly higher mortality and lower functional outcomes than patients with known diabetes or normoglycemia (3). Despite marked hyperglycemia, almost all of these patients are either never diagnosed with diabetes or do not have the hyperglycemia addressed during hospitalization (3,4). Failure to recognize and treat hyperglycemia represents a missed opportunity to reduce hospital morbidity and mortality and to initiate interventions that may delay the long-term complications of this disease (2). Some experts have suggested that all hospitalized patients be screened for hyperglycemia at admission (3).

Hospitalization in individuals with known diabetes presents a host of disruptions to his or her usual eating schedule, usual food selection, schedule for taking medication and for physical activity, and the sleep-and-wake cycle, thereby affecting glucose control and emotional state. The hospital routine is different from any type of home routine. Food trays may arrive long after the premeal insulin has been given, the food may not be appealing to the individual, and he or she may not eat enough for the amount of insulin or medication taken. In addition, individuals who routinely self-manage their diabetes may be put in a position where their management is done by others, taking away their independence. The fluctuations of glucose levels while hospitalized are often frightening to someone who has maintained glycemic control. Health care professionals should be sensitive to these issues during medical management.

Hyperglycemia can be precipitated by the body's stress response of secreting counterregulatory hormones, i.e., epinephrine, glucagon, cortisol, growth hormone. When insulin sensitivity decreases, higher doses of antihyperglycemic medications are required to correct blood glucose elevations. The disruption in normal activity and dietary intake further influences glucose control, and usual efforts to correct high blood glucose may fail. Many patients need reassurance that the treatment necessary to control glucose levels during an acute illness may differ from their usual regimen. A need for insulin during hospitalization may not mean that the patient will permanently require insulin therapy. The patient will need to understand that insulin is the most effective treatment for hyperglycemia due to increased stress or illness. However, some medications administered during an acute illness interfere with usual insulin action and/or increase insulin resistance, so caution is always warranted.

ASSESSMENT

Management of the hospitalized patient with diabetes can be challenging, with shortened inpatient stays and intensive medication regimens coupled with comorbidities and diabetes-related chronic complications. Regardless of the reason for admission or previous diabetes status, it is essential to identify suboptimally controlled diabetes and acute hyperglycemia at the time of hospital admission and to implement therapy to achieve a normoglycemic state (2). Table 31.1 identifies key information that needs to be obtained on admission (5).

Diabetes knowledge and past management of the disease (including coping skills) need to be determined. The nurse must keep in mind opportunities to improve diabetes management, particularly if suboptimal glycemic control is the underlying cause for hospitalization. Often when individuals enter the hospital, the orders for diabetes medications are based on their home regimen. However, if individuals have not been adherent in regularly and consistently taking their medications at home, then when the same dosage is administered regularly, hypoglycemia may occur. Patients with ineffective or suboptimal home regimens, as evidenced by glycated hemoglobin A_{1c} (A1C) values >7%, and frequently 8–12% or higher, experience increased counterregulatory hormones, resulting in increased insulin resistance and marked hyperglycemia. Hyperglycemia, hypoglycemic events, and chronic complications can increase the risk for falls, nosocomial skin breakdown, and infection, which may result in prolonged hospitalization and increase the length of hospital stay. Careful monitoring of blood glucose and appropriate interventions to meet target goals for glycemic levels can ensure optimal outcomes.

The American Association of Clinical Endocrinologists (AACE) and American Diabetes Association (ADA) have created guidelines for the management of the hospitalized person with diabetes. Glucose target goals for noncritical care as well as intensive care management have been set (see *Inpatient Glycemic Targets* on page 346). These recommended goals are based on a technical review examining the findings of many studies conducted in the hospital setting that evaluated glucose levels and subsequent patient outcomes, including morbidity and mortality.

RECOMMENDED LABORATORY TESTS

On admission, laboratory tests are necessary to gather baseline data about the current status of glycemic control and to evaluate the impact of diabetes on the other

Table 31.1 Baseline Diabetes Assessment

I. Initial Questions
  A. Type of diabetes
  B. Duration of diabetes
  C. Primary care physician (PCP)
  D. Primary diabetes physician, if different from PCP

II. Medical Nutrition Assessment
  A. Diet prescription
  B. Estimated compliance
  C. Weight change in past 6 mo

III. Physical Activity

IV. Medications Taken
  A. Insulin (type, amount, and frequency)
  B. Diabetes medications
  C. Other prescription medications
  D. Over the counter

V. Assessment of Control
  A. Type of meter/strips
  B. Frequency
  C. Results of home monitoring, if available
  D. A1C frequency, date of last test, and results, if available
  E. Ketones

VI. Acute Symptoms of Diabetes
  A. Hyperglycemia
    1. Thirst
    2. Frequent urination
    3. Urination during night
    4. Yeast infection
    5. History of diabetic ketoacidosis
    6. Blurred vision
  B. Hypoglycemia
    1. Episodes of sweating, shaking, pounding heart, headache, and/or confusion
    2. Frequency, timing, symptoms, and treatment

VII. Reproductive Assessment
  A. Preconception
  B. Pregnancy
  C. Menopause

VIII. Substance Abuse
  A. Tobacco
  B. Alcohol
  C. Other

IX. Barriers to Care
  A. Internal
    1. Hearing or sight impairment
    2. Cognitive dysfunction
    3. Language/literacy
    4. Physical impairment
  B. External
    1. Financial
    2. Transportation
    3. Family/significant other status

X. Chronic Complications/Comorbidities
  A. Neuromuscular/psychiatric
    1. Pain and/or numbness
    2. Depression
    3. Unusual mood dysfunction
    4. Dizziness
  B. Eye
    1. Last dilated eye exam
    2. History of diabetic eye disease
  C. Kidney/bladder
    1. History of protein in urine
    2. Kidney disease
  D. Cardiovascular
    1. Hypertension
    2. Shortness of breath
    3. Smoking
    4. Chest pain
    5. Dyslipidemia
    6. Obesity
    7. Family history
  E. Infections
    1. Recurrent infections
    2. Immunizations (flu and pneumonia)
  F. Foot and limb
    1. Numbness
    2. Foot ulcers
    3. Amputations

Reprinted with permission from American Healthways (5).

organ systems. Goals based on the ADA's Standards of Medical Care in Diabetes are published annually (6). The following list of tests routinely recommended for the hospitalized diabetes patient is not exhaustive. The reason for admission will dictate which tests need to be obtained.

THE CASE FOR GLUCOSE CONTROL

Optimal glucose control can prevent infection, support healing, and promote patient well-being. In addition, it can reduce mortality and morbidity (7). An individual's usual level of glycemic control is often disrupted by the stress of admission, the change in eating behavior, and the illness that prompted the hospitalization. Close attention must be paid to the patient's prehospital medication regimen, including any herbs or supplements the patient has taken, and to orders written for all medications, including insulin and oral diabetes drugs that the patient was taking before admission. If oral diabetes medications cannot be taken during an acute hospital period, supplemental insulin will be needed. The use of rapid-acting insulin alone is often inadequate for maintaining glycemic control. If insulin will be needed for >24 h, a basal insulin such as an intermediate- or long-acting insulin should be initiated. It is ideal to return the patient to a maintenance medication plan as soon as possible if admission or recent A1C values indicate that the prior home regimen was effective.

Blood glucose goals during hospitalization are individualized to the patient and should follow prehospitalization targets. Values >180 mg/dl (10.0 mmol/l) indicate a need to monitor glucose levels more frequently to determine the glucose trend and the need for more intensive intervention, which is typically insulin administration. Achieving these targets may require the intervention of an endocrinologist or diabetes specialist (8,9). The ADA, AACE, Endocrine Soci-

Tests Routinely Recommended for Hospitalized Patients

Laboratory Test	Purpose
Complete blood count	Assess for anemia, infection
Comprehensive serum chemistry	Assess electrolytes Assess kidney function Assess liver functions Assess nutritional status
Glycated A1C (if not done in the previous month)	Assess glucose control in past 3 months
Albumin-to-creatinine ratio (random)	Assess kidney function, cardiovascular risk
24-h urine (if indicated by the lab and hospitalization is long enough for collection)	Assess kidney function
Lipid profile	Assess cardiovascular risk

Inpatient Glycemic Targets

General medicine and surgery	<126 mg/dl (7 mmol/l) (fasting and admission)
	<200 mg/dl (11.1 mmol/l) (random)
Cardiac surgery	<150 mg/dl (8.3 mmol/l)
Critical care	<110 mg/dl (6.1 mmol/l)

From the ADA (6).

ety, and American Association of Diabetes Educators have recommended strict glycemic control, underscoring its importance in the hospital setting (9).

Myocardial Infarction

The landmark Diabetes Mellitus Insulin Glucose Infusion in Acute Myocardial Infarction (DIGAMI) study demonstrated the effect glucose control has on improved outcomes for previously diagnosed and undiagnosed patients with diabetes (7). In patients with myocardial infarction, early aggressive intervention with intravenous insulin administered when glucose levels were >198 mg/dl (>11 mmol/l), followed by subcutaneous insulin therapy four times a day for 3 months, resulted in a 30% reduction in mortality at 1 year, an average 28% reduction at 3.5 years in patients with known diabetes, and a 51% reduction in those not previously diagnosed with diabetes. Better glycemic control improved the survival rates of patients with diabetes who had a myocardial infarction.

Coronary Artery Bypass Graft

After a coronary artery bypass graft (CABG) procedure, patients with diabetes are at higher risk for fatal events, particularly individuals with suboptimal glucose control. Patients with diabetes have increased risk of low cardiac output and intra-aortic balloon pump use after CABG (10). Research has documented that for each 1-mmol/l (18-mg/dl) increase above 6.1 mmol/l (108 mg/dl) on the first postoperative day, there is a 17% increase in the risk for cardiovascular complications and sepsis for CABG patients with diabetes (11). Also, perioperative hyperglycemia is associated with longer postoperative stays, increasing hospital charges and total health care costs (12).

Improved perioperative glucose control is required to improve outcomes for patients with diabetes. CABG patients with diabetes had a significantly lower risk of death with continuous insulin infusion than those who received subcutaneous insulin. The insulin infusion provided better glucose control (10). The protective effect of continuous insulin infusion may be associated with the effective metabolic use of excess glucose to favorably alter myocardial pathways (10). Continuous insulin infusion should become a standard of care for glycemic control in patients with diabetes undergoing CABG (10).

Trauma

Trauma patients with diabetes also present a challenging balance between management of critical injuries and maintenance of glycemic control. One study found that even patients with mild hyperglycemia (>135 mg/dl [>7.5 mmol/l]) with or without diagnosed diabetes have significantly longer hospital stays, infection morbidity (e.g., urinary tract infections, wound infections, pneumonia, bacteremia), longer intensive care unit stays, and increased mortality compared with normoglycemic patients (13,14). Intensive glucose control requires close monitoring and proper intervention by the team to improve patient outcomes.

HOSPITAL GLUCOSE MONITORING

During hospitalization, capillary blood glucose monitoring (CBGM) needs to match the patient's nutritional intake and medication management for optimal glycemic control. An ideal glucose monitoring order for patients who are tolerating meals would be CBGM before meals and at bedtime. A 2-h postprandial test may be warranted if the goal is to keep blood glucose level <180 mg/dl (<10 mmol/l) at all times. Patients requiring enteral feedings and parenteral nutrition usually require CBGM monitoring every 4–6 h or as ordered. Short- or rapid-acting insulin is given before or with the meal, respectively, based on eating patterns.

Specific patient situations may warrant closer monitoring, such as hourly CBGM testing, when initiating intravenous insulin therapy. According to Clement et al. (8), although nursing acuity is high for the first few hours of insulin drip therapy, patients quickly reach target blood glucose levels and improved glucose control, and CBGM every 2–3 h may be acceptable. Patients with hypoglycemia due to sulfonylurea use, especially from those with long half-lives such as chlorpropamide, glimepiride, and glyburide, require more intensive monitoring and may need an intravenous dextrose infusion. Monitor for hypoglycemia when adjusting any pharmacological interventions (such as decreased doses of glucocorticoids), antihyperglycemic agent, or insulin.

PRACTICAL POINT

There are factors that influence the results of CBGM, including variations in hematocrit, altitude, environmental temperature and humidity, hypotension, hypoxia, peripheral perfusion, and triglyceride concentrations (15). To provide appropriate care, nurses must be aware of these factors that affect glucose monitoring and make nursing judgments accordingly. Most bedside CBGM provides results in plasma glucose values (versus whole blood) and produces results that correlate to laboratory values (15).

Management of hospitalized patients with diabetes requires careful monitoring and review of CBGM results. Hospitals depend on CBGM monitoring to evaluate glucose control in individuals with diabetes and to detect hyperglycemia in undiagnosed patients who may be at risk of developing diabetes during their illness.

This measure is analogous to an additional "vital sign" (16). Because the results from CBGM can be obtained quickly, therapeutic measures can be instituted rapidly, improving diabetes management and shortening the length of hospital stay. Use of CBGM requires proficiency testing, staff training and competency, well-defined policies and procedures, quality control procedures, and tracking (10).

Regulatory and licensing agencies mandate that hospitals and other facilities must have quality assurance programs for CBGM (17). Correlation studies comparing bedside results with laboratory values are essential elements of the quality assurance process (15). Accuracy of CBGM is an essential component in ensuring that treatment decisions are appropriate for optimal glycemic targets. For CBGM, laboratory values are the standard against which the meters are judged (15).

Frequently, individuals will bring their glucose meter into the hospital. This provides an opportunity for validating the individual's proficiency with the meter and the accuracy of the meter. It is important to evaluate an individual's monitoring technique, both initially and at regular intervals, because use of CBGM data guides treatment (18). In acute care settings, an individual's use of a personal meter must be addressed in the organization's policies and procedures. Usually, the hospital meter is used for inpatient testing, and the results are used for decisions regarding treatment changes.

MEDICATION MANAGEMENT

Regardless of whether the patient has type 1 or type 2 diabetes, maintaining glycemic control is a primary goal and a determinant in achieving positive health outcomes. The primary consideration in caring for patients with type 1 diabetes is adequate insulin replacement. Individuals with type 1 diabetes must have basal insulin across the full course of 24 h and multiple-dose injections of rapid- or short-acting insulin with meals (if they are eating). Even if patients are not eating, they may require boluses of insulin to correct the hyperglycemia produced in response to stress or illness. They may require an intravenous insulin/glucose infusion. Type 2 diabetes can be managed in the inpatient setting with diet, oral agents, insulin, or a combination (2). Most patients with type 2 diabetes who have been controlled by diet alone require medication to control hyperglycemia due to illness. Working with the nutritionist or dietitian to provide meals with adequate nutrition and meals that are consistent in both carbohydrate and calories may help maintain euglycemia and demonstrate to the patient that following a consistent and healthy meal plan can keep blood glucose levels controlled.

In the hospital, oral antihyperglycemic agents are often discontinued because they lack the flexibility and efficacy needed in an acute care setting. Metformin must be discontinued on the day of any surgical procedure and not reinitiated for at least 48 h after the procedure (see CHAPTER 5). Because metformin is metabolized by the kidney, adequate perfusion must be present for the drug to clear the system properly. Any procedure that may interfere with the clearing of the medication allows the medication to build up in the system and puts the patient at risk for developing lactic acidosis, a sometimes fatal complication. Normal renal function as determined by laboratory assessment must be established before re-initiating metformin. Therefore, insulin therapy is commonly used to manage glycemic control. However, renal insufficiency affects the onset and duration of insulin, so therapy must be individualized based on the patients' particular needs.

Also note that decreased renal clearance increases the risk of hypoglycemia associated with sulfonylurea use.

Insulin Therapy

Hospital intensive insulin management should provide basal and nutritional insulin to cover the carbohydrate in meals or enteral or parenteral nutrition as well as supplemental insulin based on a formula to correct for glycemic excursions. If the patient is not being cared for by an endocrinologist and diabetes team, a consultation with a hospital-based team or consult service to assist in the initiation of intensive management should be pursued.

There is no evidence that traditional sliding-scale regimens are an effective method for maintaining optimal glucose control in the hospital. In fact, when used alone, sliding scales may actually promote hyperglycemia (19). Short-term use of supplemental insulin may be appropriate to correct hyperglycemia. However, using the pattern management philosophy, the scheduled, nutritional, and correctional doses should be evaluated every 24–36 h and adjusted to compensate for any pattern of hyperglycemia or hypoglycemia. Using the pattern approach during the hospitalization should decrease glycemic excursions that can negatively affect clinical outcomes.

Hyperglycemia can result when there is insufficient circulating insulin. Because rapid-acting insulin analogs have a duration of action of ~4–5 h, the use of regular insulin may be more beneficial (see Table 4.2 in CHAPTER 4 for more durations of action). Regular insulin has a longer duration of action that may provide adequate circulating insulin to maintain blood glucose control. This is particularly important in managing individuals with type 1 diabetes, who require 24-h circulating insulin.

Strategies for optimal treatment are guided by two major principles: the type of diabetes and the coordination of diabetes treatment, particularly the route of insulin administration with nutritional therapy. The standard for the hospitalized NPO patient is intravenous insulin and glucose infusion (8). Several protocols exist and have been published, but studies comparing these protocols do not exist. Examples of intravenous and subcutaneous insulin protocols are available in the RESOURCES section as the ICU Glucose Management Procedure and the Subcutaneous Insulin Administration Record, respectively (8) (see also www.providence.org/resources/oregon/PDFs/Protocol80120.pdf). Standing order sets for supplemental insulin and intravenous insulin drip protocols ensure that all providers aim for ideal goals as patients deal with the glucose level variations common during hospitalization.

Transitioning from Intravenous Insulin Drips to Subcutaneous Insulin

Once an individual's health condition begins to stabilize and he or she is starting to eat, intravenous insulin is no longer necessary. If not planned and implemented carefully, the transition from intravenous to subcutaneous insulin can cause not only a major disruption in glucose control, but can also trigger diabetic ketoacidosis (DKA) in individuals with type 1 diabetes. A basal insulin should be given subcutaneously ~2–4 h before the insulin drip is discontinued, and rapid-acting insulin should be administered at least 30 min before discontinuing the intravenous drip. This prevents any interruption in circulating insulin. Careful monitoring of blood glucose levels is necessary in this transition to prevent either hyper- or hypoglycemia.

PRACTICAL POINT

In transitioning insulin therapies in a patient with type 1
diabetes, adequate circulating
insulin must be maintained. If
insulin deficits occur, the
patient is at risk for developing DKA.

Management of Patients Using Insulin Pumps

Patients who wear insulin pumps are admitted to hospitals with increasing frequency, and hospital staff must be prepared to document that glucose control is maintained. If staff nurses are not educated in pump management, a consultation with the diabetes specialist or diabetes management team should be ordered. Staff nurses should be instructed in assessing the infusion site for infection and how to disconnect the insulin pump in an emergency. Because not all staff nurses are familiar with pump management, it is in the best interest of the patient that the hospital supports a policy that allows the patient or family to maintain pump therapy (Table 31.2). However, the health care provider may offer the patient the option to change to an alternative method of insulin delivery while hospitalized. Because maintaining good metabolic control plays a critical role in achieving positive health outcomes, the insulin delivery method that best accomplishes this goal should be supported by the patient's care team. In some cases, maintaining pump therapy may not be feasible and the hospital will need to have a written protocol that allows for the conversion to another method of insulin delivery.

Management of Hypoglycemia

Treating hypoglycemia in the hospitalized patient with diabetes is a nursing intervention. All hospitals should have protocols for treating hypoglycemia (see

Table 31.2 Sample Insulin Pump Policy

POLICY/PROCEDURE		
SUBJECT: Insulin Pumps	NUMBER: M30-11	PAGE: 1 OF: 1
ORIG. 6/98	REVISED: 1/00	REVIEWED: 10/02
PREPARED BY INTERDISCIPLINARY POLICY/PROCEDURE COMMITTEE		
APPROVED BY PCMH PRESIDENT APPROVED BY VICE PRESIDENT, PATIENT CARE SERVICES		

When a patient is admitted with an insulin pump, the patient and his/her physician assume responsibility for the pump. If the patient is a pediatric patient, he or she, the parent, and physician assume responsibility for the pump. Nurses observe and document the patient's response to therapy, but they do not make any adjustment in the dose/rate of the pump.

If the patient becomes incapacitated and cannot manage the pump, the physician will order that administration of insulin by pump be discontinued. Further orders for management of the patient will be written by the physician.

Reprinted with permission from Pitt County Memorial Hospital.

RESOURCES for an example of hypoglycemia orders). These protocols should indicate the glucose level at which treatment is initiated and the type and amount of glucose to be administered to patients who are able to take oral treatment. If the patient is unable to take oral treatment for hypoglycemia, indications for the use of glucagon and intravenous dextrose should be clearly stated in the guidelines. Certain circumstances may require that the attending or resident physician be notified if the glucose level does not respond to the prescribed treatment (see also CHAPTER 7).

In hospitalized patients receiving intensive therapy for glycemic control, prevention of hypoglycemia should be an important goal. Hypoglycemia can be foreseen, and it is preventable by measures other than undertreatment of hyperglycemia (20). Hypoglycemia is normally preceded by a preventable triggering event, which usually includes a sudden change in caloric intake, e.g., transportation off ward, alteration in total parenteral nutrition or enteral feedings, or continuous venovenous hemodialysis (20). Additionally, patients who are receiving medications for hyperglycemia and have certain diseases or conditions, such as renal insufficiency, elderly age, malnutrition, liver disease, sepsis, shock, pregnancy, total parenteral nutrition, burns, congestive heart failure, stroke, hypoglycemia unawareness, tapering steroids, alcoholism, or polypharmacy, may be predisposed to hypoglycemic events.

Strategies for preventing hypoglycemia must have the following: sound understanding of the onset, peak, and duration of diabetes medications; an ongoing evaluation of the appropriateness and effectiveness of glycemic management modalities; assurances that medications are given at the correct time; and more frequent fingerstick blood glucose monitoring and dextrose replacement to maintain the glucose target (20).

Usually during oral treatment, once the customary amount of glucose (15–20 g) is administered, the nurse must remain with the patient or provide close observation and assess the response to treatment. CBGM should be performed 15–20 min after treatment. If the resulting glucose level has not returned to the target range (>70 mg/dl [3.8 mmol/l]), then treatment should be repeated. At the resolution of the hypoglycemic episode, the nurse should document the initial blood glucose levels and symptoms experienced by the patient. The amount of glucose needed to return the patient to a euglycemic state and any other pertinent information regarding dietary intake, medication, or activity that may have contributed to the hypoglycemic episode should be documented. Based on this information, adjustments in medication or diet may be necessary to prevent future hypoglycemia.

NUTRITION

Hospital nutrition services must be flexible in meeting the needs of hospitalized patients with diabetes. Diabetes control is interrupted by adjustments in nutrition orders (such as NPO, clear liquids only, and parenteral or enteral feedings) that are necessary for the treatment of other conditions. Medication adjustments need to match the altered intake to avoid acute complications, most notably hypoglycemia. Patients must be carefully monitored for glucose fluctuations resulting from changes in therapy.

Some hospitalized patients will require insulin therapy for the entire length of stay to maintain euglycemia, promote healing, and speed recovery. NPO patients, especially those with type 1 diabetes, require insulin to maintain glycemic control and avoid DKA. The long-accepted ADA and American Dietetic Association calculated calorie diets may not be appropriate (21,22). The ADA Clinical Practice Recommendations do not support the use of NCS (no concentrated sweets) or NAS (no added sugar) meal plans frequently seen in hospital settings because these infer that only sweet foods raise blood glucose. Ideally, most patients will use some version of a "consistent carbohydrate diabetes meal plan" (21,23), with the exception of patients who are counting carbohydrates and matching insulin dose with insulin-to-carbohydrate ratio(s).

Insulin pump users and those patients who follow an intensive insulin management regimen may be more comfortable with a hospital's regular meal plan so they can choose from the tray and adjust their meal bolus accordingly. Care must be taken to ensure that the carbohydrate content of the meal plan is always addressed when other diet restrictions are necessary, such as reduced sodium or protein for hypertension/renal disease and reduced cholesterol for cardiovascular disease. The nurse must work with the dietitian to retain the carbohydrate amount and distribution as patients' dietary orders progress from NPO to liquids, soft foods, and foods of regular consistency. Liquid diets, clear or full, must include 150–200 g carbohydrate/day to prevent ketogenesis (22). Options for substitutions from preprinted hospital menus give patients added choices and reduce the chance that the meal will not be eaten. Care must be taken to ensure that substitute selections are known and available to the patient.

Parenteral and enteral feedings require special monitoring, careful nutrition formula selection, and diabetes medication adjustment. If the gastrointestinal tract is intact, enteral feeding is the preferred route (24). The duration of the need for parenteral or enteral feeding will drive the formula selection. It is necessary that the formula provide adequate nutrition along with acceptable glucose control and blood lipid concentrations. With parenteral nutrition, glucose control can be maintained with subcutaneous or intravenous insulin (Table 31.3). Insulin is delivered according to calculated protocols, and necessary adjustments are made regularly (25).

Gastroparesis presents a challenge in maintaining glucose control. Expect pre- and postmeal glucose values to be variable, and there will be a tendency toward hypoglycemia. Hyperglycemia alone can cause delayed gastric emptying (26). It is important to include the patient in meal planning because he or she might know what foods work best. A nutrition consult might be indicated.

Document patient responses to meals and glucose levels. The patient may experience a feeling of fullness and/or bloating with or without nausea and vomiting (24). Hypoglycemia treatment may vary according to what the patient can tolerate.

PRACTICAL POINT

Nurses have a vital role in assisting patients to discover ways to eat healthy and maintain diabetes control. Many opportunities for explanation and clarification occur in hospitals. Meal and snack adjustments, interrupted meals, changes in meal timing, alternate feedings, and hypoglycemia treatment, all of which occur in the hospital setting, provide opportunities for patient education. Every hospital nurse must be comfortable with the principles of good nutrition and healthy food choices, so patient questions can become a teachable moment (see CHAPTER 3 for more about healthy lifestyle choices).

Table 31.3 Inpatient Diabetes Management: Enteral Nutrition

Subcutaneous insulin	
Bolus tube feedings	▪ One-half of the total daily dose as basal insulin
	AND
	One-half of the total daily dose as rapid- or short-acting insulin, divided evenly before each tube feeding.
	▪ Give only one-half of the rapid- or short-acting insulin before a night feeding, and check the 3:00 A.M. blood glucose value.
Continuous tube feedings	▪ Basal insulin once every 24 h
	OR
	Half-dose basal insulin every 12 h
	OR
	Intermediate-acting insulin divided into three to four equal doses.
	▪ Use rapid-acting insulin every 3–4 h to maintain glucose levels at target levels.
Intravenous insulin drip	▪ Usually given insulin based on the amount of carbohydrate delivered: 1 unit for every 7.5–10 g plus 1 unit/h to cover hepatic glucose production.
	▪ Note that stress factors may increase the insulin requirement three- to fivefold from hepatic glucose production and insulin resistance.

Adapted from Glister and Vigersky (25).

PATIENT TEACHING

Much debate exists concerning the most opportune time for diabetes education. Patients are no longer routinely admitted to the hospital for newly diagnosed diabetes. Guidelines are now used to determine when a patient with diabetes requires hospitalization (27). Table 31.4 lists some admission guidelines for patients with diabetes.

Diabetes education for hospital patients must be based on the individual's learning ability. For newly diagnosed patients, education may be limited to basic survival skills. However, in patients with a history of diabetes, this provides an opportunity to assess a patient's self-management skills and perhaps correct any misconceptions. Observation of blood glucose monitoring technique, insulin administration, and insulin pump skills such as changing infusion sites and delivering bolus insulin can be done during a hospitalization. Use of various patient education materials such as take-home videos, books, and pamphlets helps ensure that patients have adequate instructions to remain safe until the next contact with a primary health care provider. Patients who have a more challenging treatment regimen may benefit from consultation with a diabetes care team while in the hospital.

The nurse is crucial to implementation of the teaching plan, which must begin early in the admission to prepare the patient for self-management. In addition, the nurse can help facilitate outpatient follow-up. Whether a short stay (<24 h) or an

Table 31.4 Hospital Admission Criteria for Patients With Diabetes

Admission is necessary

Life-threatening acute metabolic complications
DKA
- Blood glucose >250 mg/dl (13.0 mmol/l)
- pH <7.3
- HCO_3 <15
- Moderate ketonuria and/or ketonemia

Hyperglycemic hyperosmolar state
- Blood glucose >600 mg/dl (33.3 mmol/l)
- Serum osmolarity >320

Hypoglycemia with neuroglycopenia
- Blood glucose <50 mg/dl (2.8 mmol/l) and treatment has not resulted in prompt recovery of sensorium
- Coma, seizures, or altered behavior from documented or suspected hypoglycemia
- Hypoglycemia caused by a sulfonylurea drug

Admission may be appropriate
- Substantial and chronic suboptimal metabolic control
- Severe chronic complications of diabetes
- Institution of continuous subcutaneous insulin infusion (insulin pump). (Some physicians or health care professionals admit patients to start insulin pump therapy because they can be closely monitored.)
- Newly diagnosed diabetes in children and adolescents
- Uncontrolled or newly diagnosed insulin requiring diabetes during pregnancy

From the ADA (27).

inpatient admission, the opportunity to provide diabetes teaching, review, and reinforcement must not be missed.

Patients With Known Diabetes

For the previously diagnosed patient, nurses must assess the current level of knowledge regarding diabetes management. Only through evaluation of the patient's current knowledge can the nurse review, reinforce, and observe self-management

Diabetes Survival Skills

- How and when to take medications
- How and when to monitor blood glucose
- Meal planning basics
- How to treat hypoglycemia
- Date of next doctor's appointment
- How to access further education as an outpatient
- Sick-day management
- When to call a physician

Reprinted with permission from American Healthways (5).

skills. Whether for a short stay (<23-h admission) or inpatient admission, diabetes review and reinforcement should be included in the plan of care.

Patients New to Insulin

Patients diagnosed with type 1 diabetes are not routinely hospitalized for the initiation and adjustment of insulin. However, patients with new-onset hyperglycemia admitted with DKA will need to begin insulin therapy during hospitalization. At times, although not ideal, the educational process must begin in the intensive care unit. Once the patient is stabilized, the remaining time spent in the hospital may be brief. Therefore, the nurse must be alert to the patient's progress and begin teaching insulin administration and self-monitoring of blood glucose as soon as the patient is able to participate. If family members are available, they should be included in these teaching sessions to support and assist the patient in this period of adjustment. The educational focus is on the survival skills needed to make the transition to the home setting. Home care referral may be needed to continue and reinforce diabetes self-management skills.

Although individuals with newly diagnosed type 2 diabetes do not depend on exogenous insulin for survival, because of the progressive nature of the disease, many of these individuals will decrease insulin production over time and require insulin for adequate blood glucose control, especially during times of stress and illness (28,29). Patients must be informed that the change to insulin is not a failure on their part and occurs due to the exhaustion of β-cell function. When teaching patients about insulin administration, the goal is for the patient to understand and successfully demonstrate the following skills, with validation by the nurse:

- insulin storage and injection preparation
- pharmacokinetics of the insulin action, peak, and duration
- injection site selection and correct injection technique
- needle safety

See CHAPTER 4 for more on insulin administration.

Newly Diagnosed Type 2 Diabetes and Pre-Diabetes

It is important that the hospitalized patient with newly diagnosed diabetes or pre-diabetes have an understanding of the seriousness of the new diagnosis and the importance of follow-up with their health care provider. The nurse should facilitate scheduling outpatient follow-up after discharge and provide the patient with the positive message that making healthy lifestyle choices now may affect the progression of their disease.

PATIENT CONCERNS

Patients with diabetes admitted to the hospital fall into two broad categories: those with optimal glucose control and those with suboptimal control. Nurses must address patient needs in each case. Patients accustomed to managing their diabetes in their own way find it difficult to relinquish control and trust the health care team to take over. These patients are often sure about what is wrong, why it is wrong, and what needs to be done to fix it. They can be adamant about when and how much insulin should be given, how often glucose should be monitored, and exactly what should be on their meal plan at every meal. The best way for nurses

---

DISCHARGE PLANNING

Discharge planning anticipates what the patient will need to continue diabetes management at home and must be initiated early in admission. By anticipating needs early, patients and their families are better informed and more confident about how they will care for themselves at home. The nurse needs to coordinate with interdisciplinary team members in planning care, teaching and reinforcing skills, and connecting with community resources for self-management support after discharge. Financial assistance, links to diabetes services and community resources, and evaluation of an existing support system minimize barriers and promote successful diabetes self-management.

---

to take advantage of the expertise that the patient brings to his or her diabetes management is to make the patient a central part of the health care team and facilitate and accommodate the patient's wishes as much as possible. When it is not possible to accommodate the patient's wishes, an understanding attitude and detailed explanations about why the care is being managed the way it is will assist the patient in accepting the new treatment plan. Reassure the patient that the medical and nursing staff are working toward achieving the best health outcome possible while resolving the current health problem and that they support the patient's timely discharge home, where the patient can return to his or her regular self-management routine.

Patients who are having difficulty making the lifestyle changes necessary to attain glycemic control present a different challenge. Nurses have a unique opportunity afforded by a hospital stay to work with the patient and discover some of the barriers to achieving better control. Unit teaching protocols, audiovisual aids, consultations with dietitians, and referrals to outside sources for ongoing education can help address educational needs. CHAPTER 21 provides additional insight into providing support to the patient struggling with the day-to-day tasks of diabetes care. Teaching with every medication administration, discussion of glucose readings, careful explanation of all tests and lab results, assistance with food choices from a menu, and solicitation of support from family and friends can all send the message that diabetes control is important and possible.

SPECIAL CONSIDERATIONS

Surgery

During their lifetimes, many patients with diabetes will require surgery. Regardless of whether the surgery is related to diabetes, managing diabetes during the pre-, intra-, and postoperative periods presents a challenge (see also "Diabetes and Surgery," a patient handout in RESOURCES). Several studies indicate that suboptimal diabetes control increases lengths of stay and rates of infection (30). The stress of surgery itself upsets control, increasing the secretion of counterregulatory hormones, inhibiting the release of endogenous insulin, and supporting ketogenesis (31). Interruption of the patient's usual management adds to this problem. Depending on the type of surgery, nutritional intake can be different from normal intake for short to extended periods. In addition, the surgical team may not be familiar with the patient's presurgery management and fail to reinitiate the treatment regimen. Long-term cardiac, renal, and neuropathic diabetes complications can put the patient at greater risk of postoperative complications. For all of these reasons, diabetes status must be carefully assessed and glucose control maintained during each hospitalization for surgery.

Whether surgery is planned or an emergency procedure, the decision regarding how to maintain glucose control depends on the type of diabetes, the type of surgery, and the length of time before the patient will be able to return to the preoperative diabetes treatment plan. For example,

- For same-day, short-stay surgery, major changes are not usually required.
- Most pump patients do not remove the pump or change their basal rates.
- Whenever possible, surgery for diabetes should be scheduled early in the day to reduce the effect on the patient's treatment plan.
- Medication management would be similar to the management used for the inpatient, except metformin, which should always be discontinued (see "Medication Management" in this chapter and Table 5.2 in CHAPTER 5).

Patients on insulin should continue their long- or intermediate-acting insulin the day before surgery. Patients may be individually advised to lower their bedtime NPH or evening Lantus dose the day prior to the admission. On the morning of surgery, one-half of the usual dose of long- or intermediate-acting insulin is given and capillary blood glucose is monitored every 2 h. A slow glucose infusion (100–125 ml/h of 5% dextrose) is given to prevent hypoglycemia, and hyperglycemia can be treated with small doses of regular insulin every 4–6 h or rapid-acting insulin every 2 h at ~0.05–0.1 units/kg. In individuals with type 2 diabetes who are not managed with insulin, oral agents should be discontinued 24 h before surgery and insulin administered if blood glucose levels are >180 mg/dl (>10.0 mmol/l).

Management of diabetes during an outpatient procedure, or *day surgery*, may be accomplished with intravenous or subcutaneous insulin in patients with type 1 or type 2 diabetes. Insulin should be used in patients with type 2 diabetes if blood glucose levels are >180 mg/dl (10.0 mmol/l). When individuals are discharged, directions should be given for frequent blood glucose monitoring with an algorithm for supplemental short- or rapid-acting insulin to be administered. Patients with type 2 diabetes who can resume their previous management should do so, but they may require supplemental short- or rapid-acting insulin to treat stress-related hyperglycemia. Instruction should be given to call the health care provider if capillary blood glucose levels are >250 mg/dl (13.9 mmol/l) (32).

Emergency Services

The acute complications of diabetes are frequently treated in the emergency room. Accurate assessment and diagnosis is critical. The symptoms of severe hypoglycemia may mimic a stroke, and a stroke may mimic severe hypoglycemia. The guidelines presented throughout this chapter also apply to the emergency department nurse. It is important for the emergency room staff to communicate with the primary care physician or diabetes health care provider regarding admissions to the emergency department. Some individuals inappropriately use emergency services to obtain supplies, including insulin. Appropriate referrals for routine services and education need to be made by the emergency department staff to alleviate improper use of emergency services and improve continuity of care.

SUMMARY

Because >6% of the U.S. population has diabetes, and ~41 million have pre-diabetes, hospital nurses in all units need to be proficient in caring for people with diabetes and hyperglycemia (33). Nurses must be familiar with the basic elements of care as well as the protocols necessary for acute care management.

Specific management protocols, order sets, treatment algorithms (for insulin drips, hypoglycemia, and hyperglycemic crises, either DKA or hyperglycemic hyperosmolar syndrome), and clinical pathways should be developed and implemented by institutions to guide the best practice for caring for the hospitalized patient with diabetes (34). With adequate training, all units can be prepared to administer intravenous insulin (2,35). The need for intravenous insulin should never be the criterion for transfer to a higher level of care. When diabetes management is seen as an integral part of the treatment of other acute medical problems, outcomes are improved and hospital stays are shortened (2). Studies provide supporting evidence about the importance of glycemic control during acute illness, and this valuable research must be incorporated into clinical practice to improve outcomes and quality of life for patients with diabetes.

REFERENCES

1. Centers for Disease Control and Prevention: *National Diabetes Fact Sheet: United States, 2003*. Atlanta, GA, Centers for Disease Control and Prevention, 2003
2. Levetan CS, Magee MF: Hospital management of diabetes. *Endocrinol Metab Clin* 29:745–770, 2000
3. Umpierrez GE, Isaacs SD, Bazargan N, You X, Thaler LM, Kitabchi AE: Hyperglycemia: an independent marker of in-hospital mortality in patients with undiagnosed diabetes. *J Clin Endocrinol Metab* 87:978–982, 2002
4. Levetan C, Passaro M, Jablonski K, Kass M, Ratner R: Unrecognized diabetes among hospitalized patients. *Diabetes Care* 21:246–249, 1998
5. American Healthways: *Inpatient Management Guidelines for People with Diabetes*. Nashville, TN, American Healthways, 2003
6. American Diabetes Association: Standards of medical care in diabetes (Position Statement). *Diabetes Care* 28 (Suppl. 1):S4–S36, 2005
7. Malmberg K: Prospective randomized study of intensive insulin treatment on long term survival after acute myocardial infarction in patients with diabetes mellitus. *BMJ* 314:1512–1518, 1997
8. Clement S, Braithwaite SS, Magee MF, Ahmann A, Smith EP, Schager RG, Hirsch IB, Diabetes in Hospitals Writing Committee: Management of diabetes and hyperglycemia in hospitals (Technical Review). *Diabetes Care* 27:553–591, 2004
9. American Association of Clinical Endocrinologists: American College of Endocrinology Consensus Development Conference on Inpatient Diabetes and Metabolic Control (Position Statement) [Internet], 2003. Available from http://www.aace.com/pub/ICC/inpatientStatement.php. Accessed 24 December 2003
10. Furnary AP, Gao G, Grunkemeier GL, Wu Y, Zerr KJ, Bookin SO, Floten HS, Starr A: Continuous insulin infusion reduces mortality in patients with

diabetes undergoing coronary artery bypass grafting. *J Thorac Cardiovasc Surg* 125:1007–1021, 2003

11. Estrada CA, Young JA, Nifong LW, Chitwood WR: Outcomes and perioperative hyperglycemia in patients with or without diabetes mellitus undergoing coronary artery bypass grafting. *Ann Thorac Surg* 75:1392–1399, 2003

12. McAlister F, Man J, Bistritz L, Amad H, Tandon P: Diabetes and coronary artery bypass surgery: an examination of perioperative glycemic control and outcomes. *Diabetes Care* 26:1518–1524, 2003

13. Yendamuri S, Fulda GJ, Tinkoff GH: Admission hyperglycemia as a prognostic indicator in trauma. *J Trauma* 55:33–38, 2003

14. Van den Berghe G, Wouters P, Weekers F, Varwaest C, Bruyninckx F, Schetz M, Vlasselaers D, Ferdinande P, Lauwers P, Bouillon R: Intensive insulin therapy in critically ill patients. *N Engl J Med* 345:1359–1367, 2001

15. Peragallo-Dittko V: Monitoring. In *A Core Curriculum for Diabetes Education*. 5th ed. Franz MJ, Ed. Chicago, American Association of Diabetes Educators, 2003, p. 189–209

16. American Diabetes Association: Bedside blood glucose monitoring in hospitals (Position Statement). *Diabetes Care* 27 (Suppl. 1):S104, 2004

17. Walker EA: Quality assurance for blood monitoring. *Nurs Clin North Am* 28:61–70, 1993

18. American Diabetes Association: Tests of glycemia in diabetes (Position Statement). *Diabetes Care* 27 (Suppl. 1):S91–S93, 2004

19. Queale W, Seidler A, Brancatti F: Glycemic control and sliding scale insulin use in medical inpatients with diabetes mellitus. *Arch Intern Med* 157:545–551, 1997

20. Braithwaite S, Buie M, Thompson C, Baldwin D, Oertel M, Robertson B, Mehrotra H: Hospital hypoglycemia: not only treatment but also prevention. *Endocr Pract* 10 (Suppl. 2):88–99, 2004

21. Valentine V: Patient with diabetes mellitus. In *Medical-Surgical Nursing: Assessment and Management of Clinical Problems*. 5th ed. Schrefer S, Ed. St. Louis, MO, Mosby, 2000, p. 1367–1405

22. Franz M: Medical nutrition therapy for diabetes. In *A Core Curriculum for Diabetes Education*. 5th ed. Franz MJ, Ed. Chicago, IL, American Association of Diabetes Educators, 2003, p. 1–58

23. American Diabetes Association: Diabetes nutrition recommendations for health care institutions (Position Statement). *Diabetes Care* 27 (Suppl. 1):S55–S57, 2004

24. Coulston AM: Enteral nutrition in patients with diabetes mellitus. *Curr Opin Clin Nutr Metab Care* 3:11–15, 2000

25. Glister B, Vigersky R: Perioperative management of type 1 diabetes mellitus. *Endocrinol Metab Clin North Am* 32:411–436, 2003

26. Rayner CK, Samson M, Jones KL, Horowitz M: Relationships of upper gastrointestinal motor and sensory function with glycemic control. *Diabetes Care* 24:371–381, 2001

27. American Diabetes Association: Hospital admission guidelines for diabetes mellitus (Position Statement). *Diabetes Care* 27 (Suppl. 1):S103, 2004

28. American Diabetes Association: Insulin administration (Position Statement). *Diabetes Care* 27 (Suppl. 1):S106–S109, 2004

29. King E, Lipps S: Illness and surgery. In *A Core Curriculum for Diabetes Education*. 5th ed. Franz MJ, Ed. Chicago, American Association of Diabetes Educators, 2003, p. 313–331

30. Schaberg DS, Norwood JM Case study: infections in diabetes mellitus. *Diabetes Spectrum* 25:37–40, 2002
31. Jacober SJ, Sowers JR: Management of diabetes in patients undergoing surgery. *Pract Diabetol* 20:7–14, 2001
32. Marks JB: Perioperative management of diabetes. *Am Fam Phys* 67:93–100, 2003
33. Centers for Disease Control and Prevention: *National Diabetes Fact Sheet: General Information and National Estimates on Diabetes in the United States, 2002.* Atlanta, GA, U.S. Department of Health and Human Services, Centers for Disease Control and Prevention, 2003
34. Quevedo S, Sullivan E, Kington R, Rogers W: Improving diabetes care in the hospital using guideline-directed orders. *Diabetes Spectrum* 14:226–233, 2001
35. Metchick LN, Petit WA, Inzucchi SE: Inpatient management of diabetes. *Am J Med* 113:317–323, 2002

Ms. English has recently retired as a Diabetes Clinical Nurse Specialist. Ms. Young is the Program Director for the Inpatient Diabetes Management Program at Pitt County Memorial Hospital, University Health Systems of Eastern Carolina, Greenville, NC.

32. Role of the Office Nurse in Diabetes Management

Kathy J. Berkowitz, APRN, BC, FNP, CDE

Over the past 20 years, the responsibility for the care of people with diabetes has shifted away from hospitals and toward primary care (1,2). Office visits have increased by 16% since 1992. At that time, the patient was seen by a physician in 95.8% of visits and a registered or licensed practical nurse in 31.3% of visits. In 2001, diabetes was among the five leading diagnoses and accounted for 3.1% of all visits (3). Expenditures for visits attributable to diabetes were $10 billion in 2002 (4), and duration of contact with the physician was between 6 and 30 min (3).

Significant opportunities exist for nurses in ambulatory care, as the emphasis in health care has shifted from acute episodic care to prevention and health maintenance. Nurses in ambulatory care have been historically underused (5). Shifting the care of patients with complex disease states to physician offices has changed and expanded ambulatory nursing practice (6). Furthermore, patient education activities have extended beyond treatment preparation instructions to include the culturally sensitive counseling of individuals and their families on lifestyle changes that prevent or mediate chronic disease.

Although the dimension of ambulatory nursing interventions has expanded, control over the encounter still primarily remains with the patient; acceptance of and implementation of health care regimens are determined by the patient. Thus, to appropriately counsel the patient with diabetes, the nurse in an ambulatory care setting needs to be competent in using technology, critical thinking, and evaluative skills and in the implementation of effective interpersonal, culturally sensitive communication (7).

MEDICAL OFFICE PRACTICE

Today, in an ambulatory setting, a nurse's function includes a diverse set of roles oriented toward collaborative practice, managing continuity of care, and using other nursing staff to triage patients and provide clinically complex care. Previously, nursing functions in small-office settings were minimal, usually involving such things as administering injections and assisting with procedures. However, as physicians began to create large specialty-group practices, organized nursing services began to emerge that focused on the abilities to respond to knowledgeable, service-oriented clients and to assist physicians in practice management (8).

ROLES AND COMPETENCIES

Nursing competency is determined by the individual nurse's education, knowledge, certification, experience, and abilities. Each nurse is responsible for identifying appropriate practice parameters within a state's nurse practice act, professional code and professional practice standards, and employer policies and for performing activities or functions in accordance with the nurse's own educational level and competence. In addition to clinical core competencies, the office nurse must demonstrate role-based competencies related to the management and coordination of patient care, supervision of unlicensed assisting personnel, management of relationships with clients and families, documentation of care provided, and support of office operations (7).

The nurse's role becomes a strong source of continuity. In specialty-practice settings such as a diabetes clinic, nurses will often work with patients and their families over extended periods while engaging in patient teaching, follow-up activities, and monitoring outcomes. They will continue to assist patients in accessing care throughout health care networks, and increasingly they will be making clients aware of their rights and negotiate on the patient's behalf when the patient is not well served (7).

TEAM RELATIONSHIPS

In partnership with the patient, nursing practice occurs within the context of a multidisciplinary team comprised of other licensed professionals, technicians, and unlicensed assisting personnel. In office settings, nurses typically work much more closely and continuously with physicians and other health care providers.

The nursing role on the ambulatory care team is limited only by the nurse's willingness to perform, levels of knowledge and competency, time restraints, and ability to negotiate the role with the team. In cases where more than one provider is able to meet patient needs, responsibilities for care will require negotiation. Areas of potential role overlap include determining which discipline performs screening assessments and who documents data regarding past history, medications, allergies, and response to treatment. As attempts to develop cost-effective delivery models occur, health care teams are being reconfigured so provider levels meet the needs of the patient without unnecessary duplication and without compromising outcomes (7). For example, nurse-managed health maintenance organizations and nurse-run clinics may be able to manage populations with diabetes more effectively and efficiently (9–15).

One factor frequently identified by office nurses is the unique collaborative relationship between the nurse and the physician. This role requires that the nurse demonstrate the ability to communicate effectively. The nurse becomes a conduit between the patient, who is self-managing his or her diabetes daily, and the physician, who may be directing care without having seen the patient, helping the two parties make decisions based on what may have been identified in a telephone assessment. Telephone communication with nurses has been shown to positively affect patient satisfaction as well as perceptions of easy access (16).

IMPROVING PATIENT CARE

Many U.S. adults with diabetes are receiving suboptimal care, and empirical data suggest that compliance with diabetes clinical practice recommendations is

---

Table 32.1 Maximizing Care at Office Visits

- Identify patients with diabetes
- Contact patients with reminder letters for appointments and list specific tests to be completed before the visit, e.g., glycated hemoglobin A_{1c}, lipids
- Encourage patients to be involved in their own care: get them to think about what they hope to accomplish and identify areas in which they may need assistance before the visit
- Facilitate the use of standardized assessment tools, encounter forms, and diabetes flow sheets to ensure that key standards of care are not overlooked
- Facilitate the use of technology, e.g., uploading blood glucose data to the Internet, faxing records, etc.

---

inadequate in primary care (17,18). There is growing evidence that, in the family physician's office, enhancing the role of the nurse can save lives and money (19).

High-quality diabetes care consists of a combination of factors: a knowledgeable staff, an involved patient empowered to improve his or her care, and an office practice system designed to help the care process. Practice systems have been identified as the richest area of improved care for most medical office practices. Most approaches have been multidisciplinary, but often the primary staff member responsible for delivering intervention and monitoring guidelines has been a nurse (20–22). Comprehensive diabetes care using a prioritized record-keeping system, such as diabetes care checklists, can help identify the important tasks that need to be performed during each office visit (23). The office nurse can serve a vital role in assisting in the development of these improved practice systems. Pre-planning for office visits can increase the quality of patient encounters and prevent excessive follow-up work (Tables 32.1 and 32.2).

PATIENT EDUCATION

Diabetes self-management education is the key to successful diabetes management. The office nurse can play a significant role in empowering patients to accept their disease and take responsibility for their health. Diabetes self-management training must start at the time of diagnosis with the initiation of survival skills

---

Table 32.2 Facilitating ADA Standards of Diabetes Care

- Ensure collection of and record results of key laboratory tests
- Measure and record blood pressure and weight at each visit
- Have the patient remove his or her shoes and socks for a foot examination
- Coordinate and document referrals for nutrition counseling and self-management training
- Coordinate and document annual referrals to an eye care specialist, dental care, or other health care professionals as appropriate
- Administer/document annual flu vaccination and pneumococcal vaccination
- Monitor smoking status/cessation referral

From ADA (24).

training and continue throughout the health care relationship. The depth of education offered to the patient in the office setting will be determined by the knowledge and skills of the nurse. Teaching opportunities generally occur at the time of the individual visit, or sometimes, several patients with similar learning needs may be offered a class in the waiting room or another identified space. Group visits can provide beneficial discussions and support while improving efficiency. Referral to a dietitian, diabetes self-management training program, or certified diabetes educator is recommended.

PRACTICAL POINT

Key Assessment Questions (see also CHAPTER 17)
- What is your goal for this visit?
- What is the most difficult issue for you in managing your diabetes?
- Are you willing to do something about it?
- What changes would you suggest to make things better?

Survival Skills Education

- Basic nutrition guidelines
- Healthy eating habits
- Role of physical activity
- Monitoring glycemic control
- Record keeping of blood glucose levels
- Medication administration and side effects
- Symptoms of and treatment for hyperglycemia and hypoglycemia
- Sick-day management
- Skin/dental care
- Emergency phone numbers and when to call for help
- Community resources/support

SUMMARY

Nurses in the office setting have a unique opportunity to help people with diabetes and their families adjust to the disease and advised lifestyle changes, improve patient care, and identify support systems and resources within the community.

REFERENCES

1. Goyder EC, McNally PG, Drucquer M, Spiers N, Botha JL: Shifting of care for diabetes from secondary to primary care 1990–5: review of general practices. *BMJ* 316:1505–1506, 1998

2. Ho M, Marger M, Beart J, Yip I, Shekelle P: Is the quality of diabetes care better in a diabetes clinic or in a general medicine clinic? *Diabetes Care* 20:472–475, 1997
3. Cherry DK, Burt CW, Woodwell DA: *National Ambulatory Medical Care Survey: 2001 Summary: Advance Data #337.* Hyattsville, MD, U.S. Department of Health and Human Services, Centers for Disease Control and Prevention, National Center for Health Statistics, 2003
4. American Diabetes Association: Economic costs of diabetes in the U.S. in 2002. *Diabetes Care* 26:917–932, 2003
5. Marszelak E: Ambulatory nursing: at the crossroads? *Nurs Health Care* 1:254–255, 1980
6. Curran C: An interview with Linda D'Angelo. *Nurs Econ* 13:193–196, 1995
7. American Academy of Ambulatory Care Nursing, American Nurses Association: *Nursing in Ambulatory Care.* Silver Spring, MD, American Nurses Publishing, 1997
8. Moore M, Geving A: Nursing's role in the ambulatory care setting. *Med Group Manage J* 37:18–24, 1990
9. Aubert R, Herman W, Waters J, Moore W, Sutton D, Peterson B, Bailey C, Koplan J: Nurse case management to improve glycemic control in diabetes patients in a health maintenance organization. *Ann Intern Med* 129: 605–612, 1998
10. Wagner E, Grothaus L, Sandhu N, Galvin M, McGregor M, Artz K, Coleman E: Chronic care clinics for diabetes in primary care. *Diabetes Care* 24:695–700, 2001
11. Pine D, Madlon-Kay D, Sauser M: Effectiveness of a nurse-based intervention in a community practice on patients' dietary fat intake and total serum cholesterol level. *Arch Fam Med* 6:129–134, 1997
12. Denver E, Barnard M, Woolfson R, Earle K: Management of uncontrolled hypertension in a nurse-led clinic compared with conventional care for patients with type 2 diabetes. *Diabetes Care* 26:2256–2260, 2003
13. Taylor C, Miller N, Reilly K, Greenwald G, Cunning D, Deeter A, Abascal L: Evaluation of a nurse-care management system to improve outcomes in patients with complicated diabetes. *Diabetes Care* 26:1058–1063, 2003
14. New J, Mason J, Freemantle N, Teasdale S, Wong L, Bruce N, Burns J, Gibson J: Specialist nurse-led intervention to treat and control hypertension and hyperlipidemia in diabetes (SPLINT). *Diabetes Care* 26:2250–2255, 2003
15. Davidson M: Effect of nurse-directed diabetes care in a minority population. *Diabetes Care* 26:2281–2287, 2003
16. Mastal M, Bulgar J, Chinault L, Donaghue J, Klein M, Kraynak M, Lusk E, McNamara M, Pray M, Roberts B, Zopp L: *Functions and Outcomes of Advice Nursing Practice* (unpublished research study). Kaiser Permanente Mid-Atlantic States Region, 1993
17. Saaddine J, Engelgau M, Beckles G, Gregg E, Thompson T, Narayan K: A diabetes report card for the United States: quality of care in the 1990s. *Ann Intern Med* 136:565–571, 2002
18. Renders C, Valk G, Griffin S, Wagner E, Eijk Van J, Assendelft W: Interventions to improve the management of diabetes in primary care, outpatient, and community settings: a systematic review. *Diabetes Care* 24: 1821–1833, 2001
19. O'Connor P: Improving diabetes care: organize your office, intensify your care. *J Am Board Fam Pract* 14:320–322, 2001

20. White B: Making diabetes checkups more fruitful. *Fam Pract Manag* 7:51–52, 2000
21. Glasgow R: Translating research to practice. *Diabetes Care* 26:2451–2456, 2003
22. Cohen S: Potential barriers to diabetes care. *Diabetes Care* 6:499–500, 1983
23. Reith P: Comprehensive diabetes care in the office. *Clinical Diabetes* 11: 109–114, 1993
24. American Diabetes Association: Standards of medical care in diabetes (Position Statement). *Diabetes Care* 28 (Suppl. 1):S4–S36, 2005

Ms. Berkowitz is the Professional Course Coordinator, Diabetes Unit, at the Grady Health System, Atlanta, GA.

33. Role of the Home Health Care Nurse

CARYL ANN O'REILLY, RN, MBA, CDE

The home health care nurse is an increasingly important member of the health care team. Patients are now discharged from hospitals and rehabilitation centers early in the episode of illness and require more sophisticated nursing management at home. The home health care nurse serves as the liaison between the health care team and the patient and his or her family and caregivers and is often the only professional who has a complete overview of the patient's medical regimen and, thus, has responsibility for the coordination of care.

NURSING ASSESSMENT

Patients are referred to home care agencies for acute episodes of care. The tool used to determine patient needs is the Outcome and Assessment Information Set (OASIS) (1). If used correctly, OASIS can give important information about the patient's functional deficits and illuminate the patient's specific needs from skilled nursing. There are 13 domains, or sections, that provide clinical information, such as patient history and integumentary, respiratory, elimination, and emotional/behavioral status. Additionally, living arrangements, support system, therapy needs related to activities of daily living (ADLs) and independent activities of daily living (IADLs), medication management, and equipment management are addressed. Patients may not always give accurate information, particularly when related to incontinence and vision. Understating the patient's status will lead to reduced payment for services as well as underservicing the patient. OASIS is required when care is initiated, interrupted, and resumed, when the patient is discharged, and when there is a significant change in health status. Managed care insurers often authorize only one or two nursing visits for assessment and teaching. Accurately identifying and documenting patient status can be the catalyst for patients to receive the care necessary to return to optimal health and functional status. OASIS provides standardized information, tracks patient outcomes, and is valuable for data collection and research potential.

The initial assessment of a patient should include the observations found in Table 33.1. Risks identified can then be evaluated and incorporated into the care plan for each patient.

Table 33.1 Initial Patient Assessment

Area of Observation	Risk

Age	■ Mental status
	  – Confusion
	  – Depression
	  – Loneliness
	■ Dehydration
	■ Neuropathy
	■ Urinary tract infection (UTI)
	■ Falls

Incontinence	■ UTI ■ Skin breakdown ■ Falls ■ Embarrassment
Visual deficit	■ Medication errors ■ Falls ■ Inability to test blood glucose
Polypharmacy	■ Drug interactions ■ Multiple physicians ■ Expense ■ Timing and action of medications ■ Hypo-/hyperglycemia

Age

Age is an important factor in patient assessment. More than 50% of people newly diagnosed with diabetes are ≥65 years of age, and most patients referred to home care are between the ages of 65 and 85 years (2). Age-related changes in the body can alter clinical presentation. With increased age, symptoms of hyperglycemia, such as polyuria, polydipsia, and polyphagia, may be absent. After congestive heart failure, diabetes is ranked second as the primary diagnosis at entry into home care and is the top diagnosis if primary and secondary diagnoses are combined.

Seniors may exhibit cognitive impairment, but this has to be evaluated carefully. Hyperglycemia, dehydration, and hypoglycemia can profoundly affect cognitive function. This may result in limitations in ADLs, undiagnosed depression, and social isolation. Normalizing blood glucose levels may restore a patient's ability to communicate and participate more fully in diabetes self-management. Too hasty a judgment by the home care nurse may overlook important, yet subtle, alterations in mental and emotional status. The mechanism associated with diabetes and cognitive impairment is unclear but may be related to episodes of hypoglycemia.

Dehydration

Dehydration is a serious complication of diabetes. Seniors lose moisture through thinning dermal layers. They do not sense thirst until they are already significantly dehydrated and may choose not to drink water because of fear of incontinence or nocturnal polyuria. Dehydration alone can increase the blood glucose level as well as medication concentrations in the blood. Also, renal threshold increases with age, compounding the problem. Patients should be encouraged to drink ≥48 oz water daily as long as there are no contraindications such as heart failure. Having a filled water bottle available, with cuing by the family or caregiver, may be helpful. Identifying the potential for dehydration, instructing the patient and/or caregiver in identifying and treating dehydration, and the response to this instruction should be documented in the patient record.

Neuropathies

Nerve damage occurs in 50% of individuals with diabetes age >60 years. Autonomic neuropathies may be difficult to detect but can have various manifestations, e.g., abnormal heart rate or orthostatic hypotension, that can be life-threatening indicators (see CHAPTER 14). It is advisable to obtain a blood pressure reading while the patient is sitting, followed by a standing reading, if the patient indicates dizziness or lightheadedness on standing. Although there is no cure for this form of neuropathy, detection and preventive measures such as compression stockings and dangling the legs before standing can prevent serious outcomes. Hypoglycemia unawareness can result from impaired glucose counterregulation and may be a hidden cause of falls. Patients with symptomatic autonomic neuropathy have a threefold greater 5-year mortality rate than diabetes patients without autonomic neuropathy (3).

Alternating bouts of constipation followed by explosive diarrhea and gastroparesis are two common forms of gastrointestinal autonomic neuropathy. They impinge on quality of life and make glucose management difficult. There are pharmacological options available to the physician; therefore, it is important that the nurse document findings and communicate these with the primary care provider.

Bladder dysfunction and urinary tract infection (UTI) are related to both diabetic neuropathy and aging. Diabetic cystopathy is chronic, predisposing patients to UTIs. It is insidious, with the only early sign being increased intervals between times of urination. This leads to enlarged bladder, atonic musculature, and incomplete emptying (4). These factors increase the probability of a UTI. The usual signs and symptoms of a UTI are frequently absent in patients with diabetes, and the diagnosis may be missed. If a urinalysis is performed, a UTI can be suspected if the nitrites are positive regardless of the presence of leukocytes. A UTI should be suspected if blood glucose levels are elevated and other possible explanations are exhausted. The patient may complain of back pain, pressure in the lower abdomen, or dribbling of urine, or say they just don't feel well. A strong urine odor or signs of incontinence, such as a urine-stained chair pad or wet socks and shoes, may be recognized. Incontinence increases the risk of UTIs, falls, embarrassment, and social isolation. Bladder training should be considered. A consult to urology may be needed to assess the need for other interventions.

Peripheral neuropathy may cause pain or numbness in the lower extremities and make it difficult for the patient to determine where the foot is in relation to the floor. Intrinsic weakness of the small muscles of the foot can alter joint mobility and affect foot mechanics (5). Patients with neuropathy develop gait abnormalities and problems with balance, which increases the risk for falling. When gait abnormality is observed, a physical therapy consultation for evaluation and recommendation should be initiated.

Foot Care

Nurses should inspect a patient's feet at every visit. Podiatric intervention can be beneficial for providing patients with orthotic footwear for off-loading pressure. Medicare provides benefits to covered individuals for routine podiatric care and therapeutic footwear. A comprehensive nursing foot examination is an important part of the initial patient assessment and should be repeated at each recertification period to evaluate the progression of diabetic foot complications and promote early detection of vascular and nerve complications of the lower extremities. This should include a visual inspection of the feet, which includes assessment of color, temperature, pulses, and hair growth. A monofilament test for detecting the insensate foot is also extremely valuable and should be incorporated into the examination if possible (see CHAPTER 15).

Primary sites for repetitive stress injuries are the metatarsal heads and the great toe. Patients who are bed bound are at risk for pressure ulcers of the heel, which are second only to sacral pressure ulcers in prevalence (5). Heels should be protected at all times from pressure that prevents vascular perfusion, which leads to ischemia and tissue death. Limb loss is more likely to occur with a heel ulcer than with a forefoot ulcer, and functional disability is also more profound (5).

Eye Care

Visual deficits should be considered if the patient has had diabetes for ≥5 years. Many patients are able to disguise the fact that they are visually impaired when they are in their own environment. Patients frequently associate loss of vision with loss of independence and will avoid its discovery as long as possible. However, it is this compromised vision that leads to errors in medication, falls, and functional deficits (see CHAPTER 10).

The home care nurse is in the position to assess patients' visual acuity by asking them to read small print, such as a medication label or phone book. Visiting nurses should also observe the patient taking blood glucose levels to assure that a proper technique is being used. If vision is impaired, the patient may benefit from adaptive equipment to assist with blood glucose monitoring and insulin administration. If impairment is significant, the patient may be eligible for referral to a low-vision center and for services through their state's Commission for the Blind. Refer the patient to a local agency, such as The Lighthouse, which works with the Commission to provide patient ADL and mobility training (see RESOURCES for more information).

Medication Management

The nurse is in the unique position of being able to identify all of the medications the patient is taking. This may require an investigative approach, however. Patients often have several physicians (podiatrist, optometrist, etc.), each of whom may be prescribing medications. Patients generally assume that each provider communicates with the others regarding medications. Patients also take a variety of over-the-counter medications and herbal supplements that may have adverse interactions with prescribed medications. Have the patient or caregiver compile a complete list of medications and supplements that are being taken. In some cases, it is best that the nurse compose this list, examining the medications and their bottles and verifying medication adherence. This list should be taken to each health care provider's office and included in the patient's chart. Another copy

Table 33.2 Diabetes and Its Comorbidities

Comorbidity	Effect	Possible Referral
Hypertension	■ One of the risk factors for diabetes ■ Increases the likelihood of end-stage renal disease and stroke ■ Increases the likelihood of vision deficits	■ Nutrition consultation ■ Exercise physiologist ■ Low-vision center ■ Adaptive equipment
Coronary artery disease	■ Provides a snapshot of the probable condition of other small vessels ■ Women are at high risk ■ Increased incidence of myocardial infarction	■ Nutrition consultation ■ Exercise/cardiac rehabilitation after coronary artery bypass graft ■ Physical therapy
Depression	■ High prevalence in diabetes ■ Variety of causes 　– Expected, requires support 　– Clinical, requires intervention	■ Social work ■ Mental health team
Wounds	■ Uncontrolled diabetes = non-healing wound ■ Foot ulcers ■ Pressure sores	■ Wound, Ostomy, and Continence Nurses Society (WOCN) ■ Physical therapy ■ Podiatry ■ Nutrition consultation
Chronic obstructive pulmonary disease and other respiratory diseases	■ Medications often increase insulin resistance ■ Increased depression and anxiety	■ Physical therapy ■ Occupational therapy ■ Social work
Skeletal disease (osteoarthritis and osteoporosis)	■ Falls ■ Dexterity deficits ■ Unusual fractures	■ Physical therapy ■ Occupational therapy

should be readily available in the event that the patient requires hospitalization or emergency care.

Medication adherence is a major factor in achieving optimal diabetes control. Patients with diabetes have multiple comorbidities, each requiring one or more pharmacological agents as treatment. Cost may be a barrier to adherence. Ask patients whether they are able to afford polypharmacy. Most patients on fixed incomes have difficulty with the costs of medication. Sometimes, they will not let the physician know that they cannot afford the medication but will share this information with the nurse. Another barrier to adherence is a lack of knowledge about the timing of medications. Ask patients what kind of insulin they are taking. Frequently, they will know the brand name but not the type of insulin. There is a general lack of understanding about the time at which certain medications should be taken and why that timing is important. Adherence is not necessarily a matter of whether a patient will do what is medically indicated, but whether they have the knowledge, cognitive skills, finances, and physical ability to do what is indicated. For patients with difficulty, the nurse can help enhance adherence in a number of ways, by putting together a pill box, for instance, or by writing out instructions for taking their medications.

Nutrition

Meal planning and good nutrition are the cornerstones of optimal diabetes control. The home care nurse, however, should guard against being the "diet police." This has a negative effect on the patient and can be very unproductive. Understand that as the coordinator of care, the home care nurse assesses the patient's status, identifies problems, and, hopefully, leaves the patient with important "take-away" lifetime self-management skills, even though there is only a brief period of interaction with the patient. Rather than trying to change years of eating habits, it is more productive to identify one or two nutrition deficits that can be altered in the short term. For example, many individuals with diabetes continue to drink sugared soda or large amounts of juice or milk. Working with patients toward modifying this habit can have dramatic effects on blood glucose control, which may encourage the patient to consider additional changes. Referral to a diabetes self-management education program or a nutrition program for ongoing nutrition counseling is important.

COMMUNICATION

The coordinator of care has the opportunity and responsibility for 360-degree communication. Changes in status, positive and negative, should be documented and communicated to the patient, physician, therapist, home health aide, or other health care team member. This ongoing dialogue keeps the team focused on the plan of care and promotes desired outcomes. *Telehealth*, health care provided over technologies such as videoconferencing, the Internet, streaming media, and satellite and wireless communications, has been used in rural and inner city communities and is also entering the realm of home care nursing (6). Changes in communication strategies in the treatment of diabetes are revolutionizing the possibilities and role for the home care nurse.

PRACTICAL POINT

Documentation Is a Priority

All aspects of nursing assessment and interventions should be carefully documented, including patient response to procedure. Any changes noted should be documented, the patient and/or caregiver should be notified, and a written report should be sent to the physician. Documentation allows consistent levels of care to be provided and ensures that the patient's health care team is always aware of any issues arising during treatment.

SUMMARY

Home care nurses are in a position to be the "first-line" professional to assess and identify problems that physicians and other health care professionals may never see or recognize. By conducting a diabetes-specific assessment, home care nurses can act as advocates for people with diabetes as they detect, intervene, and facilitate care. It is important for home care nurses to communicate their findings to the health care team and ensure that follow-up has occurred, that interventions are effective, and that the message to the patient from all professionals is consistent and understood.

REFERENCES

1. Centers for Medicare and Medicaid Services web site. Available from http://www.cms.hhs.gov/oasis. Accessed 13 November 2004
2. Visiting Nurse Service of New York, Center for Home Care Policy and Research web site. Available from http://www.vnsny.org/research/homecare.html. Accessed 13 November 2004
3. Vinik A, Erbas T, Stansberry K: Gastrointestinal, genitourinary and neurovascular disturbances in diabetes. *Diabetes Reviews* 7:358–378, 1999
4. Porter D Jr, Sherwin RS: *Ellenberg and Rifkin's Diabetes Mellitus.* 5th ed. Stamford, CT, Appleton and Lange, 2001, p. 1054–1055
5. National Diabetes Education Program: *Feet Can Last A Lifetime: Revised Kit.* Bethesda, MD, National Diabetes Education Program, 2002
6. Office for the Advancement of Telehealth web site. Available from http://telehealth.hrsa.gov. Accessed 16 October 2004

Ms. O'Reilly is a Diabetes Clinical Nurse Specialist at the Visiting Nurse Service of New York, Staten Island, NY.

34. Diabetes Care in the Nursing Home

BELINDA P. CHILDS, ARNP, MN, CDE, BC-ADM

It is estimated that one in every three people in the U.S. will reside in a long-term care facility sometime during their life. Although only 11% of our population is currently >65 years of age, that figure is expected to grow to >20% by 2020 (1). When considering the aging of the population, the increased life expectancy, and the increase in diabetes prevalence, long-term care facilities will probably play an even larger role in providing care for the individual with diabetes. The nurse's role as advocate, care provider, and educator of staff, patient, and family will be pivotal.

Of nursing home residents ≥55 years of age, 18.3% have been diagnosed with diabetes compared with 12.6% of the general population in that same age-group. Also, people with diabetes who are ≥55 years of age are twice as likely as individuals without diabetes to reside in a long-term care facility. Residents with diabetes are more likely to be younger and nonwhite compared with residents who do not have diabetes. More than 80% have cardiovascular disease, 56% have hypertension, 39% have senile dementia, and 69% have two or more chronic conditions in addition to diabetes. The nursing home resident with diabetes also has a higher incidence of kidney failure (1).

Residents with diabetes compared with residents without diabetes show greater limitations in activities of daily living in terms of their ability to bathe (91.9 vs. 88.7% for diabetes versus no diabetes, respectively), dress (82.4 vs. 78.5%), perform toileting activities (72.9 vs. 68.6%), transfer from bed to chair (70.0 vs. 65.8%), walk (76.1 vs. 71.1%), and control bowel movements (48.4 vs. 44%). The two groups were similar in having difficulty feeding (35%) and controlling urine (42%). Nursing home residents with diabetes were considered more limited in the activities of daily living than the general population with diabetes (1).

The care of the resident with diabetes is complicated by the number of chronic conditions, their limitations in daily living activities, and specific management issues related to diabetes that differ from routine nursing home care (2). In addition, providing quality care is hampered by staff shortages, staff turnover, poor pay, and lack of education and educational materials on diabetes for the residents and staff in the nursing home setting.

Diabetes care in the nursing home is carried out primarily by vocational or licensed practical nurses, medication aides, and nurse's aides. The nurse is responsible for coordination of care and development of care plans for the residents.

UNDIAGNOSED DIABETES IN THE NURSING HOME

Over 5 million Americans have undiagnosed diabetes. Type 1 and type 2 diabetes can be diagnosed at any age. The polyuria of hyperglycemia in an incontinent patient may be overlooked. The polydipsia of hyperglycemia may not be recognized because of decreased thirst sensation in elderly patients. The signs and symptoms of hyperglycemia may go unnoticed. It is important to be alert to the potential for newly diagnosed diabetes in the nursing home setting.

All staff should have some knowledge of diabetes standards of care. The team approach to the delivery of care improves the quality of care.

CLINICAL IMPLICATIONS

Diabetes care areas that need special attention include glycemic control, diabetes medications, medication interactions, glucose monitoring, medical nutrition therapy (including hydration), acute and chronic complications of diabetes, and self-management education and empowerment of the individual with diabetes (Table 34.1).

Glycemic Control

Appropriate target blood glucose levels for this population remain controversial. The American Diabetes Association (ADA) notes that "less stringent treatment goals may be appropriate for patients with limited life expectancy, the very young or older adults, and in individuals with comorbid conditions. Severe or frequent hypoglycemia is an indication for modification of treatment regimens, including setting higher glycemic goals" (3).

However, the increased risk for dehydration, infection, and acute complications, greater sensitivity to pain, urinary incontinence, decreased visual acuity, and cognition may occur as a result of elevated glucose levels. Target levels designed to control hyperglycemia and prevent symptoms and acute complications are appropriate. Medical treatment options are improving, allowing for safer management of glucose levels. If one regimen is not achieving the identified glucose targets, then alternative medication strategies are indicated.

Diabetes Medication

Key considerations with medication include appropriate timing of the diabetes medications and monitoring for side effects. Most nursing home residents will be on insulin, oral agents, or a combination (2). It is important to properly administer the medication(s). Time constraints make the administration of multiple medications to residents a challenge for the nurse who must administer medications to several patients in a timely fashion. Inappropriate administration of diabetes medication can mean the difference between hypoglycemia, euglycemia, and hyperglycemia. Inconsistent timing of medication, especially insulin, can also lead to variable patterns in blood glucose levels. The health care provider who reviews the blood glucose records must be astute in asking the right questions before

Table 34.1 Considerations for Nurses Providing Diabetes Care in Nursing Homes

Diabetes Issues	Key Considerations
Diabetes medications	
Oral agents	Is the oral diabetes medication given on time, before the meal, or with food?
	What are the side effects? Are lab results and signs and symptoms observed routinely?
Insulin	Is the type of insulin to be given with or before the meal?
	Is the insulin being stored properly?
	Is a new bottle of insulin opened every 28 days?
	Are we rotating injections? Is there a way to document?
	Is the injection subcutaneous or intramuscular?
Medication interactions	Review medication after a hospitalization
	Review for potential interactions of medications
Medical nutrition therapy	Provide adequate calories, prevent malnutrition
	Consult the dietitian if problems exist
	Regular diet is acceptable with consistent carbohydrates in meals and snacks
	Obtain blood glucose levels 2 h after meals to determine the effect of foods
	Fats do not need to be restricted in the older population
	Consider the individual
Acute complications of diabetes	Observe for signs of DKA, HHS, and LA
	Contact the health care provider immediately with signs of DKA, HHS, or LA
	Protocols for treatment of hyperglycemia and hypoglycemia are valuable
	Be cautious to not overtreat hypoglycemia
	Recheck blood glucose 15–20 min after treatment; repeat treatment if needed
Chronic complications of diabetes	Follow the ADA Standards of Medical Care in Diabetes (3) to reduce risks for blindness, strokes, and amputations
Foot and skin care	Daily inspection for individuals who cannot inspect their own feet
	Weekly nurse examination of feet
	Careful skin care, prevention of ulcers and skin tears
	Referral to podiatrist for foot care/footwear
	The resident should always wear shoes whether walking or in a wheelchair
Empowerment/ self-care	Respect the individual's history of living with diabetes
	Provide choices whenever possible
	Include the family in care

ADA, American Diabetes Association; DKA, diabetic ketoacidosis; HHS, hyperglycemic hyperosmolar syndrome; LA, lactic acidosis.

making dosage adjustments. The health care provider and long-term care staff should also consider the timing of snacks. Note the insulin action table in CHAP-TER 4 when considering times for snacks, glucose testing, and increased activity. A person should match snacks with the peak of the insulin and avoid increased activity (such as physical therapy) during these peaks. If activity is increased, then monitoring blood glucose levels and, if required, providing an extra snack might be appropriate.

A well-trained health care provider must know the ins and outs of insulin therapy before making dose adjustments. For example, a 70/30 NPH/regular insulin formulation administered after breakfast and supper may lead to high postprandial blood glucose levels but low preprandial levels. The corrective action is not an adjustment in the dose of 70/30 NPH/regular but ensuring careful administration ≥15 min (preferably 30 min) before the meal. Moreover, a different formulation may also be appropriate. Usually, the doctor is called on for dose adjustments.

Storage and administration of insulin should be reviewed. Injection sites should be rotated, and hypertrophied or scarred areas should not be used for administering insulin. Attention should be given to the technique of insulin administration. A nurse may inadvertently administer the insulin in the muscle in a lean individual, which will cause the insulin to peak sooner, placing the patient at risk for hypoglycemia, and reduce its duration of action. Routine insulin should be administered subcutaneously. Insulin bottles should be dated and discarded when they have exceeded the usage limit, which is typically every 28 days (4,5).

It is important to monitor for potential side effects from antihyperglycemic oral agents. If a resident on thiazolidinediones develops edema or increasing congestive heart failure or if the resident has an increase in creatinine and he or she is on metformin, the health care provider should be notified. CHAPTER 5 reviews the potential side effects of oral agents and recommended monitoring techniques.

Medication Interactions

Polypharmacy can be an issue for individuals with diabetes. Control of the multiple complications requires treatment with multiple medications. CHAPTER 23 discusses the issues of polypharmacy.

Diligent review of medications and observation by the nurse can prevent a resident from experiencing serious side effects. If a resident returns to the facility after a hospitalization, a careful review of medications should occur. Compare the medication list before hospitalization and the discharge list on return to the facility. Medications may have been discontinued during the hospitalization that should have been restarted on return to the nursing home facility, e.g., medications for pain, sleeping, or antiplatelet therapy. Do not assume that just because a medication is not on the discharge list that it was discontinued. It may have been overlooked. Verify the orders with the health care provider.

Glucose Monitoring

To achieve optimal glycemic control, glucose monitoring is important, regardless of the location of care. Glucose monitoring is necessary to determine the effects of food and medication as well as activity, stress, and illness. Glucose monitoring can be important in determining whether the resident's symptoms are related to hyperglycemia or hypoglycemia. It is an important tool in the management of the resident with diabetes. CHAPTER 6 is an excellent resource on self-management of diabetes.

Glucose Monitoring

Important considerations for glucose monitoring for the staff in the nursing home:
1. Wash hands in warm water to make sure there is no sucrose on the hands and to improve circulation.
2. Using alcohol is not advised because elderly patients have dry skin and alcohol increases dryness.
3. When obtaining blood from the finger, drop the resident's hand to the side to improve blood flow before sticking the finger.
4. Use the sides of the finger rather than the tips to prevent tenderness.
5. Try not to squeeze the finger (squeezing leads to bruising and soreness).
6. If you suspect hypoglycemia or hyperglycemia, test the patient's blood glucose level for verification.

Medical Nutrition Therapy

According to the ADA nutrition recommendations, providing adequate nutrition is the primary concern for residents of long-term care facilities (6). Prevention of malnourishment and malnutrition are key considerations. Experience has shown that residents eat better if they are given less-restrictive meal plans. According to the guidelines, it is appropriate to serve residents regular menus with consistent amounts of carbohydrates at each meal and snacks. The caveat of this recommendation is that there must be consistent amounts of carbohydrates such that the same amount is given each day and distributed throughout the three meals and snacks in a consistent manner. Consistency is important. Glucose monitoring and notation of foods eaten will assist in adjusting medication to control blood glucose levels.

Two other aspects of poor nutrition need to be mentioned: *1*) eating meals alone discourages appetite and *2*) dentition issues may deter patients from eating protein foods or raw fruits and vegetables that are difficult to chew. Since eating is generally a social behavior, appetite can increase when patients eat in a common dining room or have companionship while eating. Spending time with the patient during a meal can help the nurse cue in on the patient's food preferences in type and preparation style. Substitutions can then be made that will encourage nutritional balance.

Other Key Nutrition Considerations

1. Fat restriction is generally not needed in this population.
2. Residents on pureed or softened foods should receive adequate calories for nutrition.
3. Adequate hydration is also essential in the nursing home environment.

Consultation with a dietitian is essential, and individual needs and preferences should be considered when developing a nutritional plan. If the dietitian suggests changes in daily intake, the health care provider should be notified of these changes. If the individual's appetite, quantity of food, or types of food changes, increased glucose monitoring should occur and the health care provider should be notified; the antihyperglycemic medication may need to be adjusted.

Acute Complications of Diabetes

Hyperglycemia, including diabetic ketoacidosis, hyperglycemic hyperosmolar syndrome, and hypoglycemia are the most common acute complications of diabetes. The symptoms and management of these acute complications are addressed in CHAPTER 7. It is most important to try to prevent acute complications by recognizing symptoms and identifying the problem early, so treatment can be initiated as soon as possible.

The long-term care population is at increased risk for lactic acidosis (LA). LA results from inadequate oxygen delivery or utilization in individuals with serious underlying disease. The accumulation of lactic acid indicates that the balance between lactate production and utilization has been disturbed. Metformin has been associated with LA and primarily occurs in patients with renal insufficiency and/or other concomitant medical conditions associated with poor renal perfusion or hypoxia. These conditions include congestive heart failure, chronic obstructive pulmonary disease, and age >80 years (7). Nausea and vomiting and failing to offer adequate fluids may lead to dehydration and subsequently LA. An individual's health status may change, necessitating a reevaluation of their medication and safety issues.

LA will be difficult to differentiate from the other forms of critical illnesses. Conscious monitoring and notifying the health care provider of any changes in hydration, oxygen perfusion, and mental orientation may prevent an acute crisis from occurring in the nursing home.

Chronic Complications of Diabetes

Even though the prevention of diabetes complications may not seem as important in this population, maintaining function to enhance quality of life is imperative. Screening for long-term complications is recommended so that problems can be detected and treated early. The ADA guidelines should be followed (3). An annual dilated eye examination may contribute to the prevention of blindness. Assessing visual acuity and fitting with proper eyewear may prevent falls, increase quality of life, and reduce sensory deprivations. Management of hypertension reduces the incidence of strokes and kidney disease. Decreased quality of life and its associated cost of care underscores the need to provide preventive care for this population, regardless of age (2).

Foot and Skin Care

Early recognition and management of independent risk factors for foot ulcers and amputations can prevent or delay the onset of adverse outcomes (8). Individuals with diabetes are taught to do daily foot examinations, and it would seem appropriate that this recommendation be carried out in the nursing home. If the individual is unable to perform this exam, then the nursing home staff should conduct a visual inspection daily. The nurse should do a complete examination on a weekly basis (9). Many facilities have access to podiatric services and should recommend that all individuals with diabetes receive these services, particularly for nail care. Evaluation for appropriate footwear should be done by a professional. The individual should always wear shoes when walking or riding in a wheelchair to prevent foot injuries; this is especially critical for those with sensory loss.

Prevention and management of other skin ulcers and tears is also critical. Skin yeast infections are common in this population (10). Red rashy areas in the skinfolds may represent yeast infections there as well as in the groin, especially if the resident is incontinent. Keeping the long-term–care resident dry and turned frequently is imperative for skin preservation.

Empowerment and Self-Management in the Long-Term Care Facility

Nursing home residents are usually not responsible for the majority of their care. However, they can benefit from simple and new information. They deserve the opportunity to learn about their disease and have control over procedures whenever possible.

It is important for the caregiver to recognize that residents may have lived with diabetes for many years. It is important to listen to residents. They may have successfully managed this disease for years. Or this may be a new diagnosis, and they may not understand the medications, the glucose testing, or the symptoms of hypoglycemia. Allow them the opportunity to have some control over what and when they eat and of their medication, within reason. For example, the individual may direct the timing, location, and administration of the insulin injection. Encourage residents to be as physically active as they are able and assess physical activity areas for safety. Include the family in the treatment plan and listen to them. They may have insight into the resident's likes and dislikes. Older individuals with diabetes should be screened for depression and cognitive impairment (11).

SUMMARY

Nursing home residents are a special population in a special setting. This setting offers an opportunity to provide quality diabetes care. Not only will the individual's quality of life improve, but mortality, morbidity, and medical care costs will decrease (12). It is important to provide regular opportunities for continuing education for the staff. Nurses should guide the development and implementation of protocols for care, following the standards of care, and ensure that a trained staff is providing daily care for the individual with diabetes living in a nursing home/long-term care facility.

REFERENCES

1. Mayfield JA, Deb P, Potter DEB: Diabetes and long term care. In *Diabetes in America*. 2nd ed. Harris MI, Cowie CC, Stern MP, Boyko EJ, Reiber GE, Bennett PH, Eds. Washington, DC, U.S. Govt. Printing Office, 1995, p. 571–590 (NIH publ. no. 95-1468)
2. Funnell MM: Care of the nursing home resident with diabetes. *Clin Geriatr Med* 15:413–422, 1999
3. American Diabetes Association: Standards of medical care in diabetes (Position Statement). *Diabetes Care* 28 (Suppl. 1):S4–S36, 2005

4. Aventis: Insulin glargine (Lantus) [package insert]. Bridgewater, NJ, Aventis.

5. Grajower MM, Fraser CG, Holcombe JH, Daugherty ML, Harris WC, De Felippis MR, Santiago OM, Clark NG: How long should insulin be used once a vial is started? (Commentary). *Diabetes Care* 26:2665–2669, 2003

6. American Diabetes Association: Diabetes nutrition recommendations for health care institutions (Position Statement). *Diabetes Care* 27 (Suppl. 1):S55–S57, 2004

7. Clement SC: Lactic acidosis. In *Therapy for Diabetes Mellitus and Related Disorders*. 4th ed. Lebovitz HE, Ed. Alexandria, VA, American Diabetes Association, 2004, p. 100–105

8. American Diabetes Association: Preventive foot care in diabetes (Position Statement). *Diabetes Care* 27 (Suppl. 1):S63–S64, 2004

9. American Diabetes Association/American Association of Diabetes Educators: Guidelines for diabetes care in skilled nursing facilities. In *Guidelines for Diabetes Care*. New York, American Diabetes Association, 1981, p. 40–44

10. American Diabetes Association: Skin complications [Internet]. Available from http://www.diabetes.org/for-parents-and-kids/what-is-diabetes/skin-complications.jsp. Accessed 16 October 2004

11. American Geriatrics Society: New guidelines for improving the care of the older person with diabetes mellitus [Internet]. Available from http://www.americangeriatrics.org/education/diabetes_executive_summ.shtml. Accessed 10 December 2003

12. Morley JE, Kaiser FE: Unique aspects of diabetes mellitus in the elderly. *Clin Geriatr Med* 6:693–701, 1990

Ms. Childs is a Diabetes Nurse Specialist at Mid-America Diabetes Associates, Wichita, KS.

RESOURCES

Introduction

Providing comprehensive, up-to-date diabetes care and education is a challenge for the health care provider today. Keeping up with the latest treatments, standards of care, technology, and support programs available can seem overwhelming. The purpose of this section is to provide tools and resources that will be useful in your practice.

The mission of the American Diabetes Association (ADA) is to prevent and cure diabetes and improve the lives of all people affected by diabetes, and its motto is "cure, care, commitment." In addition to research, the ADA is committed to providing access to current information for health care professionals and individuals with diabetes and their families. One way that the ADA carries out this mission is through its web site (www.diabetes.org). This web site provides access to the annually updated (every January) Clinical Practice Recommendations. It is available as an annual supplement to the journal *Diabetes Care* and in its entirety on the ADA web site at http://care.diabetesjournals.org. The Clinical Practice Recommendations have been referred to extensively in this book. The Standards of Medical Care in Diabetes provide the latest guidelines for the care of people with diabetes.

Another invaluable resource that is available in its entirety from the ADA is the Resource Guide published in *Diabetes Forecast*. This resource is published in December of each year and is available online (http://www.diabetes.org/diabetes-forecast/resource-guide.jsp). The guide covers such vital information as insulin delivery systems, blood glucose meters and data management systems, products for treating low blood glucose, wound gels and prescription lotions, medical identification products, and manufacturers and exclusive distributors. Products change so frequently that studying this resource will keep the health care provider up to date on the most advanced information on technology and new therapies. Pharmaceutical companies are an excellent resource for patient education materials and most have web sites that provide patient and professional information. Pharmaceutical representatives can also frequently provide materials without charge. Addresses and web information are available through this Resource Guide. Any portion of the ADA Clinical Practice Recommendations and the Resource Guide can be printed with proper reference.

The ADA has an extensive publication list that is available online for professionals and individuals with diabetes and their families. This list is accessible online or by calling 1-800-DIABETES.

Numerous other organizations are listed in the RESOURCES section of this book, including other not-for-profit organizations. Many, including the ADA, provide information in Spanish. Most have information for professionals and the public. Some have information that can be printed for patient use. Government agencies are included, too. The National Diabetes Education Program, National Diabetes Information Clearinghouse, and Centers for Disease Control and Prevention all have information for professionals and the public that can be printed.

Resources for special populations have been listed, including those relevant for senior citizens, young people, people with disabilities, and for weight management. A web site that may identify resources for medication for your low-income or uninsured patients is also listed.

A listing of professional journals and patient-oriented magazines is provided. *Diabetes Spectrum*, *Clinical Diabetes*, *Diabetes Care*, and *Diabetes* are all publications of the ADA. *Diabetes Spectrum* translates diabetes research into practice and its readership consists primarily of nurses, dietitians, psychologists, nurse practitioners, physician's assistants, and other health care professionals. The readership of *Clinical Diabetes* is mainly directed toward primary care physicians. *Diabetes* and *Diabetes Care* present the latest in basic and clinical diabetes research. Other journals are listed as well.

Access to information on how to become a certified diabetes educator (CDE), to obtain certification through American Nurses Credentialing Center (BC-ADM), and to become a recognized diabetes education program is included.

Forms for foot exams and information management tools are available, along with other professional tools and protocols. These are examples that can be used to create forms and tools specific to the nurse's own practice. There is no one form that will work for every setting.

Several Patient Information Sheets that were previously published in *Diabetes Spectrum* or *Clinical Diabetes* are included in this RESOURCES section. They were selected because they are topics that are not frequently available in other education materials.

The use of resources is invaluable for patients and professionals alike. Knowledge is the key to understanding and improving quality of care.

Organizations and Government Agencies

These organizations and government agencies have been identified to provide additional information and to provide updated information on a number of topics. Most of these organizations provide information for both health professionals (including education) and the public. Those that do not have been indicated.

FOR HEALTH PROFESSIONALS

Organizations

American Association of Clinical Endocrinologists
(no information for people with diabetes)
1000 Riverside Ave.
Suite 205
Jacksonville, FL 32204
Phone: 904-353-7878
www.aace.com

American Association of Diabetes Educators
100 W. Monroe St.
Suite 400
Chicago, IL 60603
Phone: 800-338-3633
www.aadenet.org

American Celiac Society
59 Crystal Ave.
West Orange, NJ 07052
Phone: 973-325-8837
E-mail: amerceliacsoc@netscape.net

American Council on Exercise
(no educational materials)
4851 Paramount Dr.
San Diego, CA 92123
Phone: 800-825-3636
www.acefitness.com

American Dental Association
211 E. Chicago Ave.
Chicago, IL 60611
Phone: 312-440-2500
www.ada.org

American Diabetes Association
1701 N. Beauregard St.
Alexandria, VA 22311
Phone: 800-342-2383
www.diabetes.org

American Dietetic Association
120 S. Riverside Plaza
Suite 2000
Chicago, IL 60606
Phone: 800-877-1600
www.eatright.org

American Heart Association
National Center
7272 Greenville Ave.
Dallas, TX 75231
Phone: 800-242-8721
www.americanheart.org

American Podiatric Medical Association
9312 Old Georgetown Rd.
Bethesda, MD 20814
Phone: 800-ASK-APMA
www.apma.org

American Stroke Association
National Center
7272 Greenville Ave.
Dallas, TX 75231
Phone: 888-478-7653
www.strokeassociation.org

Celiac Sprue Association
P.O. Box 31700
Omaha, NE 68131
Phone: 877-CSA-4CSA
www.csaceliacs.org

Cystic Fibrosis Foundation
6931 Arlington Rd.
Bethesda, MD 20814
Phone: 800-344-4823
www.cff.org

Diabetes Exercise and Sports Association
8001 Montcastle Dr.
Nashville, TN 37221
Phone: 800-898-4322
www.diabetes-exercise.org

Juvenile Diabetes Research Foundation International
(no educational material)
120 Wall St.
New York, NY 10005
Phone: 800-533-2873
www.jdrf.org

National Kidney Foundation
30 E. 33rd St.
New York, NY 10016
Phone: 800-622-9010
www.kidney.org

National Lipid Education Council
www.lipidhealth.org

National Mental Health Association
2001 N. Beauregard St.
12th floor
Alexandria, VA 22311
Phone: 800-969-6642
www.nmha.org

Government Agencies

Centers for Disease Control and Prevention, Division of Diabetes Translation
P.O. Box 8728
Silver Spring, MD 20910
Phone: 877-232-3422
www.cdc.gov/diabetes

Indian Health Services, Division of Diabetes Treatment and Prevention
The Reyes Building
801 Thompson Ave.
Suite 400
Rockville, MD 20852
Phone: 505-248-4182
www.ihs.gov/medicalprograms/
    diabetes

National Diabetes Education Program
1 Diabetes Way
Bethesda, MD 20814
Phone: 800-438-5383
www.ndep.nih.gov

National Diabetes Information Clearinghouse
1 Information Way
Bethesda, MD 20892
Phone: 800-860-8747
www.diabetes.niddk.nih.gov

National Eye Institute
Information Office
31 Center Dr. MSC 2510
Bethesda, MD 20892
Phone: 301-496-5248
www.nei.nih.gov

National Institute of Diabetes and
Digestive and Kidney Diseases
National Institutes of Health
Building 31, Center Dr.
MSC 2560
Bethesda, MD 20892
www.niddk.nih.gov

U.S. Department of Health and
Human Services
200 Independence Ave. SW
Washington, DC 20201
Phone: 877-696-6775
www.hhs.gov

FOR THE PERSON
WITH DIABETES

Senior Citizens

American Association of Retired
Persons
601 E. St. NW
Washington, DC 20049
Phone: 888-687-2277
www.aarp.org

National Association of Area
Agencies on Aging
1730 Rhode Island Ave. NW
Suite 1200
Washington, DC 20036
Phone: 202-872-0888
www.n4a.org

National Institute on Aging
Bldg. 31, Room 5C27
31 Center Dr. MSC 2292
Bethesda, MD 20892
www.nia.nih.gov

Young People

American Diabetes Association
Youth Zone
1701 N. Beauregard St.
Alexandria, VA 22311
Phone: 800-232-3472
http://www.diabetes.org/youthzone/
youth-zone.jsp

American School Health
Association
7263 State Route 43
P.O. Box 708
Kent, OH 44240
Phone: 330-678-1601
www.ashaweb.org

Children With Diabetes
5689 Chancery Pl.
Hamilton, OH 45011
www.childrenwithdiabetes.org

Centers for Disease Control and
Prevention, Division of
Adolescents and School Health
1600 Clifton Rd.
Atlanta, GA 30333
Phone: 800-311-3435
www.cdc.gov/HealthyYouth/index.htm

National Association of School
Nurses
1416 Park St.
Suite A
Castle Rock, CO 80109
Phone: 866-627-6767
www.nasn.org

National Education Association
Health Information Network
1201 16th St. NW
Suite 521
Washington, DC 20036
Phone: 800-718-8387
www.neahin.org

Resources for Low-Income and
Uninsured Patients

Partnership for Prescription
Assistance
PhRMA
1100 15th St. NW
Washington, DC 20005
Phone: 202-835-3400
Fax: 202-835-3414
www.helpingpatients.org
Single point of access for >275 public
and private patient assistance
programs

For Ethnic and Racial Minorities

National Center on Minority Health and Health Disparities
National Institutes of Health
6707 Democracy Blvd.
Suite 800
MSC-5465
Bethesda, MD 20892
Phone: 301-402-1366
www.ncmhd.nih.gov

Office of Minority Health, Centers for Disease Control and Prevention
Mailstop E-67
1600 Clifton Rd. NE
Atlanta, GA 30333
Phone: 404-498-2320
www.cdc.gov/omh

Weight Management

American Obesity Association
1250 24th St. NW
Suite 300
Washington, DC 20037
Phone: 202-776-7711
www.obesity.org

Diet, Health, and Fitness Consumer Information (Federal Trade Commission)
600 Pennsylvania Ave. NW
Washington, DC 20580
Phone: 202-326-2222
www.ftc.gov/bcp/
    menu-health.htm#coned

Shape Up America
15009 Native Dancer Rd.
North Potomac, MD 20878
Phone: 240-631-6533
www.shapeup.org

Weight Control Information Network (National Institute of Diabetes and Digestive and Kidney Diseases)
1 WIN Way
Bethesda, MD 20892
Phone: 877-946-4627
www.niddk.nih.gov/health/nutrit/
    win.htm

People With Disabilities

American Foundation for the Blind
11 Penn Plaza
Suite 300
New York, NY 10001
Phone: 800-232-5463
www.afb.org

Columbia Lighthouse for the Blind
1120 20th St. NW
Suite 750 South
Washington, DC 20036
Phone: 202-454-6400
www.clb.org

Lighthouse International
111 E. 59th St.
New York, NY 10022
Phone: 800-829-0500
www.lighthouse.org

National Foundation for the Blind
1800 Johnson St.
Baltimore, MD 21230
Phone: 410-659-9314
www.nfb.com

Amputee Coalition of America
900 E Hill Ave.
Suite 285
Knoxville, TN 37915
Phone: 888-267-5669
www.amputee-coalition.org

National Center on Physical Activity and Disabilities
1640 W. Roosevelt Rd.
Chicago, IL 60608
Phone: 800-900-8086
www.ncpad.org

Identification

MedicAlert Foundation International
2323 Colorado Ave.
Turlock, CA 95382
Phone: 888-633-4298
www.medicalert.org

Publications

FOR HEALTH PROFESSIONALS

Clinical Diabetes

This quarterly journal is dedicated to improving diabetes care in primary care settings. It provides concise, clinically relevant articles on diabetes management, including pharmacological management, exercise and diet, medical legal issues, and health care delivery.

American Diabetes Association
Membership/Subscription Services
1701 N Beauregard St.
Alexandria, VA 22311
Phone: 800-232-3472 ext. 2343
http://clinical.diabetesjournals.org

Diabetes

This research-based professional journal of original diabetes research includes articles on all aspects of laboratory, animal, and human research relating to the physiology and pathophysiology of diabetes.

American Diabetes Association
Membership/Subscription Services
1701 N Beauregard St.
Alexandria, VA 22311
Phone: 800-232-3472 ext. 2343
http://diabetes.diabetesjournals.org

Diabetes Care

The world's highest circulating and most-cited journal of clinical diabetes research, including reviews, commentaries, and original articles covering clinical care, education, and nutrition, epidemiology and health services, emerging technologies and treatments, pathophysiology and complications, and pre-diabetes.

American Diabetes Association
Membership/Subscription Services
1701 N Beauregard St.
Alexandria, VA 22311
Phone: 800-232-3472 ext. 2343
http://care.diabetesjournals.org

The Diabetes Educator

The AADE's professional journal is dedicated to publishing new research in patient and provider education and advances in diabetes management.

American Association of Diabetes Educators
100 W. Monroe St.
Suite 400
Chicago, IL 60603
Phone: 800-338-3633
www.diabeteseducator.org/Products/
TDE/TDEContent.html

Diabetes Spectrum

The health care professional's tool for translating new diabetes research into clinical practice. Articles cover medical management, patient education, nutrition and behavioral science, exercise, and other topics.

American Diabetes Association
Membership/Subscription Services
1701 N Beauregard St.
Alexandria, VA 22311
Phone: 800-232-3472 ext. 2343
http://spectrum.diabetesjournals.org

FOR PEOPLE WITH DIABETES

Diabetes Forecast

The most widely circulated magazine for people with diabetes for over 50 years, covering advances in research and treatment, healthy diet, exercise, fitness, and advocacy and includes the annual Resource Guide.

American Diabetes Association
Membership Center
P.O. Box 444
Mount Morris, IL 61054
Phone: 800-806-7801
www.diabetes.org/diabetes-forecast.jsp

Diabetes Self-Management

An award-winning publication dedicated to providing up-to-date, practical self-management information for the person with diabetes.

Diabetes Self-Management
Subscription Services
P.O. Box 52890
Boulder, CO 80322
Phone: 800-234-0923
www.diabetesselfmanagement.com

Certification Programs

Education Recognition Program

American Diabetes Association
1701 N Beauregard St.
Alexandria, VA 22311
Phone: 888-232-0822
www.diabetes.org/for-health-profes-
    sionals-and-scientists/recognition/
    edrecognition.jsp

Board Certified in Advanced Diabetes Management (BC-ADM), RN, RD, Pharmacist

American Nurses Credentialing Center
8515 Georgia Ave.
Suite 400
Silver Spring, MD 20910
Phone: 800-284-2378
www.nursingworld.org/ancc/
    certification/certs.html

Certified Diabetes Educator (CDE)

National Certification Board for Diabetes Educators (NCBDE)
330 E Algonquin Rd.
Suite 4
Arlington Heights, IL 60005
Phone: 847-228-9795
www.ncbde.org

Forms

PATIENT EDUCATION TOOLS

Online Depression Screening Test: www.med.nyu.edu/psych/screens

Stress Management Tools

We all have stress. Finding ways to relieve stress and relax will make us healthier and happier. Ask yourself some simple questions.

What do you do when you feel stressed? _____

What do you do to relax? _____
(Some people like to listen to music, read a book, or talk with a friend.)

There are a number of stress management skills that you can learn and make part of your life to reduce feelings of stress.

Direct Approach	Indirect Approach
Positive Self-Talk: Telling oneself that there is hope. Seeing challenges, not defeat. Preparing oneself for success through positive input, positive affirmations, and reframing negative thoughts.	*Exercise*: Using regular, aerobic exercise to decrease the effect of stress on the body.
Communication Skills: Being able to use "I" messages. Being able to actively listen. Using "both-win" approaches to negotiation.	**Relaxation:** *Progressive Relaxation:* Deep muscle relaxation by alternatively tensing and relaxing groups of muscles.
Assertiveness Training: Being able to say "no." Being able to ask question of others, especially your medical team. Being able to express your feelings.	*Deep breathing (diaphragmatic breathing):* Abdominal rises and falls with respirations. The upper body does not move.
	Meditating: Trance-like state where noncritical focus is maintained one thought at a time.
Time Management: Learning to be more organized and efficient through good decision making and goal setting.	*Biofeedback*: Getting visual, audible, or tactile information about various body functions, such as heart rate, muscle tension, and hand temperature, in order to
Priority Setting: Making conscious choices.	learn control over that body function.
Thought Stopping: Learning not to be consumed by concerns and worries. Stopping habitual negative thought patterns.	*Nutrition*: Learning to eat healthy foods that maximize the body's energy.
Refuting Irrational Ideas: Learning to identify and refute unrealistic expectations and ideas that may have one overreacting to a situation.	*Sleep*: Prioritizing adequate sleep and developing good sleep patterns.

Adapted from Guthrie DW, Rhiley DS: Care and Control of Your Diabetes, Via Christi Regional Medical Center, Diabetes Treatment and Research Center, Wichita, KS, 2002.

PATIENT INFORMATION SHEETS

Making Time for Diabetes Care in a Woman's Busy Life
Is an Insulin Pump Right for Your Child and Family?
A Step-by-Step Approach to Complementary Therapies
Diabetes and Eating Disorders
For Great Diabetes Care, Remember Your ABCs!
How Can We Help You?
Keeping Medicine Costs Under Control
Are You at Risk for Osteoporosis?
Resources for People Who Want to Lose Weight
Be Prepared: Sick Day Management
Diabetes and Surgery
Thyroid Disease and Diabetes
Erectile Dysfunction Treatments
Guidelines for Using Vitamin, Mineral, and Herbal Supplements

Making Time for Diabetes Care in a Woman's Busy Life

Women live diverse lives. But one constant for almost all women is too little time. Most women juggle many roles and duties. It's hard to squeeze everything in—doubly hard when you have a disease such as diabetes.

Reviewing how you spend your time can help you manage better. Some diabetes tasks need to be done every day:

- Testing your blood sugar
- Taking pills or insulin and determining how much to take and when to supplement
- Recording test results and medicine doses in your log
- Exercising

Here are ways to give your diabetes the daily attention it deserves:

- Don't feel guilty about making diabetes care a top goal. Staying healthy makes it easier to be a good employee, wife, mother, and daughter.
- Make diabetes care part of your everyday routine. You'll be more likely to exercise, for example, if you have a time set aside for it.
- Make daily to-do lists. Mark the most urgent activities.
- Use memory aids:
  - ✔ Link testing and taking medicines to things you do every day at the same time, such as brushing your teeth.

- ✔ Keep your medicines and glucose meter near where you do these acts.
- ✔ Create rituals. Do things in the same order in the same place at the same time each day.
- ✔ Set a timer to remind you of your next blood test or medicine dose.
- ✔ Make a daily chart of tasks. Check off each medicine as you take it and each blood test as you do it.

Some diabetes tasks are done only when needed:

- Deciding what foods to buy, cook, and eat
- Reviewing your blood sugar records and food records
- Testing your urine for ketones
- Seeing your health care providers
- Getting lab work done
- Filling prescriptions and buying supplies
- Traveling to and from and waiting at the clinic, lab, and drugstore

Planning for these is much harder than fitting in daily tasks. They don't occur regularly. The time they require is less predictable. And many take hours instead of minutes.

Still, there are many ways to free up time for such tasks.

Start by setting personal, family, and career goals. Rank these by importance. You want to spend most of your time and effort on important goals. Then look at how you spend your time each week. Ask yourself:

- Are there ways you can spend your time more usefully? Do you watch TV shows that you don't really enjoy? Catch up on work or chores during that time instead.
- Are you using any time inefficiently? Do you go to the grocery twice a week instead of once? Planning ahead to avoid double effort can free up large blocks of time.

If you still have too little time:

- Delegate. If your husband or children have time to goof off, but you are always frantically busy, something is out of whack.
- Say "no" more often.
- Plan your schedule around your natural body clock. Do important tasks when you are most alert and energetic.
- Cut down health care visits by doubling up. Try to see the dietitian and have lab work done on the same day you visit your provider.

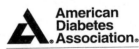

American Diabetes Association®

Cure • Care • Commitment™

8/03
Diabetes Spectrum 16:173, 2003

Is an Insulin Pump Right for Your Child and Family?

Insulin pump therapy can help people with type 1 diabetes. Pumps deliver insulin in a way that resembles the body's own release of insulin. They can improve blood sugar control, make low blood sugar (hypoglycemia) less of a problem, and lessen the risk of diabetic ketoacidosis. But pump use in children, especially very young children, is controversial. If you are considering an insulin pump for your child, read on.

How Pumps Work
Insulin pumps are about the size of a pager. They are attached to the body by a needle placed under the skin. They can remain in place for 2–3 days at a time. Pump therapy delivers rapid- or short-acting insulin continuously through the needle. The continuous insulin is called the basal rate.

In addition to providing basal insulin throughout the day, pumps are programmed to give additional insulin (bolus doses) with each meal and snack. Older children or the parents of younger children must test the blood sugar four to eight times a day to check the pump's effectiveness, adjust mealtime boluses, and correct high blood sugar levels.

So What's Not to Like?
Pumps can improve diabetes control and give children more flexibility, but very young children cannot manage their own pump use. Even older kids need a good deal of help from parents. Therefore, pump therapy requires a knowledgeable parent or caregiver to be on hand 24 hours a day, 7 days a week to help with blood sugar tests, determine mealtime insulin needs, adjust pump settings, and troubleshoot any problems.

Consider These Questions
Is your child
- willing to wear the pump?
- able to tolerate the needle-insertion process?

As your child's main caregiver, do you
- fully understand basal-bolus insulin therapy?
- know how to count carbohydrate or use some other insulin-to-food ratio?
- know how to correct for high or low blood sugar levels?
- know how to change insulin doses for changes in exercise, sick days, travel, or other special situations?
- understand how to measure ketones and what to do if they are present?

- feel sure that you can operate an insulin pump?
- have the time to care for your child's diabetes every day?
- have partnerships with school personnel and other caregivers who are willing and able to work with a pump?

Does your diabetes care team
- include a doctor, a diabetes nurse educator, a registered dietitian, a mental health professional, and other health care professionals?
- have experience using insulin pumps with young children?
- offer 24-hour telephone contact for patients who use insulin pumps?

Still Interested?
Good. Pump therapy may be a good fit for your child and family. Before making a final decision, sit down with your child's diabetes health care providers. Weigh the pros and cons for your own family situation. Consider wearing a pump yourself and having your child wear one for a few days to see what it's like. Find out all you can so that you and your child can make an informed choice.

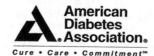
American Diabetes Association®
Cure • Care • Commitment™

A Step-by-Step Approach to Complementary Therapies

Often, the greatest levels of health and well-being can be reached when people have an integrative medical care team that is trained not only in the latest treatments and technologies, but also in how to create a healing environment for the mind, body, and spirit. Integrative care includes the best of standard medical care and complementary therapies as well as patients' full involvement in mind, body, and spirit.

The following steps can help you safely integrate complementary therapies into your health care plan.

Step 1. Identify the symptom you hope to improve.
Start a symptom diary. Record what your symptoms are, when they occur, and what makes them better or worse. For example, if you have periodic shooting pain in your legs, an entry in your symptom diary might read, "Shooting leg pain three times this evening. On a scale of 1 to 10, this pain was an 8."

Step 2. Identify possible complementary therapies.
Collect information about complementary therapies you may want to try. Discuss them with your medical team.

Ask your standard health care team:
• Is this treatment dangerous? Does it cause any side effects?
• Is it safe to combine this

with my current medical treatments?
• What should I ask when I meet with possible complementary care providers?
• What type of follow-up should I schedule with you if I use this therapy?

Step 3. Interview potential complementary therapy providers.
Expect that it will take some time and effort to find the right provider for you.

Ask potential complementary care providers:
• What do you think is causing my symptoms?
• What treatment do you recommend? What benefits can I expect from it?
• Are there any dangers or concerns associated with this treatment?
• Is it safe to combine this treatment with my current medical treatments?
• How and when will we decide whether it is working?
• What is the cost? Will my insurance pay for it? Can you help me look into this?
• What is your training? Are you licensed or certified? How do I contact the licensing agency?
• Do you need information from my medical team about my medical history and current treatments?
• Will you follow-up with my doctor about your recommendations?

Step 4. Choose a complementary therapy provider and begin treatment.
You may wish to consult your medical team before selecting a complementary care provider. Continue to keep your symptom diary as you begin complementary therapy. For example, you may record, "Reiki session on Saturday. I feel a sense of well-being and peacefulness. I felt shooting pain in my legs three times tonight, but it was less painful—a 5 on a scale of 1 to 10."

Step 5. Follow-up regularly with your complementary and standard care providers.
Review your symptom diary and the effects of the complementary treatment. Report any side effects to both your complementary and standard care providers.

To learn more about complementary and alternative therapies, contact the National Center for Complementary and Alternative Medicine (NCCAM, formerly the National Institutes of Health Office of Alternative Medicine) at 800-531-1794 or visit the NCCAM website http://altmed.od.nih.gov

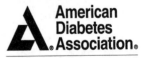
American Diabetes Association
Cure • Care • Commitment℠

Diabetes and Eating Disorders

Eating disorders are common in teenaged girls and young women. They are rarely seen in boys and men. Girls and young women with type 1 diabetes have about twice the risk of developing eating disorders as their peers without diabetes. This may be because of the weight changes that can occur with insulin therapy and good metabolic control and the extra attention people with diabetes must pay to what they eat.

The two main eating disorders are anorexia nervosa and bulimia nervosa. People with anorexia restrict their food intake to stay thin. Their perceptions of their body are often distorted. People with bulimia repeatedly eat excessive amounts of food and then induce vomiting or take laxatives to purge the food from their body.

The most common features of eating disorders in girls and young women with type 1 diabetes are:
- dissatisfaction with their body weight and shape and desire to be thinner;

- dieting or manipulation of insulin doses to control weight; and,
- binge eating.

Researchers estimate that 10–20 percent of girls in their mid-teen years and 30–40 percent of late teenaged girls and young adult women with diabetes skip or alter insulin doses to control their weight. In people with diabetes, eating disorders can lead to poor metabolic control and repeated hospitalizations for dangerously high or low blood sugar. Chronic poor blood sugar control leads to long-term complications, such as eye, kidney, and nerve damage.

Early Warning Signs
- Extremely high A1C test results
- Frequent bouts of and hospitalizations for poor blood sugar control
- Anxiety about or avoidance of being weighed
- Frequent requests to switch meal-planning approaches
- Frequent severe low blood sugar

- Widely fluctuating blood sugar levels without obvious reason
- Delay in puberty or sexual maturation or irregular or no menses
- Binging with food or alcohol at least twice a week for 3 months
- Exercise more than is necessary to stay fit
- Severe family stress

If you think that you or a loved one has an eating disorder, talk to your diabetes health care providers. They will recommend a mental health counselor who will work with the diabetes team to help you and your family deal with this problem. It is important to be nonjudgmental and supportive. It is also extremely important to seek evaluation and treatment.

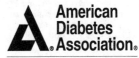

American Diabetes Association

Cure • Care • Commitment℠

For Great Diabetes Care, Remember Your ABCs!

Taking good care of your diabetes can be complex and confusing. This handy list will make remembering all the steps you need to take as easy as A B C D E F G H I!

A is for A1C.
The A1C ("A-one-C") test—short for hemoglobin A_{1c}—measures your average blood glucose (sugar) over the past 3 months.
Suggested target: Below 7
How often: At least twice a year

A is also for albuminuria.
Albuminuria means protein in the urine. A test that measures your urine microalbumin-to-creatinine ratio can detect kidney disease very early, when it can usually be stopped. This can prevent dialysis or kidney transplantation later on.
Suggested target: Below 30
How often: At least once a year

And, finally, A is for aspirin.
Taking low-dose aspirin every day can help prevent heart attacks and strokes. Children and young adults with no history of heart disease should not take aspirin without a doctor's order, nor should some older adults. Check with your doctor before starting daily aspirin.

B is for blood pressure.
High blood pressure makes your heart work too hard and can cause damage to your kidneys and eyes.
Suggested target: Below 130/80
How often: At every visit

C is for cholesterol.
Bad cholesterol, or LDL, builds up and clogs your arteries, leading to heart attacks and strokes.
Suggested LDL target: Below 100
How often: At least once a year

D is for diabetes education.
Help your doctor help you. The more you know about how food, exercise, and medicines affect your diabetes control, the better you and your doctor can work together to make any needed changes.
Suggested resources: Dietitians, nurse diabetes educators
How often: Ongoing

E is for eye exam.
Regular eye exams can catch diabetic eye disease early enough to prevent eventual blindness.
How often: At least once a year

F is for foot care
Keep an eye on your feet. If you have nerve disease and can't feel your feet, your feet can't tell you when something is wrong.

How often: Check your feet daily. Remind your doctor to check them at every visit. Get an extensive foot exam once a year.

G is for glucose (sugar) monitoring.
If you know when your blood sugar level is too high or too low, you'll know better how to treat it.
How often: Decide with your doctor.

H is for staying healthy.
For people with diabetes, getting the flu or pneumonia can lead to serious complications. Avoid them by getting vaccinated.
How often: Flu vaccine, every year; pneumonia, at least once.

I is for identifying special medical needs.
Complications are complicated. As they occur, your doctor may need to send you to various specialists. Voicing your health concerns at every visit can help your doctor spot trouble and get any extra help you need quickly.
How often: When needed

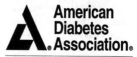

American Diabetes Association®

Cure • Care • Commitment℠

How Can We Help You?

Having a chronic illness such as diabetes can affect just about every aspect of your life. Consequently, many different problems can get in the way of your efforts to control your diabetes. Perhaps you have other illnesses or physical problems that make it hard for you to deal with your diabetes. Maybe the demanding nature of diabetes has left you feeling overwhelmed, sad, or even angry.

The good news is that your health care team can help you find ways to overcome many of the obstacles you may be facing. But they need your help to figure out exactly what types of help you may need. Here's a list of questions to ask yourself before your next visit to your health care provider to help pinpoint any problem areas you may want to discuss with your diabetes team.

Knowledge

- Do you know enough about your diabetes?
- Do you know all the members of your diabetes team?
- Are you always able to speak with and understand members of your diabetes team?
- Who or what do you believe is responsible for the cause, treatment, and progress of your diabetes?

Health and Physical Issues

- Do you have other health problems that affect your diabetes?
- Are you happy with the way your diabetes medications are working?

Stress, Feelings, and Attitudes

- Are you willing to look after your diabetes?
- Do you feel you are able to look after your own diabetes?
- Would you look after your diabetes more if you felt worse?
- What is more important than looking after your diabetes?
- Do you or your diabetes team have enough time for your diabetes?
- Are you worried, afraid, or ashamed of your diabetes?
- Are you willing to look after your diabetes fully from today?

Access

- Can you get to your diabetes team easily?
- Would you prefer your diabetes service to be closer?
- Do you have all the services you need?
- Are you happy with how these services are provided?
- Have you been unhappy with any members of the diabetes team?

- Are you happy with your diabetes education and care?
- Do you feel comfortable talking with your diabetes team?

Support

- Do you feel pressure from others not to look after your diabetes?
- Do you feel that others are holding your diabetes against you?
- Is your family helping you look after your diabetes?
- Do family demands stop you from looking after your diabetes?

Society

- Can you afford to have diabetes?
- Is there enough support for you in the community or at work?
- Should the public bear more financial responsibility for your care?
- Do people other than your family need to know more about diabetes?

There are no right or wrong answers to these questions. But there are resources to help you improve your diabetes care if you are not getting the care you need. Talk to your health care provider or call your local American Diabetes Association for more information.

Keeping Medicine Costs Under Control

The high price of medicines and supplies weighs heavily on people with diabetes. The burden can be overwhelming when you use several medicines. Here's how you can lighten the load.

Everyday Cost Cutters

- When you need an over-the-counter medicine, consider a generic instead of the name brand. Generic versions contain the same active agents but cost less. To find generic versions of a name-brand product, compare ingredient labels. Look for the same active ingredient in the same strength. Your pharmacist can help.
- Keep receipts for medical expenses, including prescription costs your insurance doesn't cover. When these are large relative to your income, some can be deducted from your income taxes.
- Scan drugstore ads for coupons.
- Check out your insurance coverage. Some health plans cover medicines. Some let you order prescriptions by mail for a reduced co-payment. If you order insulin through the mail, be sure it will be protected from getting too hot or too cold.
- Call several pharmacies to find out which one is cheapest for all your medicines put together. (For safety's sake, buy all of your medicines at one place.) If you can, check prices at online pharmacies, too.
- Limit your use of supplements and herbs to those your provider recommends. Few have been proven to have any benefit. Yet they can cost as much as—or more than—medicines proven to be safe and to work.

Working With Providers

Your diabetes team can help if you let them know you are concerned about costs.

- Ask whether adopting good health habits could cut your prescription costs. For example, exercising, quitting smoking, and limiting salt are cheaper than buying medicines to treat high blood pressure.
- Don't pressure your doctor for medicines you see in TV ads. New and heavily advertised products often cost the most.
- On the other hand, new medicines can sometimes save you money. For example, you may be taking products B and C to treat side effects of product A. If you switch from product A to new product D with milder side effects, you might be able to stop using products B and C.
- When your health care provider suggests a new medicine, ask whether there's a cheaper alternative. Providers don't always take cost into account when choosing treatments.
- Tell your provider or pharmacist you'd like to use generic medicines whenever possible.
- Check whether your insurance company has a formulary (a list of preferred products with reduced co-payments). If so, give a copy to your provider.
- Each year, review all of your medicines with your provider. Some you may no longer need. Others may now be available in cheaper generic or over-the-counter versions.
- When starting a new medicine, ask for free samples. That way, if the side effects are bad or the product doesn't work well for you, you haven't bought an entire bottle.

Specials for Seniors

- Check with your local pharmacies to see whether any offer a senior discount card.
- If your grocery or drugstore gives seniors a discount on a certain day, buy your over-the-counter products that day.
- The American Association of Retired Persons has a pharmacy service. You can get medicines and vitamins at a discount at local pharmacies or by mail.

Programs for the Needy

Programs for people with low incomes vary. Ask your diabetes team what your area has. If they don't know, talk to a social worker or your local public health or social services department.

- Some drug companies have "pharmacy assistance programs." These provide medicines for free or at a reduced price to people with low incomes.
- Some cities have free clinics or public health clinics.
- Some states have special programs to help people afford their prescriptions. These are often for low-income elderly or disabled people.

Shauna S. Roberts, PhD, is a science and medical writer in New Orleans, La.

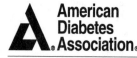

American Diabetes Association®

Cure • Care • Commitment℠

11/02
Diabetes Spectrum 15:267, 2002

Are You at Risk for Osteoporosis?

Osteoporosis is a disease that causes weak bones. This increases the risk of fractures.

What are the signs of osteoporosis?
Usually, the only symptom is a broken bone. Other noticeable signs can include height loss and curvature of the spine that occur slowly over time. Osteoporosis can cause many changes that you probably won't notice on your own but that can be identified through screening tests. It is important for people who may be at risk for osteoporosis to be screened. If osteoporosis is found, treatment should be started to avoid bone fractures.

Who is at risk?
The National Osteoporosis Foundation publishes standard risk factors. You may be at increased risk if you:
• are female or of advanced age;
• have a hormone deficiency (testosterone in men or estrogen in women);
• are a woman who had early menopause (before age 45);
• use certain medications, such as steroids or anti-seizure drugs, or take too many supplements for thyroid or vitamin A;
• eat a diet low in calcium;
• are inactive or immobile;
• smoke or use alcohol excessively;
• have parents or siblings with osteoporosis;

• have certain medical conditions, including diabetes, cystic fibrosis, malabsorption syndromes, some genetic diseases, kidney disease, thyroid disease, bulimia, or anorexia;
• have a thin body and small bone frame; or
• are white or Asian (although members of other races can also be affected).

How can I prevent osteoporosis?
Your bones grow and achieve their peak bone mass in your youth and up to age 35. During this time, you can make your bones as strong as possible by eating a healthful diet and exercising regularly.
  If you are beyond age 35, you can help prevent bone loss by getting enough calcium and vitamin D, performing weight-bearing exercises, and maintaining an overall healthy lifestyle. Speak to your health care provider about the right amount of calcium and vitamin supplements for you.
  It is also important to reduce your risk of bone fractures by preventing falls. Wear sturdy shoes, make sure your daily environment is safe, and wear hip pads if you know you already have bone loss.

How can I be tested for osteoporosis?
Bone mineral density testing provides an easy and accurate measure of your risk for osteoporosis.

Common tests include:
• dual-energy x-ray absorptiometry (DXA),
• quantitative computed tomography (QCT),
• peripheral DXA or QCT, and
• peripheral heel ultrasound
Your health care provider can provide more information about these tests.

What treatments are available?
Many different drugs are available for treating osteoporosis. Your health care provider can help you decide which one may be right for you. Commonly used drugs include:
• bisphosphonates, such as Actonel (risedronate) or Fosamax (alendronate);
• Miacalcin (a calcitonin nasal spray); and
• Evista (raloxifene)

If you think you may be at risk for developing osteoporosis, talk to your health care provider about getting screened and, if necessary, developing a treatment plan.

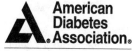

American Diabetes Association

Cure • Care • Commitment™

7/02
Clinical Diabetes 20:158, 2002

Resources for People Who Want to Lose Weight

Nonprofit Support Groups
These groups do not promote any specific weight-loss plan. rather, members following various plans meet for support.
- Overeaters Anonymous: 505-891-2664, www.oa.org
- TOPS (Take Off Pounds Sensibly): 800-932-TOPS, www.tops.org

Commercial Weight-Loss Programs
Each of these programs promotes a specific plan for losing weight.
- Diet Center: 800-656-3294, www.dietcenterworldwide.com
- Jenny Craig: 800-597-JENNY, www.jennycraig.com
- Nutrisystem: 800-321-THIN, www.nutrisystem.com
- Weight Watchers: 800-651-6000, www.weightwatchers.com

Clinical Weight-Loss Programs
Health care providers run clinical programs. they generally are very-low-calorie diets meant for people who have a lot of weight to lose.
- Health management resources: 800-418-1367, www.yourbetterhealth.com.
- Optifast: 800-662-2540, www.optifast.com

Books
- *The Commonsense Guide to Weight Loss for People With Diabetes.* By Barbara Caleen Hansen and Shauna S. Roberts. Published by the American Diabetes Association in 1998. Scientifically sound weight-loss information tailored to people with
- *Thin for Life: 10 Keys to Success from People Who Have Lost Weight and Kept It Off.* By Anne M. Fletcher. Published by Houghton Mifflin in 2003. Weight-loss methods of people who have lost and kept off at least 20 pounds.

- *Weighing the Options: Criteria for Evaluating Weight-Management Programs.* Edited by Paul R. Thomas. Published by the National Academy Press in 1995. How to find the right weight-loss program for you. Much useful information, but technical and somewhat dated.
- *Small Steps, Big Rewards: Walking Your Way to Better Health.* Published by the American Diabetes Association in 2003. Advice and tips for walking for health. Comes with a pedometer to count every step you take.

Government Web Sites Related To Weight Loss
- **Weight-Control Information Network:** www.niddk.nih.gov/health/nutrit/win.htm
- **National Institute of Diabetes and Digestive and Kidney Diseases Weight Loss and Control:** wwwniddk.nih.gov/health/nutrit/nutrit.htm
- **Federal Trade Commission Diet, Health & fitness Consumer Information:** www.ftc.gov/bcp/menu-health.htm. Brochures on many health topics, including exercise and weight loss.
- **Partnership for Healthy Weight Management:** www.consumer.gov/weightloss/bmi.htm. Here you can find out your body mass index to learn whether you weight too much.

Nutrition Information
- **American Dietetic Association Nutrition Fact Sheets:** www.eat right.org/Public/index_11722.cfm
- **Food and Drug Administration Information About Losing Weight and Maintaining a Healthy Weight:** www.cfsan.fda.gov/~dms/wh-wght.html

Diabetes Spectrum/Patient Information

- **American Diabetes Association "Weight Loss Matters" Brochures:** www.diabetes.org/health/weightloss-and-exercise/weightloss/brochures.jsp

Fitness Information
- **Shape Up America?:** www.shapeup.org. Information on becoming more fit and losing weight.
- **American College of Sports Medicine:** www.acsm.org/health%2Bfitness/ brochures.htm. Brochures on exercise equipment and other exercise topics.
- **American Running Association:** www.americanrunning.org/display industrynews.cfm. Articles on many aspects of exercise, not just running.

Finding Health Professionals and Exercise Experts
If you want expert help, start by asking your doctor for a referral. If that does not work out, here are other places to find experts.
- **American Dietetic Association:** 800-877-1600, www.eatright.org/Public/index_16304.cfm. Referrals to registered dietitians and registered dietetic technicians.
- **American Association of Diabetes Educators:** 800-338-3633, www.aade net.org/FindAnEduc/index.html. Referrals to diabetes educators.

- **American Council on Exercise:** 800-825-3636 x654, www.acefitness.org/profreg/default.aspx. Referrals to personal trainers and other certified fitness professionals.
- **American Council on Exercise:** www.acefitness.org/clublocator. Locate a health club.
- **Eating Disorder Referral and Information Center:** 800-843-7274, www.edreferral.com. Referrals to treatment centers, eating disorder specialists, telephone and online counseling, workshops, and support groups.
- **National Association of Anorexia Nervosa and Associated Disorders:** 847-831-3438, www.anad.org/site/anadweb. Provides information and referrals to support groups and health care professionals.
- **American Society of Bariatric Physicians:** 303-770-2526, www.asbp.org/locate.htm. Referrals to doctors with special training in helping people lose weight.
- **American board of Bariatric Medicine:** 303-779-0279, www.abbmcertification.org/patientinfo /physician.htm. Referrals to doctors who have passed exams testing their knowledge of obesity.
- **American society for Bariatric surgery:** 352-331-4900, www.asbs.org/html/member.html. Provides names of doctors who do obesity surgery.

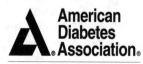

American Diabetes Association

Cure • Care • Commitment[SM]

Diabetes Spectrum/Patient Information

Be Prepared: Sick Day Management

Planning ahead can help you stay in control of your blood sugar levels during illness. Being prepared can prevent a hospitalization or emergency room visit.

Complete this checklist of "things to do" with your doctor or diabetes educator *before* you get sick. Review it once a year for changes.

❑ Know to keep taking your insulin or diabetes medications unless

_____

_____

Adjust your insulin by

_____

_____

❑ Plan to maintain a meal plan containing 150 grams of carbohydrates. Have on hand for illness the following foods, which contain 15 grams of carbohydrates each in the amounts shown.

- apple juice (1/2 cup)
- regular soda (1/2 cup)
- regular gelatin (1/2 cup)
- crackers (6 squares)

- bouillon (no calories)
- sports drink (1 cup)
- other: _____

❑ Know when to monitor your blood glucose.

_____

_____

_____

_____

❑ Know when to monitor your urine ketones:
  - When blood sugar level is greater than

  _____.

  - Regardless of blood sugar level, when vomiting or experiencing diarrhea.

Remember to check the bottle of ketone test strips for an expiration date.

❑ Know when to call your doctor or diabetes educator:
  - If your blood sugar level is greater than_____
  - If your ketones are _____for more than _____hours or if you

do not urinate for more than _____hours
  - If vomiting lasts longer than _____hours
  - If you are dehydrated. Signs of dehydration include dry tongue and difficulty breathing.
  - If surgery or a test is planned that will prevent you from eating normally
  - Any time you have a question or concern about your blood sugar level

❑ Know who to call during illness or an emergency:

Doctor_____

Daytime phone:

_____

Evening/Weekend:

_____

Diabetes educator

_____

Daytime phone:

_____

Evening/Weekend:

_____

American Diabetes Association.

Cure • Care • Commitment℠

Diabetes and Surgery

The prospect of surgery can make anyone feel worried and fearful. However, careful planning, especially for people with diabetes, can help you make your operation as safe as possible and your recovery period less stressful.

The key is to start planning well before your surgery date. This "to do" list can help you cover all the bases before your operation.

1. Meet with your primary care doctor or endocrinologist.
Work with your doctor to develop a plan for getting your blood sugar in the best possible control several weeks before you have surgery. Having good control of your blood sugar will lessen the chance of high blood sugar (hyperglycemia) or low blood sugar (hypoglycemia) reactions during your operation. Good blood sugar control also makes infections less likely and promotes healing.

Your doctor may also want to do a complete medical history and physical examination and other tests before your surgery.

2. Talk to your anesthesiologist.
This is the doctor who is responsible for monitoring your diabetes while your surgeon is performing the operation. Tell the anesthesiologist about your medical history, including details about your diabetes. Be sure to include your current medication regimen and any diabetes-related complications you have.

You may also want to discuss different types of anesthesia. Some procedures can be done with local or spinal anesthesia, allowing you to remain awake during the procedure. In such cases, recovery time is often shorter.

Other procedures require general anesthesia, which puts you to sleep during your operation. More careful monitoring of your diabetes is required during the procedure and after you undergo general anesthesia.

3. Schedule your surgery for the early morning.
Try to get the first morning time slot in the operating room. There will be less of a chance for high or low blood sugar reactions while you are waiting for your operation and are unable to eat.

4. Talk to your doctor in advance about how you will manage your diabetes immediately after your operation.
After surgery, you may need to adjust your medication or insulin doses based on your blood sugar level. Ask your doctor how you should manage your diabetes so that you can prepare in advance.

5. Get a temporary disabled parking permit, if necessary.
If you are having orthopedic surgery or another operation that will make it hard for you to walk during recovery, go to your local Department of Motor Vehicles and request the appropriate paperwork. Ask your doctor to sign it in advance so that you can get your temporary permit before your operation.

6. Fill any new prescriptions before your surgery.
Ask your doctor and surgeon whether you will need any pain medication or other prescriptions after your operation. These may include antinausea pills, laxatives, or other drugs. Ask for the prescriptions in advance, so you can have the medications ready when you need them.

7. Find out how long you will need to recover.
If you will not be eating for an extended period of time, you and your doctor will need to change your diabetes care regimen. Also, you may need to make arrangements with your workplace for an extended recovery time.

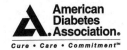

American Diabetes Association.

Cure • Care • Commitment™

Thyroid Disease and Diabetes

Diabetes and thyroid disease are both endocrine, or hormone, problems. When thyroid disease occurs in someone with diabetes, it can make blood glucose control more difficult.

The thyroid is a butterfly-shaped gland in your lower neck just beneath your skin. It regulates your body's metabolism, the processes of using and storing energy, by releasing a substance called thyroid hormone. If it produces too much thyroid hormone, your metabolism quickens (hyperthyroidism), too little and your body functions slow down (hypothyroidism).

Hyperthyroidism Symptoms
• Pounding heart
• Quick pulse
• Increased sweating
• Weight loss despite normal or increased appetite
• Shortness of breath when exercising
• Diarrhea
• Muscle weakness or tremors
• Trouble concentrating

• Change in menstrual periods
• Thick skin on the knees, elbows, and shins

Hypothyroidism Symptoms
• Fatigue
• Sluggishness
• Depression
• Feeling of being cold even when others feel warm
• Constipation
• Weight gain unrelated to increase in eating
• Low blood pressure
• Slow pulse

Effects on Diabetes
Hyperthyroidism. When your metabolism quickens, your medicines go through your body quicker. Your blood glucose level may rise because your usual dosage does not stay in your body long enough to control it.

Hyperthyroidism and low blood glucose can be hard to tell apart. If you are sweating and having tremors from hyperthyroidism, you may think you have low blood glucose and eat extra food, causing your blood glucose to rise. Using your glucose meter to

verify low blood glucose levels can help you avoid this problem.

Hypothyroidism. When your metabolism slows, your blood glucose level may drop because your diabetes medicine doesn't pass through your body as quickly as usual and so stays active longer. In hypothyroidism, it is often necessary to reduce your dose of diabetes medicines to prevent low blood glucose.

If You Think You Have Thyroid Disease
Tell your health care provider about any symptoms you have. A physical exam and simple blood tests can identify hyper- or hypothyroidism.

If you have hyperthyroidism, medicines and other treatments can help slow your metabolism by controlling the release of thyroid hormone. If you have hypothyroidism, your health care provider can prescribe thyroid hormone pills to speed up your metabolism. You will need follow-up blood tests every few months to adjust your dosage of thyroid hormone.

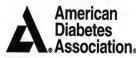

American Diabetes Association

Cure • Care • Commitment℠

Erectile Dysfunction Treatments

Erectile dysfunction (ED), former-ly called "impotence," means that a man often can't have an erection firm enough for intercourse. Men with diabetes get ED three times as often as other men.

If you think you may have ED, see your health care provider. Most cases can be treated or even cured. For example, a medical problem (such as high blood pressure) may be the cause and can be treated. Sometimes, drugs cause ED. In that case, you may be able to switch to some other drug.

ED Pills
Pills are the most common treatment for ED. Sildenafil (Viagra), vardenafil (Levitra), and tadalafil (Cialis) work by making muscles in the penis relax. Then more blood flows in.

ED pills do not cause erections by themselves. A man must also be sexually excited. The erection-helping effects of ED pills last about 4 hours with sildenafil and vardenafil and 36 hours with tadalafil.

You should not borrow these drugs from friends or buy them online. They should only be taken with your health care provider's knowledge and oversight.

Some men should never take ED pills. These include men who should not have sex for medical reasons and men who take certain drugs or have certain medical problems.

ED pills can also cause side effects. The most common are headache, flushing, upset stomach, vision changes, and erections that last longer than 4 hours.

Other ED Drugs
Alprostadil is an ED drug that comes in two forms. One form (Caverject, Caverject Impulse, or Edex) is injected into the side of the penis to increase blood flow and cause an erection within 5 to 20 minutes. Its effects last 1 hour or less. The most common side effect is pain. Other side effects include bruising, redness, numb-ness, bleeding, and irritation.

Alprostadil also comes as a pel-let that is placed within the penis. An erection then starts within 8 to 10 minutes. It lasts 30 to 60 min-utes. Side effects can include pain, aching, burning, minor bleeding, and redness.

When a man has low levels of male hormones, a doctor may pre-scribe testosterone patches. These are worn every day. Too few stud-ies have been done to know whether these patches work for ED. Injections of testosterone are also given for ED. The need for these can be determined with a blood test.

Other ED Treatments
Counseling. Stress, relationship problems, and other mental fac-tors can cause ED. Also, a man with ED may become anxious

about sex, making ED worse. So counseling may help even when ED has a physical cause.

Vacuum device. This device is placed over the penis. Then air in the device is pumped out. Blood flows into the penis and causes an erection. An elastic ring then slides onto the penis to keep the erection going after the device is removed.

Surgery. Blood vessel surgery helps some men, such as those with penis injuries. This surgery cannot help most men with dia-betes.

In another type of surgery, implants are placed in the penis. Some implants are rods that make the penis always stiff. Other implants can be inflated to cause an erection when desired.

Don't Lose Hope
In the past, many men just lived with ED. Today's treatments mean that most men with ED can get their sex lives back. The most important step is the first one: seek help by talking to your health care provider.

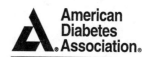

American Diabetes Association

Cure • Care • Commitment®

Permission is granted to reproduce this material for nonprofit educational purposes. Written permission is required for all other purposes.

Guidelines for Using Vitamin, Mineral, and Herbal Supplements

- **Learn about the supplements you are interested in taking.** Know the name, amounts, and effects of products you use.

- **Discuss supplements with your doctor.** Tell your health care provider about all of the medicines, herbal products, and supplements you take.

- **Keep records.** Record the doses, date started, and side effects of any supplement you use. Note your blood sugar levels while using the supplement and the effects of the supplement. Did it work?

- **Know what benefits to expect.** Long-term use of most supplements is not recommended. If a supplement is not working, stop taking it.

- **Add only one new product at a time.** It is easier to track effects if you take only one supplement at a time. If you use more than one or a combination formula, check labels to ensure that you do not exceed total dosage guidelines for individual substances.

- **Carefully follow dosage guidelines on labels.** To be cautious, start with a half dose, working up to a full dose over a week or more. Do not take greater amounts than recommended.

- **Do not combine supplements and prescription drugs without your doctor's knowledge.** Many supplements can change the way medicines work. In some cases, serious side effects can occur.

- **Never stop taking a prescribed drug without your doctor's knowledge.** Many supplements are unproven. They are not a substitute for prescription drugs you may be using.

- **Stop using supplements and contact your doctor if you notice bad side effects.** Side effects from supplements can be very serious.

- **Do not use supplements if you are pregnant or nursing or give them to young children.** The effects of many of these products on fetuses and children are not known.

- **Stop using all supplements (or check with your doctor) before surgery, anesthesia, and other medical procedures.** Several herbs can decrease the body's ability to form blood clots and could be dangerous. Others can alter the effects of anesthesia or lead to seizures.

- **Store capsules and tablets in a cool dark place at home.** Fresh herbs can be frozen in airtight containers; capsules and tablets should not be frozen.

How to Choose a Supplement

- Look for nationally known food and supplement companies.

- Look for products that have recognized symbols of quality, such as the USP, NF, TruLabel, or ConsumerLabs symbol.

- Avoid foreign products unless quality is known. Foreign products, especially those from China and India, are more likely to have dangerous contaminants.

- Avoid companies that make sensational claims or have misleading labeling.

- Look for products that have standardized extracts. Labels should clearly identify the quantities of active ingredients.

- Look for products that have an expiration date.

- Look for products that provide a toll-free customer service phone number. Call and ask if their products undergo outside testing or if there are any published studies supporting their use.

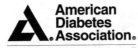

American Diabetes Association®

Cure • Care • Commitment℠

PROFESSIONAL TOOLS AND PROTOCOLS

Assessment Tools and Information Forms

Physical Assessment History

Diabetes Education Patient Self-Assessment Form

Diabetes Education—Initial Visit

Diabetes Education—Return Visit

Diabetes Education Note

Patient Diabetes Diary

Diabetes Management Plan

Diabetes Management Flowchart

Subcutaneous Insulin Administration Record

Inpatient Diabetes Management Orders—Subcutaneous Insulin

Inpatient Perioperative Glucose Management Orders

Intensive Care Unit Glucose Management Procedure

Hypoglycemia Orders

Sample Educational Objectives

Key Messages and Counseling Recommendations for Diabetes and Weight-Loss Management

Considerations When Dealing with Patients Using Atypical Antipsychotic Agents

PHYSICAL ASSESSMENT HISTORY

PLEASE ANSWER THE FOLLOWING QUESTIONS BY CHECKING THE CORRECT BOX OR FILLING IN THE UP-TO-DATE
INFORMATION. INFORMATION SHOULD RELATE TO THE LAST FEW WEEKS UNLESS OTHERWISE INDICATED.

HEALTH QUESTIONS	YES	NO	COMMENTS
ANY HEADACHES?			
ANY STUFFINESS OR PAIN IN EARS/NOSE/THROAT?			
ANY CHANGES IN VISION?			
ANY BLEEDING OR SORE GUMS?			
ANY UNUSUAL DRYNESS OF SKIN? HEEL CRACKS?			
ANY RASH OR UNUSUAL DISCOLORATION TO THE SKIN?			
FEELING TOO HOT/COLD?			
ANY CHEST PAIN OR FEELINGS OF TIGHTNESS?			
ANY NUMBNESS, TINGLING, BURNING OR PAIN IN FEET/HANDS?			
ANY PROBLEMS WITH BREATHING? SHORTNESS OF BREATH?			
ANY ABDOMINAL (STOMACH) CRAMPS?			
DIARRHEA?			
CONSTIPATION?			
ANY BURNING ON URINATION?			
PROBLEMS WITH SEXUAL FUNCTIONING?			
VAGINAL OR URETHRAL DISCHARGE?			
INCONTINENCE (LOSS OF URINE)			
ANY MUSCLE ACHES OR PAINS? BACKACHE? LEG CRAMPS?			
JOINT ACHES OR PAINS? WHERE?			
ANY DIZZINESS WHEN STANDING?			
DO YOU WEAR GLASSES?			
DO YOU WEAR DENTURES?			

LAST VISIT TO OPHTHALMOLOGIST/RETINOLOGIST:	OPTOMETRIST:
LAST VISIT TO DENTIST:	LAST VISIT TO PODIATRIST:

DO YOU FEEL YOU ARE UNDER STRESS? ❏ A LITTLE ❏ MODERATE ❏ A LOT OF PRESSURE
ARE YOU A MEMBER OF THE AMERICAN DIABETES ASSOCIATION? ❏ YES ❏ NO
IF YOU ARE ON INSULIN, WHAT SITES DO YOU USE FOR YOUR SHOTS OR INSULIN PUMP NEEDLES?
❏ ARMS ❏ LEGS ❏ ABDOMEN ❏ BACK ❏ HIPS ❏ OTHER _____
DO YOU HAVE LUMPS OR DIPS WHERE YOU GIVE YOUR SHOTS? ❏ YES ❏ NO
DO YOU HAVE SPECIFIC QUESTIONS AT THIS VISIT: _____
_____
_____
_____
_____

(continued)

SELF CARE HISTORY

NAME_____ DATE _____

To help us with your evaluation today, we would like the following information completed before your visit:

Have you changed your calories since your last visit?   ❑ YES   ❑ NO
How many calories do you eat each day?
Do you count carbohydrates?   ❑ YES   ❑ NO

LIST FOOD YOU ATE YESTERDAY *OR* USUALLY EAT IN ONE DAY

Please indicate how food was prepared. Include butter or margarine used on bread, vegetables; dressings used on salads; fried foods; sugar, milk or cream used in beverage, etc. Please list calorie/carb points for each meal and snack. Give amount or portion size for all foods eaten. Example:

What type of milk do you use?   ❑ 2%   ❑ Whole   ❑ Skim   ❑ Other _____

MEAL EXAMPLE: 1 c. 2% milk - 1 pt.;   1 c. chili - 4½ pts.;   med. apple - 1 pt.;   1 slice cheese - 1 pt.

TIME:	FOOD AMOUNT		TIME:	FOOD AMOUNT
_____	INSULIN_____ UNITS		_____	INSULIN WITH SNACKS ❑ YES ❑ NO
_____	BREAKFAST_____ CALORIE/CARB POINTS			A.M. SNACK _____ CALORIE/CARB POINTS
TIME:			TIME:	
_____	INSULIN_____ UNITS		_____	AFTERNOON SNACK _____CALORIE/CARB POINTS
_____	LUNCH _____ CALORIE/CARB POINTS			
TIME;			TIME:	
_____	INSULIN_____ UNITS		_____	EVENING INSULIN _____ UNITS
_____	SUPPER _____ CALORIE/CARB POINTS		_____	P.M. SNACK _____ CALORIE/CARB POINTS
				TOTAL CALORIE POINTS _____

Please answer the following: If female, date of last menses (period):_____

Smoke / Tobacco: ❑ Yes   ❑ No   Kind and amount per day _____

Alcohol: ❑ Yes   ❑ No   Kind and amount per week _____

Exercise: ❑ Yes   ❑ No   Kind and times per week _____
_____

Brand of Insulin: ❑ Lilly   ❑ Novolin   ❑ Aventis

Brand of Glucose Monitor _____

All Medicine with Dosage: _____
_____
_____

Reaction / Blood Sugars below 60 (Number past month) _____

Any resulting in unconsciousness: ❑ Yes   ❑ No   How many_____

This sample form is reprinted with permission from Mid-America Diabetes Associates.

DIABETES EDUCATION PATIENT SELF-ASSESSMENT FORM
(To be completed at initial visit)

Directions for filling out this form...

Your doctor has asked you to see a diabetes educator to learn more about how to take care of your diabetes. The diabetes educator will better understand your worries or concerns about diabetes after you fill out the this Diabetes Education Self-Assessment Form. This form is to be completed the first time you see the diabetes educator. Please complete all questions as best you can. If you have questions, please ask the diabetes educator during your visit.

(continued)

SECTION 1. GENERAL INFORMATION *(Please answer all questions on both sides of page)*

Today's Date: ___/___/___ Medical Record #: _____ DOB: ___/___/___

Name: _____ Referring physician or provider: _____

SECTION 2. DIABETES HEALTH STATUS

If known, please give approximate year diabetes was diagnosed _____ □ I don't know

Please give us the number of visits or days in the last 3 months that you had:

Emergency room visits or 911 calls to paramedics for high blood glucose _____ □ None

Emergency room visits or 911 calls to paramedics for low blood glucose _____ □ None

Days missed from work, school, or usual routine for diabetes _____ □ None

Hospital admissions for diabetes _____ □ None

What infections have you had within the last 3 months?

□ Head, throat, or chest □ Wound □ Vaginal (yeast) □ Foot □ Bladder □ None

SECTION 3. EXERCISE OR PHYSICAL ACTIVITY

□ Yes □ No Do you get regular physical activity or exercise? If yes, what type of exercise?_____

Frequency? _____ Length of session? _____ Usual time of day? _____

□ Yes □ No Do you adjust food, insulin, or diabetes medication for exercise?

If yes, describe _____

□ Yes □ No Do you need help in changing your physical activity or exercise?

SECTION 4. EATING OR NUTRITION

What is your height?____Weight? _____What weight are you comfortable at? _____

□ Yes □ No Has your weight changed in the past 3 months? If yes, I've □ lost or □ gained _____lbs

□ Yes □ No Was the weight change on purpose?

□ Yes □ No Have you had a diet instruction? If yes, most recent date? _____

How often do you eat or drink the following foods (answer as time per day or per week):

Fruit?_____ Juice? _____ Milk? _____ □ Fat-free □ 1% □ 2% □ Whole

Vegetables? ___ Cheese? _____ Sweets? _____ Sugar-free desserts? _____ Starches? _____

Beverages with sugar? _____ Alcohol? _____ Water? _____

How do you usually decide what to eat? □ Limit amount of fat □ Count calories

□ Count carbohydrates □ Eat anything I want □ Avoid sweets or sugar □ Follow exchange diet

□ Reduce portion sizes □ Other (please describe)_____

□ Yes □ No Do you need help or would you like a review of meal planning?

SECTION 5. MEDICATION

□ Yes □ No Do you take medications for your diabetes?

If yes, what do you take? □ Pills □ Pill and insulin □ Insulin only

If pills, what are their names and doses and when do you take them? _____

□ Yes □ No Do you have any medication allergies? If yes, what? _____

□ Yes □ No Do you take insulin? If yes, do you inject with □ a syringe? □ an insulin pen? □ an insulin pump?

What insulin do you take and when do you take it? _____

□ Yes □ No Have you ever forgotten to take your diabetes medications?

If yes, what did you do?_____

(continued)

Section 6. Monitoring Blood Glucose

☐ Yes ☐ No   **Do you check your blood glucose?** If yes, how often do you check?_____ Name of meter?_____

How do you use results? ☐ I adjust medication or insulin or food or exercise   ☐ Don't use

☐ Review with doctor or educator   ☐ Other _____

Section 7. Problem Solving for High/Low Blood Glucose and Sick Days

☐ Yes ☐ No   **Do you have low blood glucose?** If yes, what symptoms do you get? _____

At what time(s) does it tend to occur?_____ What is the cause?_____

How do you treat low blood glucose? _____

☐ Yes ☐ No   **Have you ever lost consciousness or required assistance by another person to reverse low blood glucose?**

If yes, when did it last occur? _____ How often has it occurred?_____

☐ Yes ☐ No   **Do you ever have high blood glucose?**

If yes, how do you treat high blood glucose? I change ☐ Medication ☐ Exercise ☐ Food ☐ Do nothing

What do you consider a normal blood glucose range for you? _____ ☐ I don't know

When you are sick or cannot eat your usual food, what do you do?   ☐ Drink more water

☐ Replace usual food with carbohydrates ☐ Change diabetes medication ☐ Check ketone level

☐ Contact health care provider/doctor   ☐ Check blood glucose more often ☐ Do nothing

Section 8. Risk Factor Reduction

☐ Yes ☐ No   **Do you have any of the following risk factors for diabetes complications?**

If yes, which ones ☐ High blood glucose ☐ Smoking   ☐ High cholesterol ☐ Overweight

☐ Yes ☐ No   **Do you have any of the following diabetes problems?**

☐ Eye ☐ Kidney ☐ Nerve ☐ Teeth *or* gum ☐ Foot ☐ Sexual function ☐ Other _____

How often do you check your feet? ☐ Daily   ☐ Once in awhile ☐ Rarely or never

☐ Yes ☐ No   **Do you smoke now or ever smoked in the past?** If yes, how much? _____ If quit, when?_____

☐ Yes ☐ No   **Do you drink alcohol?** If yes, how much? _____

Section 9. Living with Diabetes

☐ Yes ☐ No   **Is there much stress in your life?** If yes, explain: _____

What do you do to handle stress in your life? _____

☐ Yes ☐ No   **Do you ever get depressed?** If yes, how often? ☐ A lot ☐ Some ☐ A little

Section 10. Behavior Goals or Changes

☐ Yes ☐ No   **Do you want to change anything with your diabetes?**

If yes, please select **up to 3 things** that you want to change from the list below:

☐ Exercise more often	☐ Miss fewer medications
☐ Exercise longer	☐ Take medications on time more often
☐ Follow eating schedule better	☐ Check blood glucose more often
☐ Eat better food	☐ Miss fewer blood glucose checks
☐ Overeat less often	☐ Check blood glucose on time more often
☐ Prevent high blood glucose	☐ Get health checkups to prevent diabetes problems
☐ Treat high blood glucose	☐ Check feet daily
☐ Prevent low blood glucose	☐ Stop smoking
☐ Treat low blood glucose	☐ Lose weight
☐ Manage diabetes when sick	☐ Learn how to have a safe pregnancy
☐ Cope with diabetes	☐ Other _____
☐ Get support from my family/friends	☐ Other _____

Developed by Donna Tomky, MS, RN, CNP, CDE for the New Mexico Department of Health, Diabetes Prevention and Control Program, version 2003. Reprinted with permission.

DIABETES EDUCATION – INITIAL VISIT

Name: _____ MRN: _____ Date: _____ Age: _____

Referring/PCP: _____ Participants: ☐ Patient ☐ Family _____ ☐ Other _____

Reason for visit:	☐ Newly diagnosed	☐ Change in treatment	☐ Diabetes uncontrolled
	☐ High risk with/for complications	☐ Diabetes education	☐ Special need for 1:1 intervention

Variables affecting learning or behavior	☐ None	☐ Cultural	☐ Cognitive	☐ Emotional
	☐ Physical	☐ Language	☐ Financial	☐ Literacy
☐ Other: _____	☐ Vision	☐ Hearing	☐ Motivation	☐ Readiness

Preferred learning method ☐ Written materials ☐ Reading ☐ Discussion ☐ None stated ☐ Other: _____

Diabetes and related history Date of diagnosis: _____ ☐ Pre-diabetes ☐ Type 1 ☐ Type 2 ☐ GDM ☐ Other: _____

Symptoms/problems	☐ None	☐ Polyuria	☐ Polydipsia	☐ Polyphagia	☐ Wt change: _____
	☐ Fatigue	☐ Blurred vision	☐ Hypoglycemia	☐ Other	

Pain affecting DM management? ☐ No ☐ Yes   Pain scale (rank 0–10 _____) Pain-related visit? ☐ No ☐ Yes

Risk factors for	☐ None	☐ Age	☐ Obesity	☐ Ethnicity	☐ Chronic hyperglycemia	
diabetes or CVD	☐ Smoking	☐ Hypertension	☐ IGT history	☐ Family history	☐ Dyslipidemia	☐ GDM or >9-lb infant

Family history ☐ DM ☐ CVD ☐ Cancer ☐ Hypertension ☐ Dyslipidemia ☐ Other_____

Diabetes complications/risk assessment (Mark appropriate main category and if known, subcategories)	☐ Not reviewed ☐ No diabetes complications
	☐ Macrovascular disease --> ☐ Cardiovascular ☐ Cerebral vascular ☐ Peripheral vascular
	☐ Lower extremity -->☐ Ulceration ☐ Infection ☐ Gangrene
	☐ Nephropathy--> ☐ Microalbuminuria ☐ Macroalbuminuria ☐ Renal insufficiency ☐ ESRD ☐Transplant
	☐ Retinopathy --> ☐ Nonproliferative ☐ Proliferative ☐ Macular edema
	☐Neuropathy ---> ☐ Sexual dysfunction ☐ Gastroparesis ☐ Dysethesias
	☐ Hypoglycemia unawareness ☐ Bladder ☐ Foot deformities
	Other ------> ☐ Skin infection ☐ Dental disease ☐ Depression ☐ Other: _____
	If female --> ☐ Using birth control ☐ Not using birth control ☐ Planning pregnancy ☐ Pregnant
	☐ Sexually inactive ☐ Infertile ☐ Surgical sterilization ☐ Menopause

Past medical/surgical history	
Other current medical conditions	

CURRENT DIABETES MANAGEMENT/BEHAVIORAL ASSESSMENT

Psychosocial ☐ Not reviewed	☐ Lives alone ☐ Significant other: _____ Primary support person: _____
	# of people in household: _____ Education level: _____ Race/ethnicity:_____
	Occupation: _____ Work hours: _____ Primary language ☐ English ☐ Spanish ☐ Other _____

Risk reduction ☐ Not reviewed	Aspirin ☐ 81 mg daily ☐ 325 mg QOD ☐ None ☐ N/A	Foot exam current?	☐ No ☐ Yes ☐ Don't know
	Last dilated eye exam: _____	Flu vaccine current?	☐ No ☐ Yes ☐ Don't know
	Last dental exam: _____	Pneumonia vaccine current?	☐ No ☐ Yes ☐ Don't know
	Alcohol use? ☐ No ☐ Yes, amt?_____Tobacco use? ☐ No ☐ Yes_____	Illicit drugs?	☐ No ☐ Yes ☐ Don't know
	If female, counseled about pregnancy and diabetes? ☐ No ☐ Yes ☐ N/A		

Physical activity ☐ Not reviewed	☐ Regular exercise program	☐ Activities of daily living	☐ Limited due to physical problems
	Type: _____	Frequency: _____	Duration: _____

Nutritional management ☐ Not reviewed Change in weight? ☐ Yes _____ ☐ No _____

Usual eating: ☐ Carb counts ☐ Low fat ☐ Avoids sweets ☐ Eat anything desired ☐ Portion control Caffeine ☐ No ☐ Yes _____

Appetite: ☐ Good ☐ Fair ☐ Poor Most meals prepared in ☐ Home ☐ Home and eat out ☐ Mostly eat out or take out

24-h diet recall: Monthly food budget? ☐ Adequate ☐ Inadequate ☐ Referred to food resources

(continued)

Monitoring—Blood Glucose	Frequency of SMBG? _____	Meter? _____	Insulin storage? _____

TIME OF DAY	FASTING		LUNCH		SUPPER		BEDTIME	
BG patterns								

Diabetes medications (list)

Insulin/OHA doses								

Frequency of missed doses: Site rotation? _____ Uses sharps disposal? ☐ No ☐ Yes ☐ N/A   Other:

Drug or food allergies: ☐ None ☐ Yes (list) _____

Other medications:

Problem Solving: Acute complications/illness/hospitalizations for diabetes? ☐ No ☐ Yes (give details) ☐ Not reviewed

Wears or carries diabetes ID? ☐ No ☐ Yes Glucagon on hand and in date? ☐ No ☐ Yes ☐ Don't know ☐ N/A Checks urine ketones? ☐ No ☐ Yes ☐ N/A

Knowledge/skill deficits or behavior change requirements were identified in these areas:

☐ None identified	☐ Physical activity	☐ Nutritional management	☐ Medication
	☐ Blood glucose monitoring	☐ Problem solving	☐ Psychosocial adjustment
	☐ Risk reduction	☐ Disease process	☐ Other: _____

Objective results	Height: _____	Weight: _____	BMI: _____	Waist circumference: _____	Glucose: _____

Date	Clinical indicator	Result	BP: _____	Time since last food: _____
_____	A1C:	_____	Normal range for lab: _____	
_____	Microalbumin:	_____	If not done, is nephropathy present? ☐ No ☐ Yes	
_____	ALT:	_____	AST: _____	Foot exam findings: _____
_____	Serum creatinine:	_____		
_____	Total chol: ____ HDL: _____		LDL: _____	Triglycerides: _____

DIABETES EDUCATION INTERVENTION

Educational areas	Delivery methods	Resources	Educator's assessment
☐ Psychosocial adjustment	☐ Demonstration	☐ Audio tape	☐ Not engaged
☐ Risk reduction	☐ Discussion	☐ Computer aided	☐ Minimal knowledge gain
☐ Physical activity	☐ Computer	☐ Medical interpreter	☐ Partial knowledge or skill competence
☐ Nutritional management	☐ Lecture	☐ Video tape	☐ Verbalizes/demonstrates knowledge/skill competence
☐ Blood glucose monitoring	☐ Phone	☐ Written instructions	☐ Mastery over knowledge or skill competence
☐ Medication	☐ Other		
☐ Problem solving		☐ Printed materials →	Handouts provided: _____
☐ Disease process			_____
☐ Other			

	Behavioral strategies	Goal setting
☐ None	☐ Motivational interviewing	☐ Educator defined
☐ Self-monitoring	☐ Situational problem solving	☐ Patient defined
☐ Stimulus control	☐ Other	☐ Negotiated
☐ Cognitive reframing	☐ Other	

Management plan/behavioral goals ☐ See Diabetes Management Plan Form	Patient's confidence to change behaviors
	☐ Sure I can
	☐ Think I can
	☐ Not sure I can
	☐ Don't think I can
Length of visit in minutes: ☐ 15 ☐ 30 ☐ 45 ☐ 60 ☐ 90 ☐ 75 ☐ 120 Other: _____	Percent counseling: _____
Educator's Signature and Credentials:	**Date:**

Developed by Donna Tomky, MS, RN, CNP, CDE, for the New Mexico Department of Health, Diabetes Prevention and Control Program, version 2003. Reprinted with permission.

DIABETES EDUCATION – RETURN VISIT

Name: _____ MRN: _____ Date: _____ Age: ____

Referring/PCP: _____ Participants: ☐ Patient ☐ Family _____ ☐ Other _____

Reason for visit:	☐ Newly diagnosed	☐ Change in treatment	☐ Diabetes uncontrolled
☐ Follow-up	☐ High risk with/for complications	☐ Diabetes education	☐ Special need for 1:1 intervention

Variables affecting learning or behavior	☐ None	☐ Cultural	☐ Cognitive	☐ Emotional
	☐ Physical	☐ Language	☐ Financial	☐ Literacy
☐ Other _____	☐ Vision	☐ Hearing	☐ Motivation	☐ Readiness

Preferred learning method   ☐ Written materials   ☐ Reading   ☐ Discussion   ☐ None stated   ☐ Other: _____

Diabetes and related history Date of diagnosis: _____ ☐ Pre-diabetes ☐ Type 1 ☐ Type 2 ☐ GDM ☐ Other: _____

Symptoms/problems	☐ None	☐ Polyuria	☐ Polydipsia	☐ Polyphagia	☐ Wt change: _____
	☐ Fatigue	☐ Blurred vision	☐ Hypoglycemia	☐ Other	

Other problems _____

_____

_____

Pain affecting DM management? ☐ No ☐ Yes   Pain scale (rank 0–10 _____) Pain-related visit? ☐ No ☐ Yes

New events since last visit	☐ None

Diabetes complications/risk assessment (Mark appropriate main category and, if known, subcategories)	☐ Not reviewed ☐ No diabetes complications ☐ No change since last visit
	☐ Macrovascular disease --> ☐ Cardiovascular ☐ Cerebral vascular ☐ Peripheral vascular
	☐ Lower extremity -->☐ Ulceration ☐ Infection ☐ Gangrene
	☐ Nephropathy--> ☐ Microalbuminuria ☐ Macroalbuminuria ☐ Renal insufficiency ☐ ESRD ☐ Transplant
	☐ Retinopathy --> ☐ Nonproliferative ☐ Proliferative ☐ Macular edema
	☐Neuropathy ---> ☐ Sexual dysfunction ☐ Gastroparesis ☐ Dysethesias
	☐ Hypoglycemia unawareness ☐ Bladder ☐ Foot deformities

	Other ------>	☐ Skin infection	☐ Dental disease	☐ Depression ☐ Other: _____
	If female -->	☐ Using birth control	☐ Not using birth control	☐ Planning pregnancy ☐ Pregnant
		☐ Sexually inactive	☐ Infertile	☐ Surgical sterilization ☐ Menopause

Risk factors for CVD	☐ None	☐ Obesity	☐ Age	☐ Ethnicity	☐ Chronic hyperglycemia
		☐ Hypertension	☐ Smoking	☐ Family history	☐ Dyslipidemia

CURRENT DIABETES MANAGEMENT/BEHAVIORAL ASSESSMENT

Psychosocial ☐ Not reviewed	Changes since last visit in living situation, education, or employment? ☐ No ☐ Yes (list) _____

Risk reduction ☐ Not reviewed	Aspirin ☐ 81 mg daily ☐ 325 mg QOD ☐ None ☐ N/A	Foot exam current?	☐ No ☐ Yes ☐ Don't know
	Dilated eye exam current? ☐ No ☐ Yes ☐ Don't know	Flu vaccine current?	☐ No ☐ Yes ☐ Don't know
	Dental exam current? ☐ No ☐ Yes ☐ Don't know	Pneumonia vaccine current?	☐ No ☐ Yes ☐ Don't know
	Alcohol use? ☐ No ☐ Yes- Amt? _____Tobacco use? ☐ No ☐ Yes_____ Illicit drugs?		☐ No ☐ Yes _____
	If female, counseled about pregnancy & diabetes? ☐ No ☐ Yes ☐ N/A		

Physical activity ☐ Not reviewed	☐ Regular exercise program	☐ Activities of daily living	☐ Limited due to physical problems
	Type: _____	Frequency: _____	Duration: _____

Nutritional management: ☐ Not reviewed

Usual eating: ☐ Carb counts ☐ Low fat ☐ Avoids sweets ☐ Eat anything desired ☐ Portion control Caffeine ☐ No ☐ Yes _____

Appetite:	☐ Good	☐ Fair	☐ Poor	Most meals prepared in ☐ Home ☐ Home and eat out ☐ Mostly eat out or take out

24-h diet recall:

(continued)

Monitoring—Blood Glucose	Frequency of SMBG? _____		Meter? _____		Insulin storage? _____		
TIME OF DAY	**FASTING**		**LUNCH**		**SUPPER**		**BEDTIME**	
BG patterns								

Diabetes medications (list)								
Insulin/OHA doses								

Frequency of missed doses: Site rotation? _____   Uses sharps disposal? ☐ No ☐ Yes ☐ N/A Other:

Drug or food allergies: ☐ None ☐ Yes (list) _____
Other medications:

Problem Solving: Acute complications/illness/hospitalizations for diabetes? ☐ No ☐ Yes (give details) ☐ Not reviewed

Wears or carries diabetes ID? ☐ No ☐ Yes Glucagon on hand and in date? ☐ No ☐ Yes ☐ Don't know ☐ N/A Checks urine ketones? ☐ No ☐ Yes ☐ N/A

Knowledge/skill deficits or behavior change requirements were identified in these areas:

☐ None identified   ☐ Physical activity   ☐ Nutritional management   ☐ Medication
                       ☐ Blood glucose monitoring   ☐ Problem solving   ☐ Psychosocial adjustment
                       ☐ Risk reduction   ☐ Disease process   ☐ Other: _____

Objective results	Height: _____	Weight: _____	BMI: _____	Waist circumference: _____	Glucose: _____
Date	**Clinical indicator**	**Result**	BP: _____	Time since last food: _____	
_____	A1C:	_____	Normal range for lab: _____		
_____	Microalbumin:	_____	If not done, is nephropathy present? ☐ No ☐ Yes		
_____	ALT:	_____	AST: _____	Foot exam findings: _____	
_____	Serum creatinine: _____				
_____	Total chol: _____ HDL: _____		LDL: _____	Triglycerides: _____	

DIABETES EDUCATION INTERVENTION

Educational areas	Delivery methods	Resources	Educator's assessment
☐ Psychosocial adjustment	☐ Demonstration	☐ Audio tape	☐ Not engaged
☐ Risk reduction	☐ Discussion	☐ Computer aided	☐ Minimal knowledge gain
☐ Physical activity	☐ Computer	☐ Medical interpreter	☐ Partial knowledge or skill competence
☐ Nutritional management	☐ Lecture	☐ Video tape	☐ Verbalizes/demonstrates knowledge/skill competence
☐ Blood glucose monitoring	☐ Phone	☐ Written instructions	☐ Mastery over knowledge or skill competence
☐ Medication	☐ Other		
☐ Problem solving		☐ Printed materials →	Handouts given: _____
☐ Disease process			_____
☐ Other			

Behavioral strategies		Goal setting
☐ None	☐ Motivational interviewing	☐ Educator defined
☐ Self-monitoring	☐ Situational problem solving	☐ Patient defined
☐ Stimulus control	☐ Other	☐ Negotiated
☐ Cognitive reframing	☐ Other	

Management plan/behavioral goals ☐ See Diabetes Management Plan Form	**Patient's confidence to change behaviors**
	☐ Sure I can
	☐ Think I can
	☐ Not sure I can
	☐ Don't think I can

Length of visit in minutes: ☐ 15 ☐ 30 ☐ 45 ☐ 60 ☐ 75 ☐ 90 ☐ 120 Other: _____   Percent counseling _____

Educator's Signature and Credentials: **Date:**

Developed by Donna Tomky, MS, RN, CNP, CDE for the New Mexico Dept of Health, Diabetes Prevention and Control Program, version 2003. Reprinted with permission.

DIABETES EDUCATION NOTE

Patient name:	MRN:	Date:
Referring/PCP:	Participant(s): ☐ Patient ☐ Family_____ ☐ Other _____	
Reason for visit:		

S = "Subjective"	(Concerns, observations, and information patient reports at this visit.)
(Use back of page for additional notes)	

O ="Objective"	(Observations from meter, weight, blood pressure, or physical exam.)

☐ See Medication Flowsheet or list medications below:	Height	Weight	BMI	Waist circumference
	Cholesterol	HDL	LDL	TG
	BP	A1C	Microalbumin	

Other lab values:

Meter readings: From _____ To _____

Date	Breakfast		Lunch		Supper		Bedtime/night
	Pre	Post	Pre	Post	Pre	Post	

Physical findings/foot exam:

A = "Assessment"	(Summary of findings.)

P = "Plan"	List education/treatment plan **or** ☐ see Diabetes Management Plan form

Length of visit in minutes: ☐ 15 ☐ 30 ☐ 45 ☐ 60 ☐ 75 ☐ 90 ☐ 120 Other: _____ Percent counseling: _____

Educator's Signature and Credentials: _____ Date: _____

(continued)

(Additional Notes)	

Developed by Donna Tomky, MS, RN, CNP, CDE for the New Mexico Department of Health, Diabetes Prevention and Control Program, version 2003. Reprinted with permission.

PATIENT NAME:

Date	Day of week	Meal (Medication = Med)		Before (Blood glucose = BG)	After	What was eaten?	Amount eaten	Place eaten	Exercise (duration)
		Breakfast	Time						
			BG						
			Med						
		Lunch	Time						
			BG						
			Med						
		Supper	Time						
			BG						
			Med						
		Bedtime	Time						
			BG						
			Med						
		Breakfast	Time						
			BG						
			Med						
		Lunch	Time						
			BG						
			Med						
		Supper	Time						
			BG						
			Med						
		Bedtime	Time						
			BG						
			Med						
		Breakfast	Time						
			BG						
			Med						
		Lunch	Time						
			BG						
			Med						
		Supper	Time						
			BG						
			Med						
		Bedtime	Time						
			BG						
			Med						

DIABETES DIARY

Developed by Donna Tomky, MS, RN, CNP, CDE for the New Mexico Department of Health, Diabetes Prevention and Control Program, version 2003. Reprinted with permission.

(continued)

DIABETES DIARY

PATIENT NAME:

DATE	DAY	Morning – What was eaten? (food, amount, place eaten)	Midday – What was eaten? (food, amount, place eaten)	Evening – What was eaten? (food, amount, place eaten)	Bedtime – What was eaten? (food, amount, place eaten)
	MON	BG / Med / Time / Comments	BG / Med / Time / Comments	BG / Med / Time / Comments	BG / Med / Time / Comments
	TUES	BG / Med / Time / Comments	BG / Med / Time / Comments	BG / Med / Time / Comments	BG / Med / Time / Comments
	WED	BG / Med / Time / Comments	BG / Med / Time / Comments	BG / Med / Time / Comments	BG / Med / Time / Comments
	THURS	BG / Med / Time / Comments	BG / Med / Time / Comments	BG / Med / Time / Comments	BG / Med / Time / Comments
	FRI	BG / Med / Time / Comments	BG / Med / Time / Comments	BG / Med / Time / Comments	BG / Med / Time / Comments
	SAT	BG / Med / Time / Comments	BG / Med / Time / Comments	BG / Med / Time / Comments	BG / Med / Time / Comments
	SUN	BG / Med / Time / Comments	BG / Med / Time / Comments	BG / Med / Time / Comments	BG / Med / Time / Comments

Developed by Donna Tomky, MS, RN, CNP, CDE for the New Mexico Department of Health, Diabetes Prevention and Control Program, version 2003. Reprinted with permission.

DIABETES MANAGEMENT PLAN

Name: _____ DOB: _____ MRN: _____

Date:____/____/____		Not done	Your Goal
Your weight is:	_____ lbs	☐	
Your blood glucose (sugar) is:	_____ mg/dl	☐	Premeal _____; 2-h postmeal <____
Your A1C is:	_____ %	☐	Less than _____
Your blood pressure is:	_____/_____ mmHg	☐	Less than _____
Your total cholesterol is:	_____ mg/dl	☐	Less than _____
Your LDL cholesterol is:	_____ mg/dl	☐	Less than _____
Your HDL cholesterol is:	_____ mg/dl	☐	Greater than _____
Your triglycerides are:	_____ mg/dl	☐	Less than _____

Suggested steps to take:

_____

_____

_____

_____

_____

_____

_____

_____

_____

You need blood or urine tests for	☐ A1C (every 3–6 months) ☐ Fasting lipids "cholesterol" (annual)	☐ Urine microalbumin (annual) ☐ Other: _____
You need to make an appointment for diabetes education for	☐ Diabetes dilated eye exam (annual) ☐ Meal plan ☐ Insulin start ☐ Per diabetes educator's assessment ☐ Per assessed needs _____	☐ Podiatry for foot exam or care ☐ Blood glucose monitoring

Please schedule your next appointment in _____

I have read, understand, and have received a copy of these instructions:

_____   _____

     Patient or Guardian's Signature   Provider's Signature

White Copy – Chart   Yellow Copy – Patient

DIABETES MANAGEMENT PLAN

(continued)

General Information:

The New Mexico Department of Health Diabetes Prevention and Control Program provides a suite of tools/forms to choose from. The Diabetes Management Plan form is only one of many available to you for consistent and concise documentation of the diabetes education and/or medical care visits. The tools/forms can be used alone or in combination in educating and managing individuals with diabetes to document your assessment, intervention, and plan. This form is designed to provide both the provider and patient with a written plan to document the visit.

New Mexico Diabetes Practice Guideline 2002

This guideline is not meant to be comprehensive. It is designed to quickly summarize elements that, at a minimum, should be considered in the care plan of most individuals with diabetes.

FREQUENCY	PROCEDURE/TEST	ACTION OR GOAL
Every Visit	Interval history	Review glucose testing log, hypoglycemic episodes, current medications
	Blood pressure	<130/80 mmHg
	Weight	Obtain weight or BMI
	Foot exam	Inspect skin for signs of pressure areas and breakdown
Quarterly to Semiannually	A1C	Test 2–4 times per year, goal <7.0%
At Least Once Each Year	Assess patient knowledge of diabetes, nutrition, and self-management skills	Ensure patient needs are being met by providing or referring for self-management and/or nutrition counseling
Annually	Foot risk assessment	Check pulses, conduct monofilament exam
	Nephropathy screening	If not already diagnosed with nephropathy, screen for Microalbuminuria (normal <30 μg/mg creatinine)
	Lipid profile	LDL <100 mg/dl
		HDL >40 mg/dl in men; >50 mg/dl in women
		Triglycerides <150 mg/dl
	Retinal eye exam	

This guideline is based on the recommendations of the American Diabetes Association (ADA). For more information, including full documentation for the above clinical recommendations, consult the ADA website at www.diabetes.org or contact the ADA at 1-800-DIABETES.

This guideline should not be construed as representing standards of care or should it be considered a substitute for individualized evaluation and treatment based on clinical circumstances.

Developed by Donna Tomky, MS, RN, CNP, CDE for the New Mexico Department of Health, Diabetes Prevention and Control Program, version 2003. Reprinted with permission.

(continued)

| Example of How to Use This Form | | DIABETES MANAGEMENT PLAN | | |

Name: _John Doe Patient_ **DOB:** _____ **MRN:** __224567__

Date: _11 / 15 / 04_			Not done	Your Goal
Your weight is:	_200_	lbs	☐	
Your blood glucose (sugar) is:	_235_	mg/dl	☐	Premeal _80-120_; 2-h postmeal <_140_
Your A1C is:	_8.8_	%	☐	Less than _7.0_
Your blood pressure is:	_124 / 72_	mmHg	☐	Less than _130/80_
Your total cholesterol is:	_191_	mg/dl	☐	Less than _200_
Your LDL cholesterol is:	_135_	mg/dl	☐	Less than _100_
Your HDL cholesterol is:	_44_	mg/dl	☐	Greater than _40_
Your triglycerides are:	_230_	mg/dl	☐	Less than _200_

Suggested Steps To Take:

1. Add metformin 500 mg, take 1 pill with breakfast and supper

2. Goals selected: a) Exercise more often -- Begin walking 5-10 minutes every day

b) Prevent high blood sugars - take medication as discussed

c) Lose weight - limit carbohydrates to 60 grams per meal

3. Check blood sugar before breakfast, noon, supper, and bedtime and record results

You need blood or urine tests for	☐ A1C (every 3–6 months)	☐ Urine microalbumin (annual)
	☐ Fasting lipids "cholesterol" (annual)	☐ Other: _____
You need to make an appointment or diabetes education for	✗ Diabetes dilated eye exam (annual)	☐ Podiatry for foot exam or care
	✗ Meal plan ☐ Insulin start	☐ Blood glucose monitoring
	✗ Per diabetes educator's assessment	
	☐ Per assessed needs _____	

Please schedule your next appointment in __3 months__

I have read, understand, and have received a copy of these instructions:

_____John Doe Patient_____   _____Dr. Primary Care_____

Patient or Guardian's Signature   Provider's Signature

White Copy – Chart   Yellow Copy -- Patient

DIABETES MANAGEMENT PLAN

Developed by Donna Tomky, MS, RN, CNP, CDE for the New Mexico Department of Health, Diabetes Prevention and Control Program, version 2003. Reprinted with permission.

DIABETES MANAGEMENT FLOWCHART

This flow chart indicates minimum services / care to be provided in the continuing care of persons with diabetes according to recognized standards of care. It is not intended to preclude more intensive evaluation and management where medically indicated. Provider's initials, value, and/or date in boxes indicate service has been provided. If service not done, then either draw a line in box "— " or if done on a different visit date, add date performed.

Patient _____ DOB _____ ID # _____

OUTCOMES	Visit Date								
Height _____ Weight --> every visit (document value)									
BP --> every visit (-- document value)									
SMBG results reviewed -->every visit (document percent in target)									
Aspirin Therapy --> (document Y=yes / N=No / NI=not indicated)									
Smoking Status --> (document # of ppd or N = not smoking)?									
Acute Complications / Illness / Hospitalizations? (Y=yes/ N=no)									
# of Behavior Goals Set? --> (document total # set)									
# of Behavior Goals Met? --> (document x out y goals met)									
A1C--> every 3-6 months (document value)									
Urine Microalbumin --> at least annually (document value)									
ACE Inhibitor or ARB (document Y=yes / N=no)									
Foot Exam --> annually (document NL=normal / Abn=abnormal)									
Dilated Eye Exam -->at least annually (document date done)									
Lipids ---> Total Chol -->at least annually (document results)									
HDL-C -->at least annually (document results)									
LDL-C -->at least annually (document results)									
Triglycerides -->at least annually (document results)									
(Document treatment-->M=Meds / D=Diet / NI=Not Indicated)									
MNT-->(document D=done / amount of Carb/Meal recommended)									
Vaccinations (Adults: Influenza, Pneumovax)									
Other									
Other									
Other									
Other									

Complete provider's signature, credentials, and initials in designated area.

Signature: _____ Initials: _____ Signature: _____ Initials: _____

Signature: _____ Initials: _____ Signature: _____ Initials: _____

DIABETES MANAGEMENT FLOWCHART

Developed by Donna Tomky, MS, RN, CNP, CDE for the New Mexico Department of Health, Diabetes Prevention and Control Program, version 2003. Reprinted with permission.

⚕ LOVELACE
Albuquerque, New Mexico

INSULIN is to be administered Subcutaneous, ac and bedtime based on patient's CBG as per ordered Dose Regimen:

ORDER Date: ___ / ___ / ___ Insulin: ☐ Regular Other: _____

CBG Frequency: ☐ ac/q bedtime ☐ q6h ☐ Other _____

SELECT ONE: DOSE REGIMEN IS IN UNITS OF INSULIN

CBG	☐ **Low** Dose		☐ **Medium** Dose		☐ **High** Dose		☐ **Other**	
	NPO/ bedtime	Pre-Meal	NPO/ bedtime	Pre-Meal	NPO/ bedtime	Pre-Meal	NPO/ bedtime	Pre-Meal
Less than or Equal to 70	Hypoglycemia Protocol		Hypoglycemia Protocol		Hypoglycemia Protocol		Hypoglycemia Protocol	
71-90	0	0	0	0	0	0		
91-120	0	2	0	4	0	6		
121-150	0	3	0	5	0	8		
151-200	2	4	4	6	5	10		
201-250	3	5	5	7	7	12		
251-300	4	6	6	8	9	14		
301-350	5	7	8	10	11	16		
351-400	6	8	10	12	13	18		
Greater than 400	7	9	12	14	15	20		

BASAL INSULIN

☐ Lantus insulin _____ units Subcut q bedtime or _____ units Subcut qam

☐ NPH insulin _____ units Subcut qam _____ units Subcut q bedtime

☐ Other _____

Patients who are NPO may require a reduction in basal insulin.

INTERVENTIONS - *Diabetes Protocol Goal: daytime CBG 80-150 and bedtime CBG 100-150.*

- For any **CBG** less than or equal to 70, initiate the hypoglycemia protocol.
- If **CBG** less than 80 x 2 *within any 24 hr time period*, call MD between 0800 – 1700 hours to consider decreasing basal insulin.
- If CBG greater than 250 x 2 *within any 24 hr time period* and all readings are greater than 100, call MD between 0800 – 1700 hours to consider increasing basal insulin.

INSULIN ADMINISTRATION RECORD   *Transcribed By:* _____ /

Date:		Times to begin from 0001 hours						Signature / Title	Initials
CBG	Time								
	CBG								
	Initials								
INSULIN	Admin.Time								
	Type								
	Units								
Date:	Site								
	Admin. by								
Date:		Times to begin from 0001 hours							
CBG	Time								
	CBG								
	Initials								
INSULIN	Admin. Time								
	Type								
	Units								
Date:	Site								
	Admin. by								
Date:		Times to begin from 0001 hours							
CBG	Time								
	CBG								
	Initials								
INSULIN	Admin. Time								
	Type								
	Units								
Date:	Site								
	Admin. by								

DBT046(7/04)

SUBCUTANEOUS INSULIN ADMINISTRATION RECORD

Reprinted with permission from Lovelace.

Forms

Albuquerque, New Mexico

⚕ LOVELACE
Generic drugs will be dispensed unless otherwise ordered. Formulary substitutions will be made only with P&T approval

ALLERGIES and Adverse Drug Reactions (Describe reaction, if known): _____
_____
_____ No medications will be sent without allergy information

Date:___/___/___ Time:_____ *Note: Orders Recommended for Inpatients on Subcutaneous Insulin. Not to be used for DKA.*
1. ☐ Diabetes Education (Consult In-Patient Education)
2. CBG's - ☐ If eating, ac and bedtime ☐ If NPO, perform CBGs q 6 h ☐Other:_____
3. Admission Labs: ☐ A1C ☐ Urine Microalbumin ☐ Fasting Lipids
4. **Basal Insulin:** *Suggest using 50% of total daily insulin or weight based 0.2- 0.4 units/kg/day.*
   Patients who are NPO may require a reduction in basal insulin.
   ☐ Lantus insulin _____units Subcut at bedtime, **OR** ☐ _____Units Subcut qam **OR** ☐ Other_____
   ☐ NPH insulin _____units Subcut qam, _____ units Subcut at bedtime
   ☐ Other _____
5. **INTERVENTIONS** - *Diabetes Protocol Goal: daytime CBG 80-150 and bedtime CBG 100-150.*
   • For any CBG less than or equal to 70, initiate the hypoglycemia protocol.
   • If CBG less than 80 x 2 *within any 24 hr time period*, call MD between 0800 – 1700 hours to consider decreasing basal insulin by 10 – 30% and/or lower to the next lower dose regimen of Regular insulin.
   • If CBG greater than 250 x 2 *within any 24 hr time period* and all readings are greater than 100, call MD between 0800 – 1700 hours to consider increasing basal insulin by 10 – 30% and/or advance to next higher dose regimen of Regular Insulin.
   • **Patients who are NPO may require a reduction in basal insulin.**
6. **REGIMEN – Check below.**

NOTE: *All insulin ordered below is* **Regular insulin** *given Subcut unless otherwise specified.*

CBG	☐Low Dose *Less than 30 units of insulin per day or thin patient.*		☐Medium Dose *30 to 60 units of insulin per day or average size patient.*		☐High Dose *Greater than 60 units of insulin per day or obese patient.*		☐ OTHER	
	NPO/ bedtime	**Pre-Meal**	**NPO/** bedtime	**Pre-Meal**	**NPO/** bedtime	**Pre-Meal**	**NPO/** bedtime	**Pre-Meal**
Less than or Equal to 70	*Hypoglycemia Protocol*		*Hypoglycemia Protocol*		*Hypoglycemia Protocol*		*Hypoglycemia Protocol*	
71 - 90	0	0	0	0	0	0		
91 - 120	0	2	0	4	0	6		
121 - 150	0	3	0	5	0	8		
151 - 200	2	4	4	6	5	10		
201 - 250	3	5	5	7	7	12		
251 - 300	4	6	6	8	9	14		
301 - 350	5	7	8	10	11	16		
351 - 400	6	8	10	12	13	18		
Greater than 400	7	9	12	14	15	20		

Other:
_____
_____
_____
_____
_____
_____
_____
_____
_____
_____

Physician Signature: _____ Date: _____

DBT045 7/04

IP DIABETES MANAGEMENT ORDERS – SUBCUTANEOUS INSULIN

Reprinted with permission from Lovelace.

DATE	TIME	NOTE: specify route of administration on Medication Orders **HOUSE ORDER SET**
		Generic or therapeutic substitutions (as deemed appropriate by the Pharmacy and Therapeutics Committee) may be made unless the physician writes "NO SUBSTITUTION" on EACH medication order.

INPATIENT PERI-OPERATIVE GLUCOSE MANAGEMENT ORDERS

Pre-Operative:
1. Initiate orders for inpatients with hyperglycemia.
2. Discontinue all oral hypoglycemic agents the day of surgery.
3. Discontinue Metformin (Glucophage) the a.m. of surgery.
4. Discontinue previous insulin schedule the day of surgery.
5. If surgery start time is scheduled after 10:00 a.m., floor personnel to check blood glucose in a.m., and then every 4 hours until patients goes to surgery. If blood glucose is not within 80-120 mg/dL range, notify physician managing the diabetic aspect of the patient's care.

Intra-Operative:
6. Check blood glucose (BG) test in Pre-Op Holding Area (POHA), on arrival in OR suite if patient is transported to OR directly from the floor, or on the Ambulatory Care Unit if a.m. admit patient.
   a. For BG < 74 mg/dl, start D5/LR AT 100 ml/hr or per Anesthesia.
   b. For BG ≤ 120 mg/dl, re-check glucose q 1 hr.
   c. For BG ≥ 120 mg/dl, initiate continuous insulin IV infusion:
      50 units regular insulin in 50 ml normal saline via IV pump at 0.05 units/kg/hr.
7. Repeat blood glucose q 30-60 minutes intra-operatively.
   a. Initiate insulin infusion at any point BG ≥ 150mg/ dl.
   b. Once insulin infusion has been initiated, titrate rate to maintain blood glucose between 80-120 mg/dL.
8. Titration scales

Glucose (mg/dL)	Infusion Rate of 1-5 units/hr	Infusion Rate of 6-10 units/hr	Infusion Rate of 11-16 units/hr
< 75	DC Infusion; give D50W 10-20 ml and recheck blood glucose in 30 min. When BG > 80, restart with 50% of previous rate.		
80-120	No Changes Now If glucose continues to decrease within the desired range over 3 consecutive checks, decrease rate by 1 unit/hr		No Changes Now If glucose continues to decrease within the desired range over 3 consecutive checks, decrease rate by 2 units/hr
121-200	Increase infusion by 1 unit/hr	Increase infusion by 2 units/hr	Increase infusion by 3 units/hr
201-250	Give 2 units IVP and increase infusion by 1 unit/hr	Give 3 units IVP and increase infusion by 2 units/hr	Give 3 units IVP and increase infusion by 3 units/hr
251-300	Give 3 units IVP and increase infusion by 1 unit/hr	Give 5 units IVP and increase infusion by 2 units/hr	Give 5 units IVP and increase infusion by 3 units/hr
301-350	Give 8 units IVP and increase infusion by 1 unit/hr	Give 8 units IVP and increase infusion by 2 units/hr	Give 8 units IVP and increase infusion by 3 units/hr
351-400	Give 10 units IVP and increase infusion by 1 unit/hr	Give 10 units IVP and increase infusion by 2 units/hr	Give 10 units IVP and increase infusion by 3 units/hr

VC-1667
New 08/2003   Page 1 of 2

DRUG ALLERGIES	UNIT	ROOM #	PATIENT IDENTIFICATION
	PATIENT NAME - HAND WRITTEN		

Original - Retain on Chart   Copy - To Pharmacy
VIA CHRISTI REGIONAL MEDICAL CENTER, WICHITA, KS.
PHYSICIAN ORDER SET

(continued)

DATE	TIME	NOTE: specify route of administration on Medication Orders
		HOUSE ORDER SET
		Generic or therapeutic substitutions (as deemed appropriate by the Pharmacy and Therapeutics Committee) may be made unless the physician writes **"NO SUBSTITUTION"** on EACH medication order.

IN-PATIENT PERI-OPERATIVE GLUCOSE MANAGEMENT ORDERS

Post-Operative:

  9. Check blood glucose upon arrival to PACU or ICU.

      a.   If patient already on insulin infusion, use insulin titration scale to maintain BG between 80-120 mg/dL.

      b.   If patient not on insulin infusion, follow intra-operative parameters for starting insulin infusion based on blood glucose level.

  10. When weaning vasopressors, check blood glucose q60 minutes.

  11. Follow ICU Glucose Management Procedure Standing Orders (VC-1668).

_____

Physician's Signature

Page 2 of 2
VC-1667
New 08/2003

Approved by P&T Committee 08-14-03
Approved by PIC Committee 09-2-03

Approved by MEC Committee 09-15-03

DRUG ALLERGIES	UNIT	ROOM #	PATIENT IDENTIFICATION
	PATIENT NAME - HAND WRITTEN		

Original - Retain on Chart   Copy - To Pharmacy
VIA CHRISTI REGIONAL MEDICAL CENTER, WICHITA, KS.
PHYSICIAN ORDER SET

Reprinted with permission from Via Christi Medical Center.

DATE	TIME	
		NOTE: specify route of administration on Medication Orders **HOUSE ORDER SET**
		Generic or therapeutic substitutions (as deemed appropriate by the Pharmacy and Therapeutics Committee) may be made unless the physician writes **"NO SUBSTITUTION"** on EACH medication order.

ICU Glucose Management Procedure

1. Patient must be admitted to an Intensive Care Area.
2. Blood sugar by Accuchek and test urine ketones on initiation.
3. CBC and Basic Metabolic Panel, unless done in last 24 hours.
4. Vital signs every 2 hours X 8 hours.
5. IV Fluid: 1000 mL 0.9% normal saline to run at _____ mL/hr.
6. Human regular insulin, 50 units in 50 mL 0.9% normal saline. Start infusion at **0.05 units/kg/hour.**
7. Goal: Maintain blood glucose between 80 and 120 mg/dL.
8. Monitoring: Check glucose q1h (either capillary or blood) until stable (3 values in desired range). Checks can then be reduced to q2h X 4 checks and then q 4 hours if blood glucose remains in desired range. Restart q1h checking if any change in insulin infusion rate occurs.
9. VCRMC Hypoglycemia Orders (VC-044) on chart.

Ongoing Insulin Infusion:

Glucose (mg/dL)	Infusion Rate of 1-5 units/hr	Infusion Rate of 6-10 units/hr	Infusion Rate of 11-16 units/hr	Infusion Rate of > 16 units/hr
<75	DC Infusion; give D50W 10-20 ml and recheck blood glucose in 30 min. When BG > 80, restart with 50% of previous rate.			
80-120	**No Changes Now** If glucose continues to decrease within the desired range over 3 consecutive checks, decrease rate by 1 unit/hr		**No Changes Now** If glucose continues to decrease within the desired range over 3 consecutive checks, decrease rate by 2 units/hr	
121-200	Increase infusion by 1 unit/hr	Increase infusion by 2 units/hr	Increase infusion by 3 units/hr	Call physician for orders
201-250	Give 2 units IVP and increase infusion by 1 unit/hr	Give 3 units IVP and increase infusion by 2 units/hr	Give 3 units IVP and increase infusion by 3 units/hr	Call physician for orders
251-300	Give 3 units IVP and increase infusion by 1 unit/hr	Give 5 units IVP and increase infusion by 2 units/hr	Give 5 units IVP and increase infusion by 3 units/hr	Call physician for orders
301-350	Give 8 units IVP and increase infusion by 1 unit/hr	Give 8 units IVP and increase infusion by 2 units/hr	Give 8 units IVP and increase infusion by 3 units/hr	Call physician for orders
351-400	Give 10 units IVP and increase infusion by 1 unit/hr	Give 10 units IVP and increase infusion by 2 units/hr	Give 10 units IVP and increase infusion by 3 units/hr	Call physician for orders
> 401	Call physician	Call physician	Call physician	Call physician

_____
Physician's Signature

VC-1668
New 08/2003

Approved by P&T Committee 08-14-03
Approved by PIC Committee 9-2-03

Approved by MEC Committee 09-15-03

DRUG ALLERGIES	UNIT	ROOM #	PATIENT IDENTIFICATION
	PATIENT NAME - HAND WRITTEN		

Original - Retain on Chart   Copy - To Pharmacy
VIA CHRISTI REGIONAL MEDICAL CENTER, WICHITA, KS.
PHYSICIAN ORDER SET

Reprinted with permission from Via Christi Medical Center.

DATE	TIME	**STANDARD MEDICAL PROTOCOL**
		Generic or therapeutic substitutions (as deemed appropriate by the Pharmacy and Therapeutics Committee) may be made unless the physician writes **"NO SUBSTITUTION"** on EACH medication order. NOTE: specify route of administration on Medication Orders

HYPOGLYCEMIA

1. If patient has recurring hypoglycemia, recent diabetic ketoacidosis, gastric stasis, end stage renal disease, hepatic disease, hypoglycemia unawareness, or is malnourished, enact orders for the next level of severity and contact physician.
   IF THIS IS APPLICABLE AT ANY POINT IN THE LENGTH OF STAY, SIGN BELOW:
   _____(date, time, & signature)
2. MILD REACTION (Fully Conscious; hungry, irritable, shaky, unable to sleep, weak - do BS by meter - usually 40-60):
   A. Food (4 oz. milk or 2 graham crackers, etc.) up to 1 calorie point (75 cal.)
   B. Evaluate and recheck BS in 15-30 min. and prn. Food may be repeated x1.
   C. If BS does not elevate or symptoms worsen, treat as MODERATE REACTION.
3. MODERATE REACTION (Conscious, Can Swallow; cold, clammy, sweaty, pale, rapid pulse, mood change, confused and drowsy - do BS by meter - usually <40):
   A. Honey 1-3 tsp. or sugar 1-3 tsp. in 1-oz H_2O, or 2-oz Grape Juice in buccal mucosa several minutes, then swallow.
   B. Evaluate and recheck BS in 10-15 min. If not above 40, repeat honey, etc. x1. If above 40, 4-oz milk or 2 graham crackers, or ½ slice cheese with 2 soda crackers, etc.
   C. Evaluate symptoms. Recheck BS every 15-30 min. until BS >60.
   D. If BS does not elevate or symptoms worsen, treat as SEVERE REACTION and **notify physician.**
4. SEVERE REACTION (Unresponsive, Convulsing, Can't Swallow;):
   A. If functional IV site available, give D50, 10-20 ml IVP.
   B. If no functional IV site is available, give Glucagon IM: 1 ml >3 yr.; ½ ml <3yr. **Insert IV lock.**
   C. **AFTER** paragraph 4A or 4B, do BS by meter and **notify physician** (BS usually <40).
   D. D-50, 10-20 ml IVP repeated, or after Glucagon, to maintain BS 120-150.
   E. When patient able to swallow, re-evaluate symptoms and treat per paragraph 3 A & B.
   F. Evaluate and repeat BS every 15-30 min. until BS stabilized 120-150 x 1-2 hr.
   G. If BS cannot be maintained >60-80, start IV D10 ¼ NS @ 25-100 ml/hr. Titrate to maintain BS 120-150. Check BS every 30-60 min. **Notify physician.** DC D10 ¼ NS when BS >120-150 x 2-3 hrs. and patient eating. If BS cannot be maintained after 2-3 hrs. of D10 ¼ NS, contact physician to change IV fluids to prevent hyponatremia.
5. If NPO or unable to eat with insulin/oral agents, start IVF D10-1/4 NS @ 25-100 ml/hr and use paragraph 4G to maintain BS 120-150. **Notify physician.**
6. Treat at any BS if symptomatic with ½ to 1 calorie point (37.5-75 cal.)
7. If BS < 60 at insulin injection time, treat until BS reaches 60. When insulin injected, feed immediately: **DO NOT WAIT**
8. Do not hold insulin/oral agent without order from physician managing diabetes.
9. Notify physician managing diabetes of any change in po nutrition, IVF, TPN, tube feedings, NPO status, or corticosteroid therapy.
10. BS may be done by meter prn.
11. **PHYSICIAN:** To be notified before next insulin/oral agent is given after hypoglycemia, initial here: _____.

"Medical protocols are initiated without a specific physician order unless an order exists on the patient's record not to utilize the protocol with a particular patient."
VC-044
Chg 7/01   Approved by P&T & PIC Committees   Reviewed MEC 12/12/00

DRUG ALLERGIES	UNIT	ROOM #	PATIENT IDENTIFICATION
	PATIENT NAME - HAND WRITTEN		

Original - Retain on Chart   Copy - To Pharmacy

VIA CHRISTI REGIONAL MEDICAL CENTER, WICHITA, KS.
PHYSICIAN ORDER SET

Reprinted with permission from Via Christi Medical Center.

SAMPLE EDUCATIONAL OBJECTIVES

The following sample illustrates how one program cross-referenced their educational objectives to the curriculum content of *Type 2 Diabetes: A Curriculum for Patients and Health Professionals*. This documentation is not a requirement for programs applying for recognition. For Recognition requirements, please refer to the American Diabetes Association at www.diabetes.org/for-health-professionals-and-scientists/recognition/edrecognition.jsp#applying.

Learning and Skill Objectives	Module	Learning and Skill Objectives	Module
A. Diabetes Disease Process		f. awareness of types of fat and effects of each.	13
1. States:	1, 10	g. awareness of need to change diet with activity changes.	16
a. excess glucose in blood due to too little insulin in relationship to body needs.			
b. lifelong condition requiring treatment.		2. Has a meal plan.	14, 34, 35, 36
c. that they have type 2 diabetes.		3. Is able to:	
		a. describe personal meal plan.	
B. Psychosocial Adjustment		b. use meal plan to plan meals.	5, 14, 34, 35, 36
1. Identifies self as having diabetes.	2	c. use meal plan when eating away from home.	33, 39
2. Identifies effects of diabetes on lifestyle.	11	d. identify behaviors that help reduce risk of heart disease.	5, 14, 17
3. Identifies personal meaning of diabetes.		e. identify eating behaviors that help reduce risk of heart disease.	26
4. Identifies effects of stress on blood glucose.	30	f. plan a sick day diet.	23
5. Identifies one strategy for coping with stress/feelings related to diabetes.	11, 30	g. explain how alcohol affects blood glucose.	40
6. Identifies personal diabetes care goals.	9	h. use product labels to choose foods that fit meal plan.	37
7. Identifies desired level of support from family/friends.	12, 31	i. plan eating/behavior changes that work toward personal goals.	41
8. Informs others of ways they can be supportive.		j. calculate carbohydrate or exchange values.	35, 36, 37
9. Identifies local sources for diabetes support.	11	k. describe how to use special foods, sugar, and fat substitutes.	
C. Nutritional Management		4. Referral to dietitian.	3
1. States:	3		
a. rationale/benefits of keeping a food diary.		**D. Physical Activity**	
b. reasons for meal planning.	5, 34	1. States that exercise/activity lowers blood glucose.	15
c. rationale for eating meals on time.	4	2. Identifies personal exercise plan.	15, 32
d. rationale for reaching/maintaining desirable weight.	17	3. Identifies when not to exercise.	32
e. awareness of carbohydrate, protein, and fat content in foods.	13	4. Describes exercise snack, if needed.	16, 32

Learning and Skill Objectives	Module
5. Identifies medication adjustment for exercise.	
6. Identifies monitoring needed for exercise	
E. Medications	
■ ORAL HYPOGLYCEMIC AGENTS	
1. States:	6
a. name and dose of agent.	
b. when to take.	
c. effect on blood glucose.	
d. side effects.	
e. precautions	
■ INSULIN	
1. States:	7, 18, 19
a. type(s) and dose to take.	
b. when to take.	
c. onset, peak, and duration.	
d. effect on blood glucose.	
e. when low blood glucose is most likely to occur.	18
f. insulin adjustment plan.	
g. how to store insulin.	
2. Prepares and administers own insulin correctly.	7, 19
a. gently mixes insulin.	
b. injects air into bottle.	
c. checks for/removes bubbles.	
d. draws up correct dose.	
e. reuses and disposes of syringes/lancets correctly.	
3. Selects appropriate injection site.	7
a. selects suitable subcutaneous tissue.	
b. states rotation plan.	
4. States:	18
a. type of insulin that impacts specific blood glucose tests.	
b. need for frequent blood glucose testing.	
c. personal insulin plan and blood glucose goals.	7, 18, 19
F. Monitoring and Use of Results	
■ BLOOD GLUCOSE	
1. Demonstrates ability to test blood glucose.	8

Learning and Skill Objectives	Module
a. uses appropriate site to obtain blood samples.	
b. uses correct testing technique.	
c. accurately tests blood glucose.	
d. cares for meter and stores strips properly.	
2. States:	
a. need for monitoring.	
b. plan for monitoring blood glucose and record keeping at home.	
c. that normal blood glucose is 70–115 mg/dl.	
d. personal goal or target range.	
e. appropriate decisions to make about glucose regulation based on results.	20
f. where to obtain glucose meters and supplies.	8
3. Defines glycated HbA$_{1c}$.	20
a. states normal value.	
b. states personal goal.	
■ GLUCOSE CONTROL RELATIONSHIPS	
1. Identifies factors that influence blood glucose levels.	16
2. Identifies personal behaviors that influence blood glucose levels.	
a. relationship of food intake to blood glucose.	13, 16
b. relationship of diabetes medications to blood glucose.	6, 16, 18
c. relationship of exercise to blood glucose.	15, 18
3. States benefits of improved glucose control.	25
4. States risks of improved glucose control.	21
5. Identifies treatment methods to improve glucose control.	25
G. Acute Complications	
■ HYPOGLYCEMIA	
1. States:	11
a. meaning and other names.	

Learning and Skill Objectives	Module	Learning and Skill Objectives	Module
b. personal/common symptoms.		6. States name(s) and phone number(s) of health professional(s) to contact.	
1) occurring while awake.		a. stop smoking.	
2) occurring while asleep.		b. weight control program.	
c. causes and how to prevent.		c. social worker.	
d. when to contact a health professional.		d. visiting nurse/home health.	
e. proper action to be taken to prevent hypoglycemia		e. dietitian.	
2. Wears/carries diabetes identification.		f. diabetes support group.	
		g. education program.	
■ HYPERGLYCEMIA		h. other.	
1. States.	22	7. Describes how to care for diabetes and other chronic health problems.	45
a. meaning and other names.		8. Describes aging and its effects on diabetes care.	46
b. personal common symptoms.		9. States strategies to decrease costs of diabetes care.	48
c. causes and how to prevent.			
d. states proper action to take and when to contact provider.		**I. Chronic Complications**	
		1. States:	25
H. Risk Reduction		a. awareness of potential long-term complications and target organs.	
1. States:	23, 24	1) cardiovascular.	26
a. body areas most susceptible to infection.		2) peripheral vascular.	
b. signs/symptoms of infection and treatment measures.		3) retinopathy.	27
c. effects of smoking.	26	4) nephropathy.	28
d. need for foot care.	24	5) sensory neuropathy.	29
e. plan for personal foot care.		6) autonomic neuropathy.	
f. need for skin care.		b. symptoms indicating onset of complications and importance of early diagnosis.	
g. plan for personal skin care.		c. ways to prevent, delay, or detect complications.	
h. need for regular dental care.		d. common diabetes-related sexual concerns, dysfunctions, and treatment methods.	42, 43
i. benefits of regular medical care.	24, 45, 49		
2. States importance of plans for regular health monitoring.		**J. Problem Solving and Goal Setting**	
a. diabetes management.		1. Identifies problem-solving strategies.	9
b. ophthalmological exams.		2. Identifies personal long-term diabetes care goals.	
c. dental care.		3. Identifies personal short-term diabetes care goals.	
d. regular physical exams.		4. Identifies personal behavior change goals.	
e. others, as indicated.		5. Identifies strategies to achieve goals.	
3. Identifies personal risk factor for complications/health problems	25		
4. States how to obtain driver's license and insurance and employment rights.	47		
5. States awareness of community resources.			

Learning and Skill Objectives	Module	Learning and Skill Objectives	Module
K. Pregnancy		b. states importance of follow-up care after delivery.	
1. Preconception.			
a. states importance of normal blood glucose levels prior to pregnancy.	44	4. Blood glucose control.	
2. Pre-existing diabetes.		a. states need to maintain glucose levels in the target range throughout pregnancy.	
a. identifies importance of frequent care for changing insulin/dietary needs.		b. lists symptoms of hyperglycemia and when to call a physician.	
3. Gestational diabetes.			
a. defines as hyperglycemia related to hormonal changes during pregnancy.		c. states symptoms of hypoglycemia and how to treat.	

From American Diabetes Association: *Type 2 Diabetes: A Curriculum for Patients and Health Professionals.* Funnell MM, Arnold MS, Lasichak AJ, Barr PA, Eds. Alexandria, VA, American Diabetes Association, 2002, p. 619–622.

Key Messages and Counseling Recommendations for Diabetes and Weight-Loss Management

Topic	Key Messages for Professionals	Counseling Recommendations
Diabetes and weight	• Diabetes management—not weight management—is the first priority. • Weight loss of 5–7 kg may improve glycemic control and for some people may reduce the need for medication. However, most individuals will need medication in spite of weight loss or in the future. • Energy restriction, without weight loss, can improve glycemic control.	• Prioritize goals for both health and quality of life. Set HbA$_{1c}$, blood glucose, blood pressure, and lipid goals as appropriate. • Explain the pathophysiology of type 2 diabetes, emphasizing the progressive nature of the disease and discussing the current or eventual need for oral medication or insulin. Even if weight-loss goals are achieved, medication or insulin may be required. • Review how foods affect blood glucose levels and how to select foods and determine portion sizes for meals and snacks.
Weight-loss expectations	• Initial goal of weight-loss therapy is to reduce body weight by 5–10% from baseline. • Improved glycemic control can often increase rather than decrease weight.	• Discuss the importance of setting realistic goals in an achievable time frame. • Emphasize health and fitness rather than physical appearance. • Reinforce weight maintenance strategies after 6 months of treatment. • Be proactive about discussing weight gain as a potential side effect of intensive therapy and improved blood glucose control.
Popular diets and weight loss	• Caloric balance, not macronutrient composition, is the major determinant of weight loss. • The effect of macronutrient composition on long-term weight maintenance and adherence is unclear. • Scientifically validated and understandable information is needed for the millions of overweight and obese Americans who can attain weight loss but who struggle with weight maintenance.	• Support commitment to change. Be open to and acknowledge any positive aspects of alternative weight management approaches. • Stay abreast of current diets/trends. • Inform patients of scientific evidence (or lack thereof) supporting popular diet claims. • Discuss any side effects/contraindications associated with popular diets.
Weight-loss supplements	• Evidence does not support the use of supplements marketed for weight loss.	• Inform patients of scientific evidence (or lack therof) supporting popular diet claims. • Discuss any side effects/contraindications associated with herbs/dietary supplements.
Physical activity	• Initially, moderate levels of physical activity for 30–45 min, 3–5 days/week should be encouraged. • Adults should set a long-term goal of accumulating 30 min or more of exercise on most days, and preferably all days of the week. • Physical activity combined with a low-calorie diet is recommended because it produces weight loss that may also result in decreases in abdominal fat and increases in cardiorespiratory fitness.	• Discuss how physical activity and exercise may help improve patients' glycemic control, cardiovascular health, and psychological well-being. • Assist patients with setting realistic and achievable exercise goals. • Discuss the importance of combined diet and physical activity for weight loss and weight maintenance.

From Boucher JL, Shafer KJ, Chaffin JA: Weight loss, diets, and supplements: does anything work? *Diabetes Spectrum* 14:169–175, 2001.

Considerations When Dealing With Patients Using Atypical

Antipsychotic Agents

Atypical antipsychotics appear to increase the risk of type 2 diabetes by inducing weight gain. Hyperglycemia may resolve with discontinuation of medication.

- ❑ Monitor blood glucose levels if the patient is taking atypical antipsychotics.
- ❑ Use Diabetes Diagnosis and Classification Guidelines

Managing diabetes in patients with psychiatric disorders can be challenging.

Strategies to improve outcomes for the patient using antipsychotic agents are:
- Enlist the help of a caretaker when possible
- Use Home Health Resources
- Solicit support from community groups
- Encourage group activities for physical activity
- Set realistic goals
- Carefully treat mild hyperglycemia with medications
- Use oral agents or insulin to control severe chronic hyperglycemia
- Before using metformin, determine whether the patient will stop treatment if dehydration is likely to occur
- Before using a short-acting insulin, determine whether the patient will take medication with food
- Prescribe small quantities of insulin using prefilled syringes or insulin pens when appropriate
- Encourage patients to wear medical identification
- Review the patient's meal plan. Reduction in simple carbohydrates and simple sugar drinks may improve glucose control

For patients in whom intensive diabetes control is not realistic, other aspects of risk management may be improved:
- Treatment of hypertension
- Treatment of hyperlipidemia
- Aspirin therapy
- Regular screening for retinopathy, neuropathy, and nephropathy

Adapted from McNeely MJ: Case study: atypical antipsychotic use associated with severe hyperglycemia. *Clinical Diabetes* 20:195–196, 2002

QUICK REFERENCE GUIDES

Oral Agents
Antihypertensive Medications
Lipid-Lowering Medications

ORAL AGENTS

Trade name	Generic name	When to take	Doses	Side effects

Secretagogues (Hypoglycemia Agents) – stimulate insulin secretion from the pancreatic β-cells

(Sulfonylureas)

Trade name	Generic name	When to take	Doses	Side effects
Diabeta or Micronase	(Glyburide)	30 min before meals	1.25, 2.5, 5 mg Max: 20 mg	
Glynase	(Glyburide-press tab)	30 min before meals	1.5, 3, 6 mg Max: 12 mg	Low blood glucose Hypoglycemia
Glucotrol	(Glipizide)	30 min before meals	5, 10 mg Max: 40 mg	Weight gain
Glucotrol XL	(Glipizide)	before or with meals	5, 10 mg Max: 20 mg	
Amaryl	(Glimepiride)	before or with meals	1,2, 4 mg Max: 8 mg	

(Meglitinides)

Trade name	Generic name	When to take	Doses	Side effects
Prandin	(Repaglinide)	5-30 min before meals	0.5, 1, 2 mg Max: 16 mg	Low blood glucose Headaches
Starlix	(Nateglinide)	5-30 min before meals	120 mg, 60 mg	

Biguanides – suppress glucose production in the liver and decreases insulin resistance

Trade name	Generic name	When to take	Doses	Side effects
Glucophage	(Metformin)	Take with meals	500, 850, 1,000 mg	Nausea, diarrhea
Glucophage XR	(Metformin)	500 mg only	Max: 2,550 mg	metallic taste,
Fortamet	(Metformin)			lactic acidosis
Riomet	(Liquid Metformin)			

COMBINATION PILLS

Trade name	Generic name	When to take	Doses	Side effects
Glucovance	(Glyburide/Metformin)	Take with meals	1.25/250; 2.5/500; 5/500 mg	
Metaglip	(Glipizide/Metformin)	Take with meals	2.5/250; 5/500; 5/500	
Avandamet	(Rosiglitazone/Metformin)	Take with meals	1mg/500mg, 2/500, 4/500	

Note: Discontinued day of any procedure using iodinated contrast media or major surgery, restart 48 hours after the procedure with confirmation that renal function has returned to normal.

α-Glucosidase Inhibitors – slow down carbohydrate absorption in intestines

Trade name	Generic name	When to take	Doses	Side effects
Precose	(Acarbose)	Take with first bite of meal	25, 50, 100 mg Max: 300 mg	Nausea, diarrhea, flatulence
Glyset	(Miglitol)	Take with first bite of meal	25, 50, 100 mg Max: 300 mg	

Note: If low blood glucose level, use honey or glucose gel/tablets; do not use table or brown sugar.

Thiazolidinediones (Insulin Sensitizer) – improve peripheral insulin sensitivity

Trade name	Generic name	When to take	Doses	Side effects
Actos	(Pioglitazone)	With or without meals	15, 30, mg Max: 45 mg	Possible liver dysfunction Possible anemia, edema
Avandia	(Rosiglitazone)	With or without meals	2, 4, 6, 8 mg Max: 8 mg	

Liver function studies should be done before initiating therapy, according to prescriber's discretion within the first year and annually thereafter.

Rev: 2/03 Reprinted with permission from Via Christi Diabetes Treatment and Research Center, Wichita, KS.

Antihypertensive Medications

Brand Name	Generic Name	Starting Dose	Maximum Dose	Pearls
ACE Inhibitors				
Class side effects: Hyperkalemia, dry nonproductive cough, decrease in renal function				
Time to increase dose: 1–2 wks				
Lotensin	Benazepril	5–10 mg once a day	40 mg/day (may be divided)	**For all ACE inhibitors:**
Capoten	Captopril	25 mg b.i.d. and can double the dose up to maximum	50 mg b.i.d. or t.i.d.	Neutral metabolic affects
Vasotec	Enalapril	2.5–5.0 mg once a day	40 mg/day (may be divided)	Don't increase lipids
Monopril	Fosinopril	10 mg a day	80 mg/day (may be divided)	Don't increase orthostatic hypertension
Prinivil, Zestril	Lisinopril	5–10 mg once a day	80 mg/day	Don't aggravate coronary peripheral
Univasc	Moexipril	7.5 mg once a day, 1 h prior to meals	30 mg/day (may be divided)	vascular disease
Aceon	Perindopril	4 mg once a day	16 mg/day (may be divided)	Preserve renal function
Accupril	Quinapril	5–10 mg once a day	80 mg/day (may be divided)	
Altace	Ramipril	1.25–2.5 mg once a day	20 mg/day (may be divided)	
Mavik	Trandolapril	1 mg once a day (2 mg if African American)	4 mg/day	
Angiotensin Receptor Blockers				
Class side effects: Dizziness, cough (less than ACE inhibitors)				**For all angiotensin receptor blockers:**
Time to increase dose: 1–2 wks				Similar effects as ACE inhibitors for kidneys
Atacand	Candesartan	16 mg once a day	>32 mg/day no benefit	
Teveten	Eprosartan	600 mg/day (may be divided)	>800 mg/day no experience	
Avapro	Irbesartan	150 mg once a day	300 mg once a day	
Cozaar	Losartan	25–50 mg once a day	100 mg/day (may be divided)	
Micardis	Telmisartan	40 mg once a day	80 mg/day	Candesartan: Nausea may be reduced by taking with food
Diovan	Valsartan	80 mg once a day	320 mg once a day	
Benicar	Olmesartan	20 mg once a day	40 mg once a day	Olmesartan: Titration is 2–4 wks
β-Blockers				
Class side effects: Increased triglycerides, decreased HDL cholesterol, masks symptoms of hypoglycemia, hyperglycemia/hypoglycemia (inhibits insulin secretion, generates insulin resistance)				
ISA (intrinsic sympathomimetic activity): Do not decrease cardiac output, do not induce glucose intolerance				
b1 (β-1 receptor selectivity): Do not provoke bronchospams, do not reduce insulin secretion and glycogenolysis, selectivity diminishes at higher doses				
Time to increase dose: 1–2 wks				
Sectral	Acebutolol (b1, ISA)	200–400 mg q.d. (may be divided)	800 mg/day	**For all β-blockers:**
Tenormin	Atenolol (b1)	25–50 mg once a day	>100 mg/day, no benefit	Documented increase survival in diabetes and coronary artery disease
Kerlone	Betaxolol (b1)	5–10 mg once a day	>20 mg/day, no benefit	
Zebeta	Bisoprolol (b1)	2.5–5.0 mg once a day	20 mg once a day	
Cartrol	Carteolol (ISA)	2.5 mg once a day	>10 mg/day, no benefit	U.K. Prospective Diabetes Study: decrease stroke, heart failure
Lopressor, Toprol	Metoprolol (b1)	50–100 mg q.d. (may divide)	400 mg/day	
Corgard	Nadolol	20–40 mg once a day	320 mg/day	Hypoglycemic symptoms masked
Levatol	Penbutolol (ISA)	10–20 mg once a day	80 mg/day, no benefit	
Visken	Pindolol (ISA)	5 mg b.i.d.	60 mg/day	
Inderal	Propranolol	40 mg b.i.d. or 80 mg once a day (SR)	640 mg/day	
Blocadren	Timolol	10 mg b.i.d.	60 mg/day	
Coreg	Carvedilol	6.25 mg b.i.d. for hypertension	50 mg/day	Carvedilol: FDA approved for heart failure—3.125 mg b.i.d. in heart failure

Diuretics

Thiazides

Class side effects: Hyperglycemia (insulin resistance) at higher doses, hyperlipidemia, hypercalcemia, hypokalemia, hypomagnesemia, hyperuricemia, hyponatremia, sexual dysfunction

Diuril	Chlorothiazide	0.5–1.0 g/day (may be divided)	2 g/day	**For all thiazide diuretics:**
Hygroton	Chlorthalidone	12.5–25.0 mg/day in A.M. with food	>25 mg/day, no benefit	Low doses have additive effect
Hydrodiuril	Hydrochlorothiazide	12.5-25 mg/day (may be divided)	>50 mg/day, no benefit	<25 mg shouldn't cause increased insulin resistance
Diucardin	Hydroflumethiazide	25-50 mg q.d. to b.i.d.	200 mg/day	
Lozol	Indapamide	1.25 mg A.M.; can double dose to increase	5 mg/day	May increase lipids
Enduron	Methyclothiazide	2.5–5.0 mg once a day	5 mg/day	
Zaroxolyn	Metolazone	2.5–5.0 mg once a day	5 mg/day	
Hydromox	Quinethazone	50–100 mg once a day	150–200 mg/day	

Loop

Class side effects: No glucose or lipid changes, hypocalcemia, hypokalemia, hypomagnesemia, hyperuricemia, hyponatremia, sexual dysfunction

Lasix	Furosemide	40 mg b.i.d., reduce dose of other agents at least 50%	240 mg/day	
Demadex	Torsemide	5 mg once a day	10 mg once a day	

Calcium Channel Blockers

Dihydropyridines

Class side effects: Reflex tachycardia, edema, palpitations, headache, dizziness

Time to increase dose: 10–14 days

Norvasc	Amlodipine	2.5–5.0 mg once a day	10 mg once a day	**For all dihydropyridine calcium channel blockers:**
Plendil	Felodipine	5 mg once a day	10 mg/day	
DynaCirc	Isradipine	2.5 mg b.i.d., increase by 5-mg/day increments	>10 mg/day no benefit	Often used as second agent with ACE inhibitors
				Metabolically neutral
Procardia XL, Adalatt CC	Nifedipine	30-60 mg once a day, take Adalat CC on an empty stomach	>120 mg/day (Procardia XL), >90 mg/day (Adalat CC)	Not recommended in congestive heart failure, edema, tachycardia
Sular	Nisoldipine	20 mg once a day, increase by 10-mg increments	60 mg once a day	Nisoldipine: Avoid taking with high-fat meal and grapefruit

Nondihydropyridines

Class side effects: Dizziness, Headache, decreased heart rate

Time to increase dose: 10–14 days

Dilacor XR	Diltiazem	180–240 mg once a day	540 mg/day	
Cardizem CD	Diltiazem	180–240 mg once a day	>360 mg/day, no experience	
Cardizem SR	Diltiazem	60–120 mg b.i.d.	360 mg/day	
Calan, Isoptin, Covera, Verelan	Verapamil	120–240 mg/day (may be divided)	>360 mg/day, no benefit	Verapamil: Take slow release with food

Combinations

Aldoril	Methyldopa/hydrochlorothiazide	Maxzide, Dyazide	Hydrochlorothiazide/triamterene
Avalide	Irbesartan/hydrochlorothiazide	Moduretic	Amiloride/hydrochlorothiazide
Diovan HCT	valsartan/hydrochlorothiazide	Prinzide	Lisinopril/hydrochlorothiazide
Hyzaar	Losartan/hydrochlorothiazide	Tarka	Trandolapril/verapamil ER
Inderide	Propranolol/hydrochlorothiazide	Tenoretic	Atenolol/chlorthalidone
Lexxel	Enalapril/felodipine ER	Uniretic	Moexipril/hydrochlorothiazide
Lopressor HCT	Metoprolol/hydrochlorothiazide	Vaseretic	Enalapril/hydrochlorothiazide
Lotensin	Benazepril/hydrochlorothiazide	Zestoretic	Lisinopril/hydrochlorothiazide
Lotrel	Amlodipine/benazepril	Ziac	Bisoprolol/hydrochlorothiazide

From the individual package inserts and the 2004 Physicians' Desk Reference, 59th ed., Montvale, NJ, Medical Economics Company, 2004. Compiled as part of the Professional Education Program for Nurses on Hyperlipidemia and Hypertension Teleconference, May–June 2003. Hinnen DH, Childs BP, Marynuick M, Vu J: Pharmaceutical treatment of hypertension and dyslipidemia in people with diabetes: an educator's perspective. Part 1: Hypertension. *Diabetes Spectrum* 17:60–64, 2004

Lipid-Lowering Medications

Brand Name	Generic Name	Starting Dose	Maximum Dose	Pearls	
HMG-CoA Reductase Inhibitors					
Indications for use: Lowering LDL, raising HDL					
Class side effects: Headache, GI upset, myalgia, rash, dizziness, insomnia, elevated transaminase, myopathy, rhabdomyolysis with renal dysfunction					
Monitor liver function before therapy and 12 wks after start of therapy. Decrease if serum transaminase is >3× normal level. Discontinue if myopathy or elevated creatine phosphokinase occurs or if there is a predisposition to renal failure. Avoid concomitant gemfibrozil.					
Contraindications: Active or chronic liver disease					
Crestor	Rosuvastatin	10 mg	40 mg	Daily	**For all HMG-CoA reductase inhibitors:** Avoid grapefruit or grapefruit juice while on this product
Lescol XL	Fluvastatin	20 mg	80 mg	Give at bedtime	
Lipitor	Atorvastatin	10 mg	80 mg	Daily	
Pravachol	Pravastatin	10–20 mg	40 mg	Daily	
Mevacor	Lovastatin	10–20 mg	80 mg	Give with evening meal	
Zocor	Simvastatin	20–40 mg	80 mg	Give at bedtime	
Nicotinic Acid Derivative and HMG-CoA Reductase Inhibitor					
Class side effects: Flushing, headache, pain, pruritus, dyspepsia, flu syndrome, rash, asthenia, hyperglycemia, hypotension					
Advicor	Niacin/Lovastatin	500 mg/20 mg	1,000 mg/20 mg		
Fibric Acid Derivatives					
Indications for use: Hypertriglyceridemia, additional LDL-lowering effect					
Class side effects: GI upset, abdominal pain, dyspepsia, gallstones, myopathy, increased risk of hepatotoxicity					
Lopid	Gemfibrozil	600 mg b.i.d.	600 mg b.i.d.	Take 30 min before eating. Drug interaction: warfarin (monitor patient)	
Tricor	Fenofibrate	67 mg b.i.d., unless switching from another agent, start 200 mg	200 mg q.d.	Also has LDL-lowering effect, drug-to-drug interaction with warfarin (monitor patient). If combined with bile acid sequestrants, give 1 h before or 4–6 h after	
Nicotinic Acid					
Indication for use: Combined dyslipidemia					
Class side effects: Flushing (tolerance improved over time), nausea, vomiting, flatulence, pruritis, peptic ulcer, heptatoxicity, hyperuricemia, gout, hyperglycemia (dose related)					
Obtain baseline uric acid, liver function tests (alanine aminotransferase, aspartate aminotransferase), 6–8 wks after reaching 1,500 mg, 6–8 wks after maximum dose and periodically thereafter.					
Contraindications: Liver disease, renal disease					
Niacin	Crystalline nicotinic acid	250 mg q.d. (usual dose is 1.5–3.0 g in divided doses b.i.d. or t.i.d.)	4.5 g	Flushing and pruritus more common with immediate-release niacin but may abate with time; administer acetylsalicylic acid (325 mg) and with food; monitor glucose levels, uric acid levels in patients with gout. Slow dose increase every 4–7 days until 2 g, then every 2–4 wks until 3 g, if lipid profile not improved. Available over the counter.	
Niacin time release	Sustained-release nicotinic acid	500 mg (usual dose 1–2 g)	2 g, divided doses	Monitor blood glucose, uric acid levels in patients with gout. Slow dose increase every 1.5 wks. Available over the counter.	
Niaspan	Extended-release nicotinic acid	500 mg (usual dose 1–2 g)	2 g, single dose	Rare fulminant hepatitis reported in some SR formulations. Slow dose increase every 1–2 wks.	
If switching from crystalline nicotinic acid to a sustained-release nicotinic acid, use smaller dose to decrease risk of hepatoxicity. Titrate up slowly.					
Bile Acid Sequestrant					
Indications for use: Reducing LDL					
Class side effects: Constipation, fecal impaction, aggravation of hemorrhoids, GI disturbance, osteoporosis, vitamin A, D, or K or folic acid deficiencies, increased bleeding, hypochloremic acidosis, rash, oral or anal irritation					
Contraindications: Dys-β-lipoproteinemia or triglycerides >400 mg/dl					
Colestid	Colestipol	2 g once daily or b.i.d.	tablets 6 g/packets 30 g		
Questran Light	Cholestyramine	1–2 scoops/packets q.d.	6 scoops/packets		
2-Axetidionone: Indicated for lowering LDL					
Contraindications: Liver disease, pregnancy					
Zetia	Ezetimibe	10 mg daily	10 mg daily	Use as monotherapy or as complement to statin. Take 2 h before or 4 h after a bile sequestrant.	
Combination Medication					
Vytorin	Ezemtimibe/simvastatin	10/10, 10/20, 10/40, 10/80 max 10/80		First combined cholesterol lowering agent	

COMBINATIONS: There is an increased risk of myopathy and rhabdomyoloysis with all combination therapy.
Caution: Monitor liver function tests and creatine kinase.
Statins and fibrates: Effective for combined dyslipidemia; insure renal function, limit dose of the statin when combining; check creatine kinase level at baseline and recheck if symptoms of muscle soreness present.
Statins and nicotinic acid: Effective for atherogenic dyslipidemia, increases HDL. Use smaller dose of nicotinic acid.
Fibrates and nicotinic acid: Not well studied.
Fibrates and bile acid sequestrants: Administer fibrate 1 h before or 4–6 h after taking bile acid sequestrant.

From individual package inserts and the 2003 Physicians' Desk Reference, 58th ed., Montvale, NJ, Medical Economics Company, 2003.

Index

Macular degeneration, 118–119
Macular edema, 117
Magnesium salts, 256
Magnetic therapy, 228
Mallet toes, 173
Maturity-onset diabetes of the young (MODY), 8, 286
Mauriac syndrome, 288
Meal planning. *See* Medical nutrition therapy (MNT); Nutritional care
MedicAlert Foundation International, 389
Medical nutrition therapy (MNT), 16, 21–25. *See also* Nutritional care
  carbohydrates and, 23–24
  for children, 289–296
  fat intake, reducing, 24–25
  goals for, 24
  in nursing homes, 376*t*, 378–379
  nutritional outcomes research, 23*t*
  physical activity and, 25
  portion control, 24
  process of, 23–25
  tool box approach, 25, 26*t*
  weight, healthy, 25
Medications. *See also* Polypharmacy
  antihypertensive, 253–255, 443–444
  cardiac, 97*t*
  combinations of, 444, 445
  costs, controlling, 402
  diabetes. *See* Insulin; Oral antidiabetic agents
  drug-induced diabetes, 8, 320–322
  for elderly patients, 312, 313, 316
  for hospital patients, 348–351
  interactions among, 253–257, 376*t*, 377
  lipid-lowering, 97*t*, 445
  in nursing homes, 375–377
  quick reference guides, 442–445
Meglitinides, 50–51, 128
Menstruation, blood glucose control and, 279
Metabolic syndrome, 13, 14*t*, 52, 287*t*
Metformin/Glucophage, 15*t*, 53*t*
  cystic fibrosis–related diabetes (CFRD) and, 326
  for children, 298
  heart failure and, 98
  liver function tests and, 331
  pregnancy risk and, 280

surgery and, 348
Mexican Americans, 213
Microalbuminuria, 126–127, 326
Micronase, 50*t*
Middle Easterners, 274
Miglitol/Glyset, 55*t*
Mild nonproliferative diabetic retinopathy, 116
Mineral supplements, 410
Minidose glucagon, 302
Moderate nonproliferative diabetic retinopathy, 116
Motivational interviewing, 204, 205*t*
Motor neuropathy, 158, 166–167
Mucosal diseases, 140–141
Myocardial infarction (MI), 91, 92
  acute, 98–99
  glycemic control and, 346
Myocardial ischemia, 91–92, 96

N

Nateglinide/Starlix, 50*t*
National Association of Area Agencies on Aging, 388
National Association of School Nurses, 388
National Center for Complementary and Alternative Medicine (NCCAM), 223, 225–226
National Center on Minority Health and Health Disparities, 389
National Center on Physical Activity and Disabilities, 389
National Certification Board for Diabetes Educators (NCBDE), 195, 392
National Cholesterol Education Program (NCEP), 13, 14*t*, 21
National Cholesterol Education Program Adult Treatment Panel III, 14*t*
National Diabetes Education Program (NDEP), 387
National Diabetes Information Clearinghouse (NDIC), 194, 387
National Education Association, Health Information Network, 388
National Eye Institute, 387
National Foundation for the Blind, 389

About the American Diabetes Association

The American Diabetes Association is the nation's leading voluntary health organization supporting diabetes research, information, and advocacy. Its mission is to prevent and cure diabetes and to improve the lives of all people affected by diabetes. The American Diabetes Association is the leading publisher of comprehensive diabetes information. Its huge library of practical and authoritative books for people with diabetes covers every aspect of self-care—cooking and nutrition, fitness, weight control, medications, complications, emotional issues, and general self-care.

To order American Diabetes Association books: Call 1-800-232-6733 or log on to http://store.diabetes.org

To join the American Diabetes Association: Call 1-800-806-7801 or log on to www.diabetes.org/membership

For more information about diabetes or ADA programs and services: Call 1-800-342-2383. E-mail: AskADA@diabetes.org or log on to www.diabetes.org

To locate an ADA/NCQA Recognized Provider of quality diabetes care in your area: www.ncqa.org/dprp

To find an ADA Recognized Education Program in your area: Call 1-888-232-0822. www.diabetes.org/for-health-professionals-and-scientists/recognition/edrecognition.jsp

To join the fight to increase funding for diabetes research, end discrimination, and improve insurance coverage: Call 1-800-342-2383. www.diabetes.org/advocacy-and-legalresources/advocacy.jsp

To find out how you can get involved with the programs in your community: Call 1-800-342-2383. See below for program Web addresses.

- *American Diabetes Month:* educational activities aimed at those diagnosed with diabetes—month of November. www.diabetes.org/communityprograms-and-localevents/americandiabetesmonth.jsp
- *American Diabetes Alert:* annual public awareness campaign to find the undiagnosed—held the fourth Tuesday in March. www.diabetes.org/communityprograms-and-local events/americandiabetesalert.jsp
- *The Diabetes Assistance & Resources Program (DAR):* diabetes awareness program targeted to the Latino community. www.diabetes.org/communityprograms-and-local events/latinos.jsp
- *African American Program:* diabetes awareness program targeted to the African American community. www.diabetes.org/communityprograms-and-localevents/african americans.jsp
- *Awakening the Spirit: Pathways to Diabetes Prevention & Control:* diabetes awareness program targeted to the Native American community. www.diabetes.org/community programs-and-localevents/nativeamericans.jsp

To find out about an important research project regarding type 2 diabetes: www.diabetes.org/diabetes-research/research-home.jsp

To obtain information on making a planned gift or charitable bequest: Call 1-888-700-7029. www.wpg.cc/stl/CDA/homepage/1,1006,509,00.html

To make a donation or memorial contribution: Call 1-800-342-2383. www.diabetes.org/support-the-cause/make-a-donation.jsp